An Annotated Bibliography of HEALTH ECONOMICS

English Language Sources

A companion volume, including material from Austria, Belgium, Denmark, Finland, France, Germany, Italy, Luxembourg, the Netherlands, Norway, Sweden and Switzerland is also being produced by the Sandoz Institute for Health and Socio-Economic Studies, Geneva.

An Annotated Bibliography of HEALTH ECONOMICS

A. J. CULYER
Reader in Economics, Assistant Director, Institute of Social and Economic Research, University of York

JACK WISEMAN
Professor of Applied Economics, Director, Institute of Social and Economic Research, University of York

ARTHUR WALKER
Research Fellow, Institute of Social and Economic Research, University of York

St. Martin's Press
NEW YORK

Printed in Great Britain

ISBN 0–312–03873–9
Library of Congress Catalog Card No. 77-79018

First published in the United States of America in 1977

Contents

Preface

The justification of a bibliography must be first that a subject-matter exists, and second that there is need to facilitate access to the material for an existing body of scholars. The present volume has been prepared in the belief that these conditions now pertain in respect of the economics of health.

As a specialist field of study, the economics of health has had only a relatively short life. As an examination of the section *General Works* will confirm, there do not yet exist definitive texts to which the student can be directed to obtain a first but comprehensive coverage of the subject-matter, in the fashion that such information might be obtained in such areas as, say, public finance or the theory of the firm. Moreover, health economics is located in the spectrum of economics specialisms within the broader band of the economics of human resources: itself a new development (or re-development) in the period since the Second World War, and still awaiting a definitive general text.

As a specialism, then, health economics shares some of the characteristics of human resources studies, but also exhibits interesting features of its own. It shares with (e.g.) the economics of education, arguably the best-developed of the human resources studies, a concern with the quality of the human factor of production and with economic activities influencing that quality; in this context there are clear affinities with the economics of labour. It shares with human resources studies generally a concern with the measurement and evaluation of output, and a special attitude to problems of income distribution and redistribution. But the health output problem has its own peculiarities, both in respect of what it is ('better health'?) and in respect of how it should be valued. The provision of health is also unusual in that some of the agents of changes in health conditions (e.g. doctors) also have a special role in the identification and evaluation of the conditions themselves. Finally, the very fact that man has a finite expectation of life, and that there are obvious, though subtle, relations between mortality, morbidity, and the arrangements for delivery of, and access to, health care, means that members of society see the provision of

vii

health care as 'different'. They do not appraise the 'efficiency' of arrangements for the delivery of health care by the criteria that they might accept for, say, the provision of radio sets.

Perhaps enough has been said, in a Preface, to provide an impression of the nature and problems of health economics; those who want more will be encouraged to buy the bibliography. We must now say something about the contents. It is characteristic of the recent emergence of health economics as a specialist field of study that the literature should be scattered over a variety of sources, some of which are not wholly, or indeed primarily, journals specialised in economics. Summarily, at the time of writing the status of health economics as an academic discipline in English-speaking countries could be described as follows: there are a relatively few institutions with a specialised facility in research and graduate study in health economics. Outside these few specialised groups, individual scholars are to be found with a complete (or, more commonly, a partial) commitment to research in health economics, and, consequentially to graduate studies (and to a lesser extent, some specialist teaching for mature undergraduates) in this special area. The directly 'academic' written output, oriented generally but not exclusively towards journals concerned with economics, comes from this sector.

Another interest group is to be found in governments and their agencies. The concern here is to find solutions to practical policy problems: how to provide, or intervene in the provision of health services; how to control the size and growth of public expenditures on health; and so on. There are two related characteristics of the written results of this kind of 'public' activity that are of practical concern for us. First, much of the material appears in official documents whose prime concern may or may not be with the *economic* problems of health as we would define them. Second, in so far as the enquiry concerned does have an economic dimension, it has become increasingly common for members of the academic group described above to become involved in one way or another. We shall return to this question shortly, when discussing coverage.

Finally, relevant written material originates from people who are themselves employed in the health sector, but are working on economic problems. The economic problems of health care delivery are not of course new, though their specialised study by economists may be. Many non-economists seeking to solve problems of practical concern to them have become involved in research with an economic dimension. A good example would be the kind of medical study that sets out to compare alternative ways of treating a defined condition, but finds itself involved in problems of comparative costs (do the different methods use the 'same resources'?) and of output evaluation (are there differences in prognosis?) The relevant group in the health sector can conveniently be further sub-divided into those who do not regard themselves as economists but are working on problems with economic characteristics, and economists working on health problems within the health sector, commonly with other specialists. The publications of both sub-groups are as likely to appear in non-economic (particularly medical) as in economic journals. The very existence of this group is a reason for the production of a bibliography that brings together their own contributions and the 'academic' ones appearing in journals directly concerned with economics. As with government publications, the output of this group raises classification problems: there are many studies whose origin is medical but whose output is wholly or (more usually) partly economic. The non-economist researcher needs guidance when he discovers, e.g., that 'cost' is not a simple or un-ambiguous concept; the economist working in a medical context needs access to a specialist literature. (In the U.K., the Health Economists' Study Group, administered from the University of York, was set up in recognition of the need for a single forum for people working on health economics problems inside and outside universities. Only a minority of the membership are affiliated to university departments of economics.)

Our coverage, therefore, has necessarily been determined by the content of publications rather than by their source. This, of course, leaves us vulnerable to criticism: we are sure to have missed some sources and hence some publications. But it seems to us that such a procedure was the only practically possible one. We hope that our friends will bring omissions to our notice. Meanwhile, there is no bibliography of health economics: and we would rather be remembered as the producers of the first Model T Ford than as the producers of the first Cadillac. Cadillacs are for second editions. Our journal search embraced not only the periodicals listed under *Abbreviations*, but also others of potential relevance, which have not been included because no appropriate material was discovered.

Coverage is concerned not only with the field of search, but also with the criteria for inclusion. The general principle here has been that the publication should make some significant contribution to the *economics* of a health problem, that is, that it should be concerned in some way with a resource-use problem: cost, scarcity, method of delivery, pricing, investment, or whatever. This gives us a focus. We are concerned with the great questions of health economics: the yield to investment in health, valuation of output, 'economic efficiency' of systems of provision, the 'demand' and 'need' for health services, and so on. But this general principle does not entirely solve the practical problem of all bibliographies: where to stop. In this regard, we have limited ourselves in the following ways. First, the publication must have an identifiable 'economic' content. Second, it must be in English. This is a limitation of necessity. It seems probable, given the way the subject has developed, that an English-language bibliography will comprehend the major developments in the subject. But work has been going on and been published in other languages, and we would have liked to extend our coverage to them. While our own work was in progress, we learned that the Sandoz Institute were planning an essentially similar bibliography covering the major languages. We have since collaborated in respect of such matters as organisation, definitions, etc., and the Sandoz publication can thus be regarded as a 'sister' publication to our own. It is our mutual intention that the two publications should eventually be integrated.

The treatment of government publications also requires further explanation. The list of conceptually relevant publications of this kind is an extraordinarily long one. For reasons both of choice and necessity, we have restricted our coverage. The guiding principle has been that, unless an official publication is *predominantly* concerned with issues of direct relevance, it has not been included. This prevents the text from being dominated, for example, by the large number of essentially medically-oriented fact-finding publications generated by such bodies as the U.S. Department of Health, Education and Welfare. Thus, the 'frontier' of selection is to be found in such publications as the U.K. Todd Report on medical manpower (Royal Commission on Medical Education 1965–8, Cmnd. 3569, London: HMSO, 1968) which is essentially about medical education but provides information of interest to health economists. Our principle of exclusion is related to our view, earlier expressed, that economists become involved in relevant projects of this kind, and so the material of interest to economists subsequently turns up in the non-government publications which *are* classified here. (For example, the Guillebaud Committee set up to investigate the U.K. National Health Service stimulated pioneering work on the costs of health services, and many U.S. academic publications have been written under contract with the U.S. Department of Health, Education and Welfare.) The principle is not of course a rigid one: if readers find that it has led to the omission of relevant publications and hence diminished the value of the work, we would be glad to hear from them so that subsequent editions can remedy the deficiency.

Finally, we have excluded unpublished documents, dissertations, discussion papers and, save in special cases, publications in relatively ephemeral sources such as weeklies.

Our approach to classification of material is implied by our attitude to coverage. Our concern is with the *economics* of health: we have accordingly eschewed any kind of 'institutional' taxonomy in favour of one that follows the broad divisions of economic analysis – essentially, demand for health, supply of health, output and valuation of health services, financing and planning of health services, financing and planning of health service provision. Such a taxonomy is in any case indicated by the intended readership. It is hoped that the bibliography will be helpful to all researchers with problems that have an economic dimension. But some general (if elementary) knowledge of economics is needed for such a problem to be recognised, and the bibliography assumes such a knowledge in the reader.

Within this classification, entries are in broad chronological order within sections. The choice between a chronological and an alphabetical (author) order must always be difficult. In our case, the decision was much influenced by the recent development of the specialism, to which we have already referred. The benefit to readers in having available an encapsulated description of the development of thought on particular topics seemed to us likely to outweigh any possible advantages from an alphabetical listing – the more so in that readers wishing to trace the work of a particular author can do so by way of the alphabetical (author) index at the end of the volume. The cross-referencing of entries is based on the same assumptions: the 'linkages' that are identified are those that economists with a specialist knowledge of the field might be expected to make (or, more honestly, the 'linkages' that the authors as members of such a specialist group themselves would make). Once again, cross-referencing must involve arbitrary decisions: one could invent intellectual 'linkages' between *all* items in the bibliography. We recognise this by including in our commentary on sections an indication of the other related topics to which readers with particular interests might like to refer.

Even more than other academic works, the production of a bibliography draws upon the benefits from the advice of others. We acknowledge our debt to the many colleagues interested in health economics who have contributed to the production of this volume, and in particular to the (overlapping) membership of three groups: our economist colleagues at the University of York, the academic and research staff members of the Health Economics Group at the University of York, and the members of the Health Economists' Study Group. Acknowledgement must also be made of the indirect but valuable support of the Social Science Research Council, which finances the latter group and some of the research in health economics at York, and of The Nuffield Provincial Hospitals Trust, whose priming support was instrumental in establishing health economics as a specialist research interest at York.

Within this general acknowledgement, certain individuals at the University of York have made a personal contribution that places us in their debt: John Cullis, Mike Drummond, Bob Lavers, Chris Trinder, Peter West, Dave Whynes and Ken Wright, all present or past Research Fellows at the Institute of Social and Economic Research, and Alan Williams of the Department of Economics and Related Studies.

We are also greatly indebted to Miss Barbara Dodds and her secretarial colleagues for the efficient organisation and preparation of a difficult manuscript.

Finally, but by no means least important, we have to acknowledge our financial sponsors, without whose support the study could not have been undertaken. The bibliography was prepared with the help of a research grant from the U.K. Department of Health and Social Security to the Health Economics Group at the University of York. We are grateful to the Department for their imagination in supporting a venture whose contribution to their own ends must of necessity be indirect (though we would hope not therefore insubstantial), and for their generosity in respect of publication arrangements.

System of Classification

1 Entries are classified by topic in Sections, and within Sections are listed in date order. Entries are numbered consecutively from the beginning of the bibliography to the end.

2 Numbers appearing in brackets in Section Introductions identify a relevant entry in the text.

3 The system of cross-referencing of entries is as follows:

    (a) Cross-references are given at the end of entries in numerical order.

    (b) Numbers in roman type refer to another entry of the same item. This entry will be annotated.

    (c) Numbers in italics refer to other entries concerned with closely related topics. All such cross-references are to annotated entries.

The following entry provides an illustration:

7 R. W. CONLEY, 'A benefit-cost analysis of the vocational rehabilitation programme'
JHR, Spring, 1969, 4(1), pp. 226–52.
{Annotation}
See 652, 1353.

The reader referring to item 652 will find an annotated version of a related book, also (as it happens) by Conley. Item 1353 is a separate reference to the same article as item 687. At 687, the article is annotated in the context of cost–benefit analysis, at 1353 in the context of income redistribution.

4 Readers will appreciate that when an item is not annotated, the roman cross-references indicate where a description of the item is to be found.

Abbreviations

AAAPSS	Annals of the American Academy of Political and Social Science
AE	Applied Economics
AEH	Archives of Environmental Health
AEP	Australian Economic Papers
AER	American Economic Review
AGP	Annals of General Practice
AJE	American Journal of Epidemiology
AJP	American Journal of Psychiatry
AJPH	American Journal of Public Health
AJTMH	American Journal of Tropical Medicine and Hygiene
Am.Beh.Scientist	American Behavioral Scientist
Amer.Econ.	American Economist
AMH	Administration in Mental Health
Ann.Intern.Med.	Annals of Internal Medicine
APMR	Archives of Physical Medicine and Rehabilitation
AS	Applied Statistics
ASBMT	Annales de la Société Belge de Médicine Tropicale
Aus.Ec.Rev.	Australian Economic Review
BCRRS	Blue Cross Reports Research Series
BDJ	British Dental Journal
BER	Bulletin of Economic Research
BHJ	British Hospital Journal and Social Service Review
BISI	Bulletin of the International Statistical Institute
BJHM	British Journal of Hospital Medicine
BJP	British Journal of Psychiatry
BJPSM	British Journal of Preventive and Social Medicine
BMA	British Medical Association
BMB	British Medical Bulletin
BMJ	British Medical Journal
BOUIES	Bulletin of the Oxford University Institute of Economics and Statistics
Bull.N.Y.Acad. Med.	Bulletin of the New York Academy of Medicine
CJE	Canadian Journal of Economics
CJPH	Canadian Journal of Public Health
CMAJ	Canadian Medical Association Journal

DD	Development Digest
EBB	Economic and Business Bulletin
EC	Economica
EDCC	Economic Development and Cultural Change
EG	Economic Geography
EJ	Economic Journal
ER	Economic Record
GC	Growth and Change
HA	Hospital Administration (Chicago)
HB	Health Bulletin (Edinburgh)
HLR	Harvard Law Review
HM	Hospital Management
The Hospital	The Hospital and Health Services Review
Hospitals	Hospitals (Chicago)
Hosp.Pract.	Hospital Practice
HP	Hospital Progress
HSF	Hospital Services Finance
HSMHA Health Rep.	Health Services and Mental Health Administration Health Reports
HSR	Health Services Research
HT	Health Trends
IJE	International Journal of Epidemiology
IJHS	International Journal of Health Services
IJMS	Israeli Journal of Medical Science
ILR	International Labour Review
ILRR	Industrial and Labour Relations Review
Indian J.Med.Res.	Indian Journal of Medical Research
Indian J.Tuberc.	Indian Journal of Tuberculosis
IR	Indian Relations
ISSR	International Social Security Review
JACHA	Journal of the American College Health Association
JADA	Journal of the American Dental Association
JAMA	Journal of the American Medical Association
JASA	Journal of the American Statistical Association
JB	Journal of Business
J.Biosoc.Sci.	Journal of Biosocial Science
JCD	Journal of Chronic Diseases
JCGP	Journal of the College of General Practitioners
JDS	Journal of Development Studies
JEB	Journal of Economics and Business
JEI	Journal of Economic Issues
JET	Journal of Economic Theory
JHHB	Journal of Health and Human Behaviour
JHR	Journal of Human Resources

JHSB	Journal of Health and Social Behaviour
JLE	Journal of Law and Economics
JME	Journal of Medical Education
JNMD	Journal of Nervous and Mental Disease
JPE	Journal of Political Economy
JRCGP	Journal of the Royal College of General Practitioners
JRI	Journal of Risk and Insurance
JRSH	Journal of the Royal Society of Health
JRSS A	Journal of the Royal Statistical Society, Series A
J.Saf.Res.	Journal of Safety Research
JSP	Journal of Social Policy
JTEP	Journal of Transport Economics and Policy
Law Contemp. Probl.	Law and Contemporary Problems
LBR	Lloyds Bank Review
Man.School	Manchester School
Mayo Clin.Proc.	Mayo Clinic Proceedings
MC	Medical Care
MCR	Medical Care Review
ME	Medical Economics
Ment.Hyg.	Mental Hygiene
Meth.Inform. Med.	Methods of Information in Medicine
MH	Modern Hospital
Miss.Val.J.Bus. Econ.	Mississippi Valley Journal of Business and Economics
MJA	Medical Journal of Australia
MMFQ	Milbank Memorial Fund Quarterly
Mon.Lab.Rev.	Monthly Labour Review
MS	Management Science
MSMJ	Maryland State Medical Journal
NEJM	New England Journal of Medicine
NJEB	Nebraska Journal of Economics and Business
NR	Nursing Research
NTJ	National Tax Journal
OEP	Oxford Economic Papers
OG	Obstetrics and Gynecology
OHE	Office of Health Economics (London)
OR	Operations Research
ORQ	Operational Research Quarterly
PF	Public Finance
PFQ	Public Finance Quarterly
PHR	Public Health Reports
PI	The Public Interest
Population Studs.	Population Studies

PP	Public Policy
PPA	Philosophy and Public Affairs
PS	Political Studies
QJE	Quarterly Journal of Economics
QREB	Quarterly Review of Economics and Business
Rev.Econ.Cond. Ital.	Review of Economic Conditions in Italy
Rev.Econ.Stats.	Review of Economics and Statistics
RIW	Review of Income and Wealth
RL	Rehabilitation Literature
RSE	Review of Social Economics
SEA	Social and Economic Administration
SEJ	Southern Economic Journal
SGO	Surgery, Gynaecology and Obstetrics
SJE	Swedish Journal of Economics
SJPE	Scottish Journal of Political Economy
Soc.-Econ.Plan. Sciences	Socio-Economic Planning Sciences
SP	Social Psychiatry
SSB	Society Security Bulletin
SSM	Social Science and Medicine
SSQ	Social Science Quarterly
ST	Social Trends
USDHEW	United States Department of Health, Education and Welfare
WEJ	Western Economic Journal
WHO Bulletin	Bulletin of the World Health Organisation
WHO Chronicle	World Health Organisation Chronicle
W.Hosp.	World Hospitals
YB	Yorkshire Bulletin
YEE	Yale Economic Essays
YLJ	Yale Law Journal
YJBM	Yale Journal of Biology and Medicine

1 General Works

The purpose of this section is to give the reader an introduction to, and overview of, the field of study. For reasons explained in the Preface, the selection of entries for such a section is not straightforward: there are no works that are genuinely comprehensive, in the sense that they cover all or the greater part of the subject-matter classified in the bibliography. Consequently, it would be too restrictive to limit ourselves to 'guidebooks' and survey papers. Within the general principle that the work should be of sufficient breadth to justify the title 'general', therefore, we have included all works meeting one or both of two criteria: the work is concerned to define or examine the scope of health economics, or it illustrates how the tools of economic analysis may be applied to a general set of problems in the health care field.

Four papers attempting to define the subject-matter of 'health economics' are included: Mushkin (2, 9), Ginzberg (5) and Rothenberg (10). These will be useful to the reader wishing to discover what the subject is about. Among the longer texts, the works of Klarman (11), Ruchlin and Rogers (39) and Fuchs (43) come closest to being comprehensive. Fuchs, which is the most recent of these, is deficient only in that the treatment is intentionally elementary in an attempt to interest non-economists in the economist's approach. Campbell (23) and Donabedian (35) offer more limited coverage but deal in greater depth with the material they cover. To some extent, these two works are complementary, Campbell being strong on finance and organisation (principally in the United States) while these are the major gap in Donabedian's work.

There are a number of introductory and survey papers: Fuchs (12), P. J. Feldstein (15), Bowen and Jeffers (22), Abel-Smith (40) and M. S. Feldstein (42). The paper by M. S. Feldstein is a review of all of the major areas of empirical work and provides one of the most thought-provoking introductions to the field. The two papers by Bowen and Jeffers (26) and Levy (29) survey the current state of research in health economics in U.S.A. and France respectively. Two other studies of the U.S. health care systems – Somers and Somers (3) and Harris (6) – warrant inclusion as early studies of the health system that occupies most of the health economists in the world today.

Also included in this section are the general entries of four sets of conference proceedings – Mushkin (8), Klarman (18), Hauser (28) and Perlman (44); two sets of readings – Fuchs (27) and Cooper and Culyer (33); and nine collections of essays – McLachlan (ed.) (7, 13, 16, 20, 24, 25, 30, 37, 38). Most of the papers in these various compilations are separately annotated under the relevant sections of the bibliography.

Finally, we include a full list of the collection of short papers *Studies on Current Health Problems* issued by the Office of Health Economics (4). The attention of the reader is drawn to this collection since, although individual papers deal only with specific topics, the set provides an excellent conspectus of current issues.

1951

1 AMERICAN ECONOMIC ASSOCIATION, 'Economics of medical care'
AER, May, 1951, 41(2), pp. 617–96.
A session of the annual meeting of the AEA devoted to the economics of medical care. Six papers were presented:
Part I   The Problem
E. Ginzberg, 'Perspective on the economics of medical care', pp. 617–25.
F. Goldmann, 'Major areas of achievement and deficiency', pp. 626–32.
H. E. Klarman, 'Requirements for physicians', pp. 633–45.
Part II   Alternative
S. E. Harris, 'The British health experiment: the first two years of the National Health Service', pp. 652–66.
C. A. Kulp, 'Voluntary and compulsory medical care insurance', pp. 667–75.
J. Rothenberg, 'Welfare implications of alternative methods of financing medical care', pp. 676–87.
See 57, 984, 1084, 1152.

1958

2 S. J. MUSHKIN, 'Towards a definition of health economics'
PHR, September, 1958, 73(9), pp. 785–93.

An introductory article tracing the development of health economics as a discipline concerned with resource allocation rather than a discipline concerned simply with money and its relationship to medicine. The scope of health economics must not, however, be drawn so broadly that it shades into all other fields of economic inquiry, and its task is seen to be 'to appraise the efficiency of the organisation of health services, and to suggest ways of improving this organisation'.

1961

3 H. M. SOMERS, A. R. SOMERS, *Doctors, Patients, and Health Insurance*
Washington D.C.: The Brookings Institution, 1961, pp. xx, 576.

A major work. Although now fifteen years old, most of the issues treated remain issues today. Further, although this is a study of the American health-care system many of the subjects treated are of relevance to other systems. The book has six main sections: the first looks at medical progress and the emergence of scientific medicine; succeeding sections are entitled, the technological revolution in medicine, the revolution of rising expectations in consumer demand, the changing medical market place, private health insurance programmes, pressures and problems, and the changing doctor–patient relationship. A seventh section provides a summary and looks at critical areas for policy.

1962

4 OFFICE OF HEALTH ECONOMICS, *Studies on Current Health Problems*
London: Office of Health Economics, 1962–

A series of short booklets (20–40 pages) covering a wide variety of health topics. 51 had been produced by the end of 1974 and they continue to appear at the rate of three or four a year. A fairly high proportion deal with specific disease problems, and typically provide an outline of the nature of the disease, the history of its diagnosis, incidence, treatment, and costs to the National Health Service. Other topics that have been the subject of more than one booklet are general practice and the hospital service in Great Britain. A clear guide to the reorganisation of the National Health Service is also included in the series.

1   Progress against Tuberculosis
2   The Lives of Our Children: a study in childhood mortality
3   Hospital Costs in Perspective
4   Pneumonia in Decline
5   Health Services in Western Europe
6   The Price of Poliomyelitis
7   The Personal Health Services
8   The Venereal Diseases
9   Infants at Risk
10 The Costs of Medical Care
11 The Finance of Medical Research
12 New Frontiers in Health
13 The Pattern of Diabetes
14 The Pharmacist in Society
15 The Cost of Mental Care
16 Work Lost Through Sickness
17 The Local Health Services
18 Progress in Mental Health
19 The Common Illness of our Time (heart disease)
20 Medical Manpower
21 Disorders Which Shorten Life (mortality 15–44)
22 Efficiency in the Hospital Service
23 Malnutrition in the 1960s?
24 Pharmaceutical Research: the case for growth in Britain
25 Drug Addiction
26 Old Age (mortality and morbidity 64+)
27 Without Prescription (self medication)
28 General Practice Today
29 The Dental Service
30 Obesity and Disease
31 The Age of Maturity
32 Antibiotics in Animal Husbandry
33 The Ophthalmic Service
34 Alcohol Abuse
35 Building for Health
36 Off Sick
37 Prospects in Health
38 Epilepsy in Society
39 Hypertension
40 Family Planning in Britain
41 Migraine
42 Hospital Purchasing
43 Medicine and Society

44 Medical Care in Developing Countries
45 Rheumatism and Arthritis in Britain
46 Skin Disorders
47 Mental Handicap
48 The NHS Reorganisation
49 The Work of Primary Medical Care
50 Vaccination
51 Parkinson's Disease
See 195, 1054.

1964

5 E. GINZBERG, 'Medical economics – more than curves and computers'
   In S. J. Mushkin (Chairman) *The Economics of Health and Medical Care*, pp. 14–18 (8).
   A brief review of the field, a number of propositions that have been given inadequate consideration, the major problem areas, and some views about health-care policy.

5 S. E. HARRIS, *The Economics of American Medicine*
   New York: The Macmillan Company, 1964, pp. xvi, 508.
   The volume tackles a wide variety of issues. The emphasis is on the examination of the United States institutional base, and wherever possible illustrative statistics are provided. The opening section identifies the 'crucial issues' in health and medical economics that are to be dealt with in the succeeding chapters. Sections are included on the rising price of medical services, rising medical expenditures, and the economics of drugs. Medical manpower is dealt with in two sections: one section considers the total supply and distribution of physicians, physician productivity and physician remuneration; the final section of the book is a study of medical schools in the United States – variations in cost, sources of finance, and the role of the government in their finance. A long section of the book deals with hospitals, their costs, pricing policy and financing. Two sections of the book consider finance and organisation of health-care systems: one looks at compulsory programmes such as the British National Health Service and Medicare, the other at voluntary health insurance programmes.

7 G. MCLACHLAN (ed.) *Problems and Progress in Medical Care, Essays on Current Research, First Series*
   London: Oxford University Press, for Nuffield Provincial Hospitals

Trust, 1964, pp. xii, 368.

The first volume in a series of nine (up to 1974). It presents results of research sponsored by the Nuffield Provincial Hospitals Trust. The material is the product of a variety of socio-medical disciplines. The contents are as follows:

R. F. L. Logan, 'Studies in the spectrum of medical care', pp. 3–51.

R. W. Revans, 'The morale and effectiveness of general hospitals', pp. 55–69.

I. Jones, A. Barr, C. Butler, M. J. Tobin, J. O. F. Davies, 'Operational research in nursing', (five studies), pp. 73–111.

R. Scott, 'The family doctor diagnostic centre', pp. 115–32.

J. Collins, 'The social work content of general medical services', pp. 135–69.

C. W. M. Wilson, J. B. Banks, R. E. A. Mapes, S. M. T. Karte, 'The assessment of prescribing: a study in operational research', pp. 173–201.

A. Jones, H. L. Miles, 'The Anglesey mental health survey', pp. 205–63.

B. M. Mandelbrote, 'Mental illness in hospital and community: developments and outcome', pp. 267–90.

E. G. Oram, M. C. Knowles, 'The chronic mentally ill – movements in a rural area: 1900–1961', pp. 293–316.

G. F. Rehin, H. Houghton, F. M. Martin, 'Mental health social work in hospitals and local authorities: a comparison of the work situations', pp. 319–51.

K. Jones, A. Tillotson, 'The population of epileptic colonies', pp. 355–68.

8   S. J. MUSHKIN (Chairman), *The Economics of Health and Medical Care*
Ann Arbor: University of Michigan, 1964, pp. viii, 321.

The proceedings of a conference on the economics of medical care held at the University of Michigan in 1962. Seventeen papers on the following six broad topics were presented:

1   The Role of the Economist in the Health Services Industry
2   Organisation and Financing of Health Services
3   Demand, Costs, and Prices of Health Care
4   The Microeconomics of Health Care
5   Investment in Health
6   Agenda for Research

See 5, 9, 10, 47, 67, 158, 180, 366, 368, 650, 951, 952, 1098, 1166, 1167, 1168.

9   S. J. MUSHKIN, 'Why health economics?'
In S. J. Mushkin (Chairman) *The Economics of Health and Medical Care*, pp. 3–13 (8).

The attention given by economists in the early 1960s to health resulted, it is suggested, from the interest in economic growth, the growing importance of the public sector, the increasing share of national resources being devoted to health, and the fact that the health industry is in transition. Policy problems are viewed as being largely the result of the previous ten years' medical developments, and the growth in capacity to provide health care. The chief problems to be faced are, it is argued, those connected with the allocation of real resources.

J. ROTHENBERG, 'Agenda for research in the economics of health'
In S. J. Mushkin (Chairman) *The Economics of Health and Medical Care*, pp. 309–16 (8).

A long list of topics, the paper was added after the conference to round off the book of readings.

1965

H. E. KLARMAN, *The Economics of Health*
New York: Columbia University Press, 1965, pp. viii, 200.

The book is an attempt both to interest economists in the health field and to acquaint the layman with the economist's approach to health problems. The opening chapter offers a definition of health economics, an outline of the health care industry, and a discussion of the distinctive economic characteristics of health and medical services. The middle chapters consider the factors influencing private demand for care, demand by business, philanthropy and government, the supply of medical manpower, the supply of hospital services, and the organisation and regulation of care. The book closes with an examination of three problem areas: the construction and use of the medical care price index, the calculation of the costs and benefits of health programmes, and the problem of determining what a society can afford to spend on health care. There is no empirical work in the book.

1966

V. R. FUCHS, 'The contribution of health services to the American economy'
MMFQ, October, 1966, 44(2), pp. 65–101. Also in V. R. Fuchs (ed.) *Essays in the Economics of Health and Medical Care*, pp. 3–38 (27) and M. H. Cooper, A. J. Culyer (eds.) *Health Economics*, pp. 135–71 (33).

A survey article showing the approach of the economist to the health-care field. The article examines the contribution of health services, discusses how health care is different from other goods, the nature of health and the factors that contribute to it, indexes of health, and the relation between health services and health. The need to measure the output of the health industry is stressed throughout. A substantial bibliography is provided.

13   G. McLachlan (ed.) *Problems and Progress in Medical Care, Essays on Current Research, Second Series*
London: Oxford University Press, for Nuffield Provincial Hospitals Trust, 1966, pp. xi, 338.

Eleven papers, mostly non-economic, organised in three sections, constitute the second volume in this series.

Part I   Studies of Hospital Out-patient Services

1   R. Scott, M. Gilmore, 'The Edinburgh hospitals', pp. 3–41.

2   J. Chamberlain, 'Two non-teaching hospitals in South-East England', pp. 43–76.

3   E. M. Backett, G. Sumner, J. Kilpatrick, I. Dingwall-Forsyth, 'Hospitals in the North-East Scotland region', pp. 77–122.

4   J. Butterfield, M. Wadsworth, 'A London teaching hospital', pp. 123–52.

Part II   Studies of Function and Organisation

5   R. Z. Apte, 'The transitional hostel in the rehabilitation of the mentally ill', pp. 155–85.

6   W. Carson, T. W. Maver, 'Cost-effectiveness and the engineering services in hospitals', pp. 187–205.

7   D. J. Newell, A. Zinovieff, L. W. Hunt, 'The evaluation of an experimental pre-discharge ward', pp. 207–33.

8   C. J. H. Mann, 'An experiment in communication between GPs and hospital staff', pp. 235–48.

Part III   Examining the Bases of Policy

9   R. Shegog, 'The future of the maternity services: a suitable case for study', pp. 251–76.

10   E. G. Knox, 'Cervical cytology: a scrutiny of the evidence', pp. 277–309.

11   N. D. Richards, A. J. Willcocks, 'The level of dental health: the field for study', pp. 311–38.

1968

14   P. Bierman, E. J. Connors, E. Flook, R. R. Huntley, T. McCarthy, P. J. Sanazaro, 'Health services research in Great Britain'
MMFQ, January, 1968, 46(1, part 1), pp. 9–102.

The majority of the work surveyed is social medicine, operations research and social administration, work that has in many cases provided the background for more recent economic studies. Health services research in Great Britain and the U.S.A. is compared. A bibliography of 175 items is included.

15   P. J. Feldstein, 'Applying economic concepts to hospital care'
HA, Winter, 1968, 13(1), pp. 68–89.

A simple introduction to the application of economics in the medical care field, and an outline of some basic economic concepts and the sort of questions they can be used to deal with.

G. McLachlan (ed.) *Problems and Progress in Medical Care, Essays on Current Research, Third Series*
London: Oxford University Press, for Nuffield Provincial Hospitals Trust, 1968, pp. x, 170.

Seven papers are included in the third volume in this series, although only three, on manpower, have an economic bias.
1 J. R. Ashford, F. S. W. Brimblecombe, J. G. Fryer, 'Birth weight and perinatal mortality in England and Wales 1956–65', pp. 1–30.
2 S. L. Morrison, 'Medical manpower in the National Health Service', pp. 31–50.
3 R. Shannon, 'Manpower planning in the National Health Service', pp. 51–62.
4 A. J. Willcocks, 'The staffing of the maternity services', pp. 63–90.
5 N. W. Timms, 'Child guidance service: a pilot study', pp. 91–114.
6 H. Houghton, 'Problems of hospital communication: an experimental study', pp. 115–44.
7 R. F. A. Shegog, 'Reviewing some applications of computer to medicine: a tale of two philosophies', pp. 145–70.
See 211, 213.

1970

M. Blaug, *An Introduction to the Economics of Education*
Hardmondsworth, England: Penguin Books Ltd., 1970, pp. xx, 363.

A survey of a closely related field. An appendix is included on the similarities and differences between health and education. The sections on manpower forecasting and rate of return to education calculations are also of particular interest to health economists.

H. E. Klarman (ed.) *Empirical Studies in Health Economics*
Baltimore: The Johns Hopkins Press, 1970, pp. x, 433.

The proceedings of the Second Conference on the Economics of Health held at Baltimore in 1968 (S. J. Mushkin (Chairman) *The Economics of Health and Medical Care*, records the first conference). Eighteen papers are included in this volume, arranged under five broad headings:
1 Population, Health, and Programme Planning

2   Demand Analysis
3   Structure of Industry
4   Productivity and Cost
5   Factors of Production
Klarman provides an introduction, entitled 'Trends and tendencies in health economics', pp. 3–14.
See 8, 90, 97, 98, 228, 241, 246, 426, 427, 429, 434, 437, 442, 571, 869, 960, 963, 1389.

19 J. R. LAVE, L. B. LAVE, 'Medical care and its delivery: an economic appraisal'
Law Contemp.Probl., Spring, 1970, 35(2), pp. 252–66.
A brief survey of many of the issues and the difficulties involved in determining the correct allocation of resources to health care.

20 G. MCLACHLAN (ed.) *Problems and Progress in Medical Care, Essays on Current Research, Fourth Series*
London: Oxford University Press, for Nuffield Provincial Hospitals Trust, 1970, pp. x, 204.
Six papers are included in this volume, although only the first and third concern themselves directly with economic issues:
1   G. Forsyth, R. G. Thomas, S. P. Jones, 'Planning in practice: a half-term report', pp. 1–28.
2   G. A. Neligen, 'Prescriptive screening of children', pp. 29–44.
3   D. R. Wilson, J. E. McLachlan, 'Supporting service centres', pp. 45–96.
4   E. G. Knox, J. W. Dale, 'The operational syntax of medical records', pp. 97–144.
5   A. Smith, I. D. Richards, M. Nicholson, E. Gronick, 'The Glasgow linked system of child health records', pp. 145–78.
6   B. Watkin, M. Taylor, 'An experiment in management education for nurses', pp. 179–204.

21 G. F. ROHRLICH (ed.) *Social Economics for the 1970s*
New York: Dunellen Publishing Company, 1970, p. 189.
Problems and policies to deal with them in the U.S.A. in the fields of social security health care and manpower development are discussed in this volume. The book is divided into four parts. The first and fourth parts by Rohrlich review the field of social economics and social policy, and consider draft legislation awaiting consideration by Congress. The second part of the book provides a historical and conceptual background to the policy areas and includes an article by G. Piel entitled 'Improving the Nation's health: joint leverage for economic and social adjustment'. The third part of the book deals with existing or specific proposed programmes and includes an article by H. M.

Somers entitled 'Delivery of health care: do we know where we are going?', which looks at trends in costs and utilisation, at quality of care, and at health facilities planning.

1971

H. R. BOWEN, J. R. JEFFERS, *The Economics of Health Services*
New York: General Learning Press, 1971, p. 24.

After outlining the basic characteristics of the health system of the U.S.A., its activities, total expenditures, resources and sources of finance, the paper moves on to consider some of the basic questions which have occupied health economists. The questions dealt with include: what, if any, are the special characteristics of health services? what are the goals of the health services industry, and how successful is it in fulfilling them? Finally, public policy in the U.S.A. in the health services industry is examined. It is concluded that a major overhaul of the U.S. health services industry is needed.

R. R. CAMPBELL, *Economics of Health and Public Policy*
Washington D.C.: American Enterprise Institute for Public Policy Research, 1971, p. 108.

This slim volume is intended to provide background material necessary for understanding the health industry, and to enable the reader to assess for himself the many proposals for changing the United States health system. Six short sections deal respectively with the availability and organisation of health service resources, third-party payments (their role and effects), levels of health in the United States, the markets for emergency and non-emergency care, methods of allocating care, and finally policy considerations and suggested alternatives in organising and financing medical care.

G. McLACHLAN (ed.) *Problems and Progress in Medical Care, Essays on Current Research, Fifth Series*
London: Oxford University Press, for Nuffield Provincial Hospitals Trust, 1971, pp. viii, 174.

Seven papers on a very diverse set of topics:
1   R. G. S. Brown, C. Walker, 'The distribution of medical manpower', pp. 1–44.
2   J. D. Pole, 'Mass radiography: a cost–benefit approach', pp. 45–56.
3   G. R. Andrews, N. R. Cowan, W. F. Anderson, 'The practice of geriatric medicine in the community', pp. 57–86.

4   M. Shepherd, 'Childhood behaviour, mental health, and medical services', pp. 87–106.
5   M. Capes, 'The care and treatment of the adolescent psychiatric patient', pp. 107–18.
6   T. McKeown, 'Health and humanism', pp. 119–36.
7   W. J. McNerney, 'Financing and delivery of health services in Britain', pp. 137–74.
See 250, 720.

25   G. McLACHLAN (ed.) *Portfolio for Health, Problems and Progress in Medical Care, Essays on Current Research, Sixth Series*
London: Oxford University Press, for Nuffield Provincial Hospitals Trust, 1971, pp. xiv, 301.

Sub-titled 'The Role and Programme of the Department of Health and Social Security in Health Services Research', the volume is divided into three parts. The first part is a paper by R. H. L. Cohen explaining the Department's role in research and development; the third part provides a list of the Department's current activities. The long second part of the volume consists of twenty-three papers, most of them fairly short, on selected activities and problems. Of particular interest to economists are the papers by G. K. Matthew, 'Measuring need and evaluating services', and by J. M. G. Wilson, 'Screening in the early detection of disease'.
See 108, 725.

1972

26   H. R. BOWEN, J. R. JEFFERS, 'The economics of health services in the United States'
In M. M. Hauser (ed.) *The Economics of Medical Care*, pp. 280–303 (28).

An outline of the principal areas of current study, and a discussion of some notable pieces of research. The studies discussed cover manpower, economies of scale in hospitals and physician practice, the organisation of medical practice, Medicare and finance, cost–benefit and cost-effectiveness of disease, and health indicators. Some examples of the basic statistics on health services being collected in the U.S.A. are also presented.

27   V. R. FUCHS (ed.) *Essays in the Economics of Health and Medical Care*
New York: National Bureau of Economic Research, 1972, pp. xxii, 239.

A collection of nine papers arranged in four sections:
1 An economist's view of health and medical care
2 Medical care – demand and supply
3 The production of health
4 Spatial variations in mortality rates
The individual studies in the volume relate to the United States health system.
See 12, 49, 98, 127, 162, 278, 418.

M. M. HAUSER (ed.) *The Economics of Medical Care*
London: George Allen and Unwin Ltd., 1972, pp. 334.

The proceedings of a conference held at the University of York in 1970. Fifteen papers on five topics are included in the volume, with two further papers outlining some of the problems for health economics. A comprehensive survey of the issues raised in the conference is provided by Hauser. The topics covered are as follows:
1 Efficiency and Equality in Medical Care Provision
2 Economic Analysis as a Means of Programme Assessment
3 Efficiency and Planning in Hospital Care
4 Social Accounting and Operational Research in Medical Care
5 International Studies
See 26, 29, 128, 461, 477, 481, 485, 748, 754, 1032, 1127, 1134, 1135, 1136, 1404.

M. E. LEVY, 'French studies on health economics: a survey'
In M. M. Hauser (ed.) *The Economics of Medical Care*, pp. 269–79 (28).

A survey of recent French studies in the field of health economics. The studies cover needs for health care, needs for facilities, the demand for care and the influences upon demand, the costs of illness, the optimal size of departments within hospitals, cost–benefit analyses of tuberculosis, mental health, and health screening, and the value of human life.

G. MCLACHLAN (ed.) *Problems and Progress in Medical Care, Essays on Current Research, Seventh Series*
London: Oxford University Press, for Nuffield Provincial Hospitals Trust, 1972.

A collection of nine papers; the first three and the seventh are of particular interest to economists.
1 A. J. Culyer, 'The "market" versus the "state" in medical care – a minority report on an empty academic box', pp. 1–31.
2 R. J. Lavers, M. Rees, 'The distinction award system in England and Wales', pp. 33–68.

3   J. Bradshaw, 'A taxonomy of social need', pp. 69–82.
4   J. G. Rosen, K. Jones, C. M. Taylor, 'Profile of the male nurse. A research report', pp. 83–92.
5   C. M. Taylor, 'From person to patient. A pilot study of hospital admission procedures', pp. 93–112.
6   B. M. Oatey, 'Rural communities in the welfare state. Social policy reappraised', pp. 113–30.
7   P. Gedling, D. J. Newell, 'Hospital beds for the elderly', pp. 131–45.
8   K. R. Gilhome, D. J. Newell, 'Community services for the elderly', pp. 147–62.
9   L. Rosenbloom, 'Postgraduate medical education in developmental pediatrics', pp. 163–200.
See 115, 283, 474, 1030.

31   OPEN UNIVERSITY, *Health* (Block V, Parts 1–5)
Bletchley, Bucks: The Open University Press, 1972, p. 197.

Part of an Open University course 'Decision making in Britain'. In examining the British National Health Service most of the issues that have occupied social scientists studying health and health care are touched upon.
See 1133.

1973

32   B. ABEL-SMITH, B. BENJAMIN, W. W. HOLLAND, J. W. PEARSON, D. F. J. PIACHAUD, O. GOLDSMITH, J. D. POLE, *Accounting For Health*
London: King Edward's Hospital Fund, 1973, p. 63.

The report of a King's Fund Working Party, it examines the role of economic principles in improving the use of health service resources. Sections of the report examine the evaluation of outcomes, data sources and their limitations, and activity units.

33   M. H. COOPER, A. J. CULYER (eds.) *Health Economics*
Harmondsworth, England: Penguin Books Ltd., 1973, p. 396.

A collection of fifteen major papers arranged in four sections: economic efficiency, improving decisions, hospitals and the value of human lives.
See 12, 46, 246, 375, 403, 435, 676, 827, 829, 830, 954, 1006, 1017, 1161, 1380.

34   A. J. CULYER, *The Economics of Social Policy*
London: Martin Robertson and Company Ltd., 1973, pp. xii, 268.

The book examines the role of economics in formulating and evaluating social policy. Health topics specifically discussed include health planning, output measurement, and drug abuse.

5 A. DONABEDIAN, *Aspects of Medical Care Administration: Specifying Requirements for Health Care*
Cambridge, Massachusetts: Harvard University Press, 1973, p. 649.

A massive work, not as the title might suggest a work on management, but a work that is 'abstract and conceptual', designed 'to foster a particular way of thinking about medical care problems'. There are only five chapters, but these are subdivided. Extensive bibliographies follow each chapter. The first chapter examines different value positions and the way they affect thinking and choices about medical care provision, and also at the distinctive characteristics of medical care. Chapter two examines organisational objectives. Chapter three is entitled 'The assessment of need' and examines the concept of need and the problems of measuring need defined in terms of health status. The fourth chapter, the longest in the book, looks at supply, the problems of measuring output and productivity, economies of scale in hospital and ambulatory care. The final chapter looks at the problems of estimating the requirement for services and resources, at methods based on demand, methods based on need, and methods that project supply and compare them to requirements.
See 134, 296, 504, 621, 911, 1019, 1414, 1489.

6 P. J. FELDSTEIN, *Financing Dental Care: An Economic Analysis*
Lexington: D.C. Heath and Company, 1973, pp. xvii, 260.

While the subject of this volume is dental care, the problems tackled are similar to those found in the health-care field generally; similarly the body of techniques used to tackle the problems are of more general application. The study is divided into six parts. The first part, entitled 'Needs in dental health care', presents a schematic model of the dental care sector showing how the various parts interrelate. The second part examines the demand for personal dental care, its growth over time and the role of insurance; both cross-section and time series analyses of per capita expenditures on dental care are carried out. The third part of the study considers the supply of dental care, the nature of the dental firm, the factors influencing the use of auxiliary personnel, the determinants of long-run supply, and the problem of improving the distribution of dentists. Estimates of the rate of return to dental education made by Hansen and Maurizi are included in an appendix. The fourth section examines the demand for and supply of educational facilities in the dental sector and includes an empirical examination of economies of scale in dental education. The fifth section presents an econometric model for forecasting and policy evaluation in the dental sector, which is specified at three levels: the market for dental visits; the market for dental manpower; and the market for dental manpower training facilities. The final section considers the role of government in the financing and provision of dental services, and besides theoretical discussion estimates are made of the probable utilisation, costs and effects of alternative national insurance plans for dental care.

37   G. McLachlan (ed.) *Portfolio for Health 2, Problems and Progress in Medical Care, Essays on Current Research, Eighth Series*
London: Oxford University Press for Nuffield Provincial Hospitals Trust, 1973, pp. xx, 463.

A second volume examining the work and activities of the Department of Health and Social Security in health services research. The format is similar to the sixth series volume: an introductory section by R. H. L. Cohen, the Chief Scientist of DHSS; a second section of twenty-six papers, the first sixteen on research directions, mainly medical, the last ten looking at the work of specific research units; and a final section listing research units and projects supported by DHSS and details of the publications of these research units.

38   G. McLachlan (ed.) *The Future – and Present Indicatives, Problems and Progress in Medical Care, Essays on Current Research, Ninth Series*
London: Oxford University Press, for Nuffield Provincial Hospitals Trust, 1973, pp. xii, 193.

Six papers are included in the ninth volume in this series; the second, third and sixth papers are of particular interest to economists.
1   Sir G. Godber, 'Future developments in epidemiology', pp. 1–15.
2   E. G. Knox, 'A simulation system for screening procedures', pp. 17–55.
3   J. R. Ashford, G. Ferster, D. M. Makuc, 'An approach to resource allocation in the reorganised National Health Service', pp. 57–90.
4   M. R. Alderson, 'Information systems in the unified Health Service', pp. 91–136.
5   J. M. Yates, 'Information for the management of clinical work in hospitals', pp. 137–55.
6   C. R. Hearn, 'Evaluation of patients' nursing needs: prediction of staffing', pp. 157–93.
See 302, 1412.

39   H. S. Ruchlin, D. C. Rogers, *Economics and Health Care*
Springfield, Illinois: Charles C. Thomas Publisher, 1973, pp. xvii, 317.

A comprehensive textbook designed to acquaint health administrators with the application of economics to the health field. To aid this purpose a chapter is included on economic methodology, as are expositions of the theory of demand, production, neo-classical growth theory, and investment criteria; two appendices are included on statistical and mathematical tools. The ten chapters that form the core of the book cover most of the major topics of health economics: national income accounting and health care, the medical care price index, the demand for care, production and cost studies, investment and cost–benefit analysis, economic growth and health planning, and finally a chapter on the financing of health care. Incorporated in three of the chapters are research studies undertaken by other economists: Rosenthal on the demand for hospital facilities, Cohen, Baligh and Laughhunn on hospitals, Weisbrod on poliomyelitis, and Klarman, Francis and Rosenthal on renal disease. Bibliographies of supplementary reading are provided for each chapter. *See* 1259.

1974

B. ABEL-SMITH, 'Economics of health and disease'
Encyclopaedia Britannica, 1974, 8, pp. 689–93.
A brief review of the problems with which health economics attempts to deal. The bulk of the paper is concerned with finance of health care, payment of medical personnel and international comparisons of health expenditure.

A. J. CULYER (ed.) *Economic Policies and Social Goals*
London: Martin Robertson and Company Ltd., 1974, p. 349.
Fourteen papers by past and present York economists covering a variety of social policy issues and the theoretical/methodological problems underlying social policy economics. Four papers by A. Williams, J. Wiseman and J. Cullis, R. L. Akehurst and K. G. Wright, deal with health economics problems.
See 155, 791, 949, 1365, 1370.

M. S. FELDSTEIN, 'Econometric studies of health economics'
In M. D. Intriligator, D. A. Kendrick (eds.) *Frontiers of Quantitative Economics*, Amsterdam: North-Holland, 1974, Vol. 2, pp. 377–447.
Provides a survey of the empirical work done in health economics in the last decade. The survey is divided into four main parts: the market for hospital services, the market for physicians' services, the economics of health insurance, and some problems of the econometric method.
See 149, 319, 534, 591, 1265.

V. R. FUCHS, *Who Shall Live? Health, Economics, and Social Choice*
New York: Basic Books Inc., 1974, pp. vii, 168.
An outline and analysis of the problems facing the American, and many other health-care systems. The book is intended primarily for non-economists, and

the central theme developed in the book is 'the necessity of choice at both the individual and social levels'. Other topics considered are the role of the physician as a decision-taker, the doctor shortage, the impact of different methods of payment for medical care and the relationship between health and medical care. Chapters are also included on hospitals and the drug industry.

44   M. PERLMAN (ed.) *The Economics of Health and Medical Care*
London: Macmillan Press Ltd., 1974, pp. xx, 547.

The proceedings of the conference held by the International Economic Association in Tokyo in 1973. Twenty-five papers, arranged in five sections, together with summaries of the discussions that the papers stimulated, are presented. The principal findings of the papers are outlined in Perlman's introduction, and each paper is preceded by a brief author summary.
See 54, 55, 56, 150, 318, 331, 529, 533, 552, 594, 628, 792, 936, 940, 947, 981, 983, 1047, 1081, 1141, 1142, 1143, 1270, 1422, 1424.

2 Demand/Need for Health

In this section we have separated the general 'human capital' approach to the demand for health from work on the demand/need for health services. The human capital approach examines the demand for health as such, the value of health or cost of ill-health, how health is a factor affecting the 'household production function' and how health can be produced, with explicit recognition that inputs other than medical services contribute towards the production of health. The other work in this section is concerned with questions relating to the demand for health services. This is clearly in part a derived demand (derived from the demand for health itself) but studies typically investigate other interdependencies too, such as the relationship between social, economic and medical factors in determining the pattern of demand and supply for health services.

(a)   The Human Capital/Investment Approach

The earlier pieces of work cited in this section form part of a long tradition: Dublin and Lotka (45) and Fein (50) document the major contributions to this tradition dating back over the previous two centuries. The tradition reaches greater sophistication, and particularly empirical sophistication as a result of better data sources, with the work of Fein, Mushkin and Weisbrod. (More of their empirical work is included in Section 4(a).) The work of Becker on education (48) is included because it is the origin, and remains the most thorough discussion, of much of the conceptual apparatus of human capital theory.

The later work in this section draws on Becker's work on demand theory/time allocation. The major work is undoubtedly that of Grossman (51, 52).

1946

45   L. I. DUBLIN, A. J. LOTKA, *The Money Value of a Man*
New York: Ronald Press, 1946, pp. xvii, 214.

The second chapter of the book provides a survey of attempts to measure the money value of a man from the work of Sir William Petty to twentieth-century publications on the human capital costs of war.
See 823.

1962

46   S. J. MUSHKIN, 'Health as an investment'
JPE, October, 1962, 70 (5 part 2), pp. 129–57. Also in M. H. Cooper, A. J. Culyer (eds.) *Health Economics*, pp. 93–134 (33).

The paper begins with an examination of the similarities and differences between investment in education and investment in health. The problem of measuring capital formation resulting from improved health care is discussed, and estimates made of the magnitude of such capital formation in the United States. The paper concludes with a study of the different approaches used in studies that estimate the value of human capital created through health programmes.

1963

47   S. J. MUSHKIN, B. A. WEISBROD, 'Investment in health – lifetime health expenditures on the 1960 work force'
Kyklos, 1963, 16(4), pp. 583–98. Also in S. J. Mushkin (Chairman) *The Economics of Health and Medical Care*, pp. 257–70 (8).

An estimate is made of the value of resources, private and public, devoted to the health of the 1960 U.S. work force since their birth. Estimates are also made of average health expenditure over the lifetime of different age groups. The aggregate health stock, as the total expenditure figure is termed, is compared with the aggregate education stock, and with the stock of physical capital.

1964

8   G. S. BECKER, *Human Capital*
New York: National Bureau of Economic Research, 1964, pp. xvi, 187.
A classic work, concerned principally with education. There are nevertheless numerous observations of relevance to investment in health, for instance the discussion of the relation between on-the-job and outside-the-job investments in health, diet and other factors, (pp. 33–6).

1969

9   R. AUSTER, I. LEVESON, D. SARACHEK, 'The production of health: an exploratory study'
JHR, Fall, 1969, 4(4), pp. 411–36. Also in V. R. Fuchs (ed.) *Essays in the Economics of Health and Medical Care*, pp. 135–58 (27).
The primary purpose of the paper is to estimate the elasticity of health with respect to medical services. This is achieved by examining by means of a regression model the impact of a number of factors on the age-adjusted death rate of whites and non-whites in the United States: income, education, proportion of the population in manufacturing, alcohol consumption per capita, cigarette consumption per capita, health expenditures per capita, and presence of a medical school. A second model disaggregates the medical care component into four separate parts. Both models indicated that a 1 per cent increase in medical services was associated with a reduction in mortality of about 0.1 per cent.

1971

0   R. FEIN, 'On measuring economic benefits of health programmes'
In G. McLachlan, T. McKeown (eds.) *Medical History and Medical Care*, London: Oxford University Press, 1971, pp. 181–220.
See 711.

1972

51   M. GROSSMAN, 'On the concept of health capital and the demand for health'
JPE, March–April, 1972, 80(2), pp. 223–55.
A model of the demand for the commodity 'good health' is developed. The model has its origins in the new approach to consumer behaviour in which consumers produce 'commodities' with inputs of market goods and their own time. The model assumes that consumers inherit a stock of health capital that depreciates over their lifetime, and that this stock can be augmented by investment. Variations in health and demand for medical care are explained in the model by variations in the demand for, and supply of, health capital. The implications of increases in the rate of depreciation of the stock of health with age, and the effects of wage rate and education charges on the demand for, and supply of, health capital are explored.

52   M. GROSSMAN, *The Demand for Health: A Theoretical and Empirical Investigation*
New York: National Bureau of Economic Research, 1972, pp. xvii, 155.
A model of the demand for health, developed from the new theory of consumer behaviour, is constructed. Besides examining the theoretical implications of the model and exploring the effects of changes in such elements as education and wage rates on the demand for health and medical care, the monograph also includes some empirical analysis, and estimates are made of demand curves for health and medical care and gross investment production functions.

53   A. G. HOLTMANN, 'Prices, time, and technology in the medical care market'
JHR, Spring, 1972, 7(2), pp. 179–90.
The implications of Becker's model of consumer behaviour, which takes account of the cost of time in consumption, are examined. The effects of wage and price changes and technical changes on the demand for care are analysed.

1974

54   V. R. FUCHS, 'Some economic aspects of mortality in developed countries'
In M. Perlman (ed.) *The Economics of Health and Medical Care*, pp. 174–93 (44).
Examination of cross-section, and some time series data, reveals that the traditional negative association between mortality and income per capita is disappearing in the developed countries. Changes in the availability of medical care, holding the state of the art constant, likewise appear to make only a small

contribution to life expectancy. Differences in mortality must be explained by reference to 'life style'. The demand for life and the ability to produce it vary among populations (some illustrative examples are given). Knowledge of the underlying production and demand functions is necessary for an understanding of longevity.

5 M. GROSSMAN, L. BENHAM, 'Health, hours and wages'
In M. Perlman (ed.) *The Economics of Health and Medical Care*, pp. 205–33 (44).

The household production function model of demand theory is used to construct a three-equation model to examine the effects of health on wages and weeks worked. Results indicated that health had positive effects on wages and weeks worked. Treating health as an endogenous variable strengthened the effect of health on market productivity.

6 J. P. NEWHOUSE, C. E. PHELPS, 'Price and income elasticities for medical care services'
In M. Perlman (ed.) *The Economics of Health and Medical Care*, pp. 139–61 (44).

The paper extends the work of Grossman (1972) on investment in health by allowing for multiple medical inputs in the production of health, introducing reimbursement insurance, which alters the net price of care, and allowing the choice of different 'styles' of care. Demand curves are then estimated from 1963 United States household survey data.
See 52.

(b) Demand and Need for Health Care

From the beginning of their interest in health systems, economists have shown awareness that, at least from the normative point of view, the traditional individualistic basis of demand analysis left much to be desired. Whether the notion of 'need' adequately transcended the limitations of 'demand' has been much debated with particular emphasis on whether 'paternalism' is involved and on the technological characteristics of need. The modern approach tends to be to treat the interests of third parties as a kind of 'merit want' relationship or as the consequence of direct interdependence between utility functions.

On the positive side emphasis has increasingly been placed upon the agency role of physicians – a crucial aspect of the doctor–patient relationship being seen as the professional's responsibility to interpret (and then supply) the 'needs' of the patient. In empirical work this has led to recognition of the fact that price changes may, in addition to having the expected negative relationship with the patient's preferred rate of consumption, have a positive relationship with the physician's assessment of need. Thus, a rise in price may cause patients to move upwards along a demand curve *and* cause physicians to shift that curve to the right.

Both these aspects (normative and positive) have induced scepticism about the efficiency of market operations, the former because of the difficulty of ensuring that externalities are reckoned with, the latter because of the interdependency of supply and demand. Unfortunately, no clear guidance emerges for the public sector either. On the one hand attention tends to focus on the 'merit good', 'externality', dimensions to the exclusion of the patient's preferences, while, on the other hand, there are no obvious means of distinguishing the effects of professional judgements about patients' needs from the effects of professional self-interest.

It is now generally recognised that professional assessments of 'need' not only largely determine 'demand' (other things being equal) but that these judgements are a mixture of both technical considerations and the results of social conditioning. The consequences for utilisation studies, efficient allocation of resources and physician monitoring are, however, only just beginning to be explored.

Articles dealing with the central issues include Klarman (57), Boulding (73), Culyer *et al.* (101), Evans *et al.* (135) and Williams (155).

1951

57 H. E. KLARMAN, 'Requirements for physicians'
   AER, May, 1951, 41(2), pp. 633–45.

   An early discussion of need rather than economic criteria as a basis for determining requirements for medical care. It is suggested that need can best be established by studying utilisation of medical services by a group who receive comprehensive care for moderate insurance premiums.

1958

E. G. JACO (ed.) *Patients, Physicians and Illness*
New York: The Free Press, 1958, p. 600.

A collection of fifty-five papers, mostly non-economic, but a number of papers deal with social, cultural and economic aspects of health and disease, in particular B. J. Stern on 'Socio-economic aspects of heart disease', J. M. Ellis on 'Socio-economic differentials in mortality from chronic diseases', and P. S. Lawrence on 'Chronic illness and socio-economic status'.

L. S. ROSENFELD, A. DONABEDIAN, J. KATZ, 'Unmet need for medical care' *NEJM*, February 20th, 1958, 258(8), pp. 369–76.

A study attempting to measure the ratio of unmet to met need for medical care in each of five socio-economic groups in Boston. Five indices of unmet need are used in the study relating to perinatal mortality, the amount of prenatal care, prenatal dental visits, the presence of untreated symptoms considered by doctors to be important enough to warrant medical care, and the number of dental visits.

1961

H. M. SOMERS, A. R. SOMERS, *Doctors, Patients and Health Insurance*
Washington D.C.: The Brookings Institution, 1961, pp. xx, 576.
See 3.

1964

M. S. FELDSTEIN, 'Hospital planning and the demand for care'
BOUIES, November, 1964, 26(4), pp. 361–8.
See 363.

P. J. FELDSTEIN, W. J. CARR, 'The effect of income on medical care spending'
American Statistical Association Proceedings, Social Statistics Section, 1964, 7, pp. 93–105.

Examination of data on medical care spending and income unadjusted for transitory components revealed an income elasticity of demand in 1950 of 0.7; allowance for the transitory component in income raised this figure to 1.0. An estimate for 1960 with allowances for transitory components and increased health insurance enrolment suggested an income elasticity of 0.883, although the authors thought that this estimate was likely to be slightly low. See also the comments by H. E. Klarman, J. Rothenberg, pp. 106–12.

63 S. JUDEK, *Medical Manpower in Canada*
Ottawa: Royal Commission on Health Services, Queens Printer, 1964, pp. xx, 413.
See 182.

64 R. F. L. LOGAN, 'Assessment of sickness and health in the community: needs and methods'
MC, July–September, 1964, 2(3), pp. 173–90, and *MC*, October–December, 1964, 2(4), pp. 218–25.
Of interest to economists chiefly as a survey of available data and their deficiencies for assessing sickness and health in the community. It is concluded that mortality is an inadequate yardstick of health, and that more varied measures of morbidity are needed to assist in the allocation of resources. The problems of measuring morbidity are discussed, and the difference between demand and need, the problem of the 'iceberg' and the influence of information and facilities upon it. Various sources of information on morbidity are then examined and their strengths and limitations discussed.

65 D. J. NEWELL, 'Problems in estimating the demand for hospital beds'
JCD, September, 1964, 17(9), pp. 749–59.
See 346, 352, 369, 370, 371, 474, 484.

66 G. D. ROSENTHAL, *The Demand for General Hospital Facilities*
Chicago: American Hospital Association, Hospital Monograph Series No. 14, 1964, pp. 101.
The study is divided into three sections. The first short section provides a review of the growth of the hospital system in the United States, and examines various methods that have been used to estimate bed needs. The second section develops a method for estimating bed needs based on a demand model that estimates hospital utilization for an area from socio-demographic and economic characteristics. The theoretical model developed is used to estimate the demand for patient days of care in the United States for 1950 and 1960; these estimates are then used to provide estimates of the beds needed per 1000 population in the separate states. The third section of the study deals with the implications of the estimated relationships for the distribution of facilities throughout the United States. The influence of the supply of facilities on

demand is examined, and while the two are clearly interrelated the study indicates that demand merits a separate and more careful consideration than some writers would allow. The final chapter makes a number of qualifications of the analysis and suggests directions for future research.

7 G. WIRICK, R. BARLOW, 'The economic and social determinants of the demand for health services'
In S. J. Mushkin (Chairman) *The Economics of Health and Medical Care*, pp. 95–124 (8).

A model of the individual's demand for medical care is constructed. This model views the formulation of demand as taking place in several stages: existence of real physiological need, perception of real or supposed physiological needs, willingness to meet felt needs by securing care, and ability to secure care. Multivariate methods are then used in a statistical analysis of Michigan population survey data to assess the importance of a number of factors in this process of demand formulation: age, income, family income, insurance coverage, response to minor symptoms, education etc.

1965

8 B. BENJAMIN, *Social and Economic Factors Affecting Mortality*
The Hague: Mouton and Company, 1965, pp. x, 88.

A review of the problems of sorting out the influence of social, economic and environmental factors on mortality and morbidity. A large number of studies are reviewed and a good bibliography is provided.

9 M. S. FELDSTEIN, N. R. BUTLER, 'Analysis of factors affecting perinatal mortality: a multivariate statistical approach'
BJPSM, 1965, 19, pp. 128–34.

An examination of the effects on perinatal mortality of maternal age, parity and social class. The interdependence found between the three factors makes mortality rates for specific age groups, parities and social classes of little value.

0 M. S. FELDSTEIN, 'A method of evaluating perinatal mortality risk'
BJPSM, 1965, 19, pp. 135–9.

A multiple regression model is developed for evaluating perinatal mortality risks and identifying cases most likely to benefit from intensive antenatal care or hospital delivery. The risk prediction model is developed on the basis of two factors: mother's age and parity.

71   H. E. KLARMAN, *The Economics of Health*
New York: Columbia University Press, 1965, pp. viii, 200.
See 11.

72   G. D. ROSENTHAL, 'Factors affecting the utilization of short-term general hospitals'
AJPH, November, 1965, 55(11), pp. 1734–40.
See 1438.

1966

73   K. E. BOULDING, 'The concept of need for health services'
MMFQ, October, 1966, 44(2), pp. 202–21.
The concept of need with which the paper is mainly concerned is need based on professional choice. This concept of need is seen to rest upon some definition of homeostasis (state maintenance). The question of which state of the individual is to be maintained is discussed; the conclusion reached is that it is probably culturally determined, a matter of 'social definition'. Other concepts of need for health services are briefly discussed.

74   J. C. G. BURNHAM, 'Estimation of hospital bed requirements'
W. Hosp., 1966, 2, pp. 110–18.
See 384.

75   M. S. FELDSTEIN, 'A binary variable multiple regression method of analysing factors affecting perinatal mortality and other outcomes of pregnancy'
JRSS A, 1966, 129(1), pp. 61–73.
A multiple regression method of analysing classificatory survey data is developed. The method is used to analyse the effects of age, parity and social class and the interactions between these factors on perinatal mortality.

76   P. J. FELDSTEIN, 'Research on the demand for health services'
MMFQ, July, 1966, 44(3), pp. 128–65.
Sets out an economic framework to explain variations in the demand for health services, and then presents a survey of existing literature and research showing where it fits into the framework. The need to consider usage of all components of care in considering usage variations in medical care is stressed (usage is seen as a product of the interaction of demand and supply).

D. C. PAIGE, K. JONES, *Health and Welfare Services in Britain in 1975.*
Cambridge: Cambridge University Press for the National Institute of
Economic and Social Research, Occasional Papers 22, 1966, p. 142.

A comprehensive set of projections is provided for the development of the
different sectors of the health and welfare services in Great Britain up to 1975.
The projections are based upon a growth rate for the economy as a whole of 3.5
per cent per year. The factors seen as affecting the total demand for health and
welfare services were the rate of growth, age structure and marital status of the
population, the rate of medical and sociological advance, the effect of rising
incomes and the distribution of income on the demand for social services, and
the extent of present unsatisfied demand.
See 1101.

G. C. WIRICK, 'A multiple equation model of demand for health care'
HSR, Winter, 1966, 1(3), pp. 301–46.

A simultaneous equation model is used to examine the effects of physical need,
realisation of need, financial resources, motivation to obtain care, and
availability of services on the demands for different types of medical care.

1967

T. D. BAKER, M. PERLMAN, *Health Manpower in a Developing Economy*
Baltimore: Johns Hopkins Press, 1967, pp. xi, 203.
See 198, *212, 220.*

M. H. BRENNER, 'Economic change and mental hospitalization, New York
State, 1910–1960'
SP, November, 1967, 2(4), pp. 180–8.

An examination of the evidence of fluctuations in mental hospital admissions
and fluctuations in the employment index in New York State over the period
1910–60. This study extends the earlier work on hospitalisation for functional
psychosis, and looks at male and female first admissions for five categories of
psychosis, and at first admissions for 34 ethnic groups. It was found that the
two ethnic groups where pattern of mental hospitalisation was most sensitive to
economic change were among the highest groups in socio-economic status,
while the two least sensitive were among the lowest in socio-economic status.

R. FEIN, *The Doctor Shortage: An Economic Diagnosis*
Washington D.C.: The Brookings Institutions, 1967, pp. xi, 199.
See 201.

82   M. S. FELDSTEIN, *Economic Analysis for Health Service Efficiency*
Amsterdam: North-Holland Publishing Company, 1967, pp. xii, 322.
See in particular the section on the 'inadequacy of the manifest demand
approach' in chapter 7, on the supply and use of hospital inpatient care.
See 392.

83   M. S. FELDSTEIN, 'An aggregate planning model of the health care sector'
MC, November–December, 1967, 5(6), pp. 369–81. Also in M. H.
Cooper, A. J. Culyer (eds.) *Health Economics*, pp. 210–29 (33).
See 1380, *1381.*

1968

84   R. ANDERSEN, *A Behavioural Model of Families' Use of Health Services*
Chicago: Center for Health Administration Studies, Research Series
No. 25, 1968, pp. xi, 111.

85   M. H. BRENNER, W. MANDELL, S. BLACKMAN, R. M. SILBERSTEIN,
'Economic conditions and mental hospitalization for functional psychosis'
JNMD, 1968, 145(5), pp. 371–84.
A study using aggregate data to consider the effects of economic downturns as
precipitators of hospitalisation for mental illness. As expected, increased
unemployment was associated with increased first admissions for the three
diagnoses looked at in the study; the data also showed different first admissions
patterns by sex. A survey is provided of other literature on the subject, and a
substantial bibliography included.

86   J. S. BULMAN, N. D. RICHARDS, G. L. SLACK, A. J. WILLCOCKS, *Demand
and Need for Dental Care*
Oxford: Oxford University Press, 1968, pp. viii, 103.
A report to the Nuffield Provincial Hospitals Trust of a study of the dental
state of the population in two areas, Salisbury and Darlington, the former area
being relatively well supplied the latter badly supplied with dentists. Data are
provided on dental care needed, dental care sought by social class, and the
attitudes of the population to dental health.

7 V. R. FUCHS, 'The growing demand for medical care'
NEJM, July 25th, 1968, 279(192), pp. 190–5. Also in V. R. Fuchs (ed.)
Essays in the Economics of Health and Medical Care, pp. 61–8 (27).
See 162.

1969

8 R. M. BAILEY, 'An economist's view of the health services industry'
Inquiry, March, 1969, 6(1), pp. 3–18.

A discussion of the effects of price and income changes on the demand for
medical care. It is argued that income/price changes have a large effect on the
demand for curative services and some effect on the demand for preventive
services.

9 K-K. RO, 'Patient characteristics, hospital characteristics, and hospital
use'
MC, July–August, 1969, 7(4), pp. 295–312. Also in V. R. Fuchs (ed.)
Essays in the Economics of Health and Medical Care, pp. 69–96 (27).
See 418.

1970

10 R. ANDERSEN, L. BENHAM, 'Factors affecting the relationship between
family income and medical care consumption'
In H. E. Klarman (ed.) *Empirical Studies in Health Economics*, pp.
73–95 (18).

An econometric examination of the relationship between family income, and
medical and dental care expenditures. The underlying hypothesis tested is that
the income elasticity of demand for medical care may be altered significantly if
account is taken of factors other than current family income and consumption
of medical and dental services, e.g. permanent income, preventive care.
Comment by M. Grossman.

11 J. R. ASHFORD, N. G. PEARSON, 'Who uses the health services and why?'
JRSS A, 1970, 133(3), pp. 295–357.

A study of the demand for medical care in a large community met by general
practice and hospitals. All consultations and hospital admissions and dis-

charges were recorded for a calendar year for a population of 70,000 living in or around Exeter. The recorded morbidity is examined in relation to personal characteristics derived from general practice records and a special census. An approach to the mathematical modelling of the operation of the health system is discussed.

92 P. J. FELDSTEIN, S. KELMAN, 'A framework for an econometric model of the medical care sector'
In H. E. Klarman (ed.) *Empirical Studies in Health Economics*, pp. 171–90 (18).
See 1389.

93 I. LEVESON, 'The demand for neighbourhood medical care'
Inquiry, December, 1970, 7(4), pp. 17–24.
The paper first considers the determinants of the demand for medical care in the aggregate, paying particular attention to the roles of social benefit, health, insurance and education. The choice of a particular source of medical care and the factors that affect this choice, with particular reference to the demand for ambulatory care, are then considered.

94 G. N. MONSMA, 'Marginal revenue and the demand for physicians' services'
In H. E. Klarman (ed.), *Empirical Studies in Health Economics*, pp. 145–60 (18).
See 241.

95 V. NAVARRO, 'Methodology on regional planning of personal health services: a case study: Sweden'
MC, September–October, 1970, 8(5), pp. 386–94.
See 1391.

96 J. P. NEWHOUSE, 'Determinants of days lost from work due to sickness'
In H. E. Klarman (ed.) *Empirical Studies in Health Economics*, pp. 59–70 (18).
See 869.

97 G. D. ROSENTHAL, 'Price elasticity of demand for short-term general hospital services'
In H. E. Klarman (ed.) *Empirical Studies in Health Economics*, pp. 101–17 (18).

An econometric study to determine the impact on the length of stay in hospital of two price variables – cash outlay as a percentage of total bill and average daily room charge. See also the comment by V. R. Fuchs, pp. 118–20.

M. SILVER, 'An economic analysis of variations in medical expenses and work loss rates'
In H. E. Klarman (ed.) *Empirical Studies in Health Economics*, pp. 121–40 (18). Also in V. R. Fuchs (ed.) *Essays in the Economics of Health and Medical Care*, pp. 97–118 (27).
An empirical study, in which the main piece of empirical analysis is a calculation of the income elasticity of demand for medical care as a whole and for its components. The overall elasticity is 1.2, a figure higher than that found in other studies. One section of the study is an attempt to ascertain whether work loss rate can be used as a measure of health; this is achieved by testing hypotheses that suggest that variations in work days lost are a reflection of differences in economic variables rather than in the objective state of health. The results are not conclusive but the evidence does suggest that differences in unadjusted work loss days may be unreliable measures of variations in health status. See also the comment by R. Fein, pp. 141–4.

1971

N. B. BELLOC, L. BRESLOW, J. R. HOCHSTIM, 'Measurement of physical health in a general population survey'
AJE, 1971, 93(5), pp. 328–36.
A measurement of health based on a population survey. Respondents were arranged on the basis of their responses along a spectrum from inability to work/or care for personal needs, to no complaints and a high level of energy. The spectrum was then summarised and that figure, the mean 'ridit', used for comparing sub-groups within the population.

R. R. CAMPBELL, *Economics of Health and Public Policy*
Washington D.C.: American Enterprise Institute for Public Policy Research, 1971, p. 108.
See 23.

A. J. CULYER, R. J. LAVERS, A. WILLIAMS, 'Social indicators: health'
ST, 1971, 2, pp. 31–42.
See 877.

102 I. J. FAHS, T. CHOI, K. BARCHAS, P. ZAKARIASEN, 'Indicators of need for health care personnel: the concept of need, alternative measures employed to determine need, and a suggested model'
MC, March–April, 1971, 9(2), pp. 144–51.
See 253.

103 M. S. FELDSTEIN, 'Hospital cost inflation: a study of non-profit price dynamics'
AER, December, 1971, 61(5), pp. 835–72.
See 447.

104 A. I. HARRIS, J. R. BUCKLE, C. R. W. SMITH, E. HEAD, E. COX, *Handicapped and Impaired in Great Britain*
London: HMSO, Office of Population Censuses and Surveys, Parts I and II, 1971, Part III, 1972, p. 600.
See 891.

105 J. R. JEFFERS, M. BOGNANNO, J. C. BARTLETT, 'On the demand versus need for medical services and the concept of shortage'
AJPH, January, 1971, 61(1), pp. 46–63.
Distinctions are drawn between consumer and medical concepts of need, between need and demand, and between various concepts of shortage that they imply.

106 H. JOSEPH, 'Empirical research on the demand for health care'
Inquiry, March, 1971, 8(1), pp. 61–71.
A survey of nine major pieces of empirical work on the demand for health care.

107 L. B. LAVE, E. P. SESKIN, 'Health and air pollution'
SJE, March, 1971, 73(1), pp. 76–95.
One of a series of papers using multiple regression analysis to investigate the relationship between air pollution and mortality and morbidity. In this particular study data from 117 U.S. cities were analysed, and variables on occupational mix were incorporated in the regression equation. The addition of occupational mix did not reduce the estimated air pollution coefficients. A substantial association between air pollution and mortality was shown to exist.

108 G. K. MATTHEW, 'Measuring need and evaluating services'
In G. McLachlan (ed.) *Portfolio for Health, Problems and Progress in Medical Care, Essays on Current Research, Sixth Series*, pp. 27–46 (25).

The first part of the paper looks at recent work attempting to assess need, and considers epidemiological, clinical and planning problems associated with the concept of need.

G. A. POPOV, *Principles of Health Planning in the U.S.S.R.*
Geneva: World Health Organisation, Public Health Papers No. 43, 1971, p. 172.
See 1401.

J. A. RAFFERTY, 'Patterns of hospital use: an analysis of short-run variations'
JPE, January–February, 1971, 79(1), pp. 154–65.
See 455.

D. E. YETT, L. DRABEK, M. D. INTRILIGATOR, 'A macro-econometric model for regional health planning'
EBB, Fall, 1971, 24(1), pp. 1–21.
Two broad types of variables are used in the model to explain the demand for the different types of health service: the size of the community's population and its demographic characteristics, and financial variables representing both cost and ability to pay. Some preliminary estimates of the demand for hospital care are included.
See 1403.

1972

J. G. ANDERSON, 'Causal model of a health services system'
HSR, Spring, 1972, 7(1), pp. 23–42.
Path analysis is used to construct a model of the process by which socio-economic and demographic characteristics affect the health status of the population of New Mexico. Health status is measured by mortality rates from accidents, suicide and cirrhosis of the liver, but a number of other mortality and morbidity measures have been successfully used with the model.

S. E. BERKI, *Hospital Economics*
Lexington, Massachusetts: Lexington Books, D. C. Heath and Company, 1972, pp. xxi, 270.
The sixth chapter of the book deals with demand for and utilisation of care. A

demand model is presented that stresses the multiple nature of demands for medical care, and examines various kinds of demand such as 'felt need' and doctor-generated utilisation; all of the demands presuppose the existence of some level of health status disequilibrium that leads to their formation. The rest of the chapter is devoted to a critical review of empirical demand studies. *See* 462.

114   I. D. BOGATYREV, 'Establishing standards for outpatient and inpatient care'
IJHS, February, 1972, 2(1), pp. 45–9.
Morbidity statistics based on examination of 54,000 people from different communities in the U.S.S.R. are used to estimate the number of hospital beds per 1000 population required in different specialities.

115   J. BRADSHAW, 'A taxonomy of social need'
In G. McLachlan (ed.) *Problems and Progress in Medical Care, Essays on Current Research, Seventh Series*, pp. 69–82 (30).
Four separate definitions of need are used by administrators and researchers: felt need, expressed need, comparative need, and normative need. The meanings of these definitions and the overlap between them are examined. Twelve possible situations result – from one extreme where all definitions overlap to a situation where there is an absence of need by all definitions. The taxonomy is discussed in relation to housing need.

116   B. S. COOPER, N. L. WORTHINGTON, 'Medical care spending for three age groups'
SSB, May, 1972, 35(5), pp. 3–16.
One of a series of articles appearing annually in the May issue of the Social Security Bulletin. Information is presented on total medical care expenditure, by type of expenditure, advance of funds, for three age groups (under 19 years, 19–64 years, over 64 years) in the U.S.A. for the fiscal years 1966–71.

117   A. J. CULYER, R. J. LAVERS, A. WILLIAMS, 'Health Indicators'
In A. Shonfield, S. Shaw (eds.) *Social Indicators and Social Policy*, London: Heinemann Educational Books, for the Social Science Research Council, 1972, pp. 94–118.
See 877.

118   K. DAVIS, L. B. RUSSELL, 'The substitution of hospital outpatient care for inpatient care'
Rev.Econ.Stats., May, 1972, 54(2), pp. 109–20.

Demand functions for outpatient and inpatient care were estimated by regression analysis of data from 48 states. The price elasticity of demand for outpatient care was high (-1.0); similarly price elasticity of demand for inpatient care was quite high (-0.32 to -0.46); inpatient demand was also responsive to outpatient price (elasticity -0.25). The demand for outpatient care was shown to be sensitive to the inpatient occupancy rate. Some tentative estimates suggested that total hospital costs could be reduced by changing the relative price of the two types of care.

H. G. Dove, C. G. Richie, 'Predicting hospital admissions by state'
Inquiry, September, 1972, 9(3), pp. 51–6.
A stepwise regression model is developed to predict hospital admissions by state. The predictive capability of the model was tested by applying the regression coefficients to data from subsequent years that had not been used in the development of the original equations.

V. R. Fuchs, M. J. Kramer, *Determinants of Expenditures for Physicians' Services in the United States 1948–68*
Washington D.C.: U.S. Department of Health, Education and Welfare, National Center for Health Services Research and Development, DHEW Publication No. (HSM) 73–3013, December, 1972, p. 63.
The study is divided into two parts. The first part is a statistical decomposition of the rate of change in expenditures and related variables over the period 1948–68. The period is divided into three sub-periods 1948–56, 1956–66 and 1966–68; the rates of change in expenditures per capita, quantity per capita and quantity per physician were substantially different between the different sub-periods. The influence of changes in price, insurance coverage, income, demographic structure, number and type of physicians, and medical technology on the differences between the sub-periods are examined. The second part of the study is a cross-section analysis of differences between states using 1966 data. The aim of the second part of the study is to analyse the behaviour of physicians and patients netting out the impact of technological change. The major findings of the study were that supply factors (technology, physicians) appeared to be decisive in determining utilisation of and expenditures for physicians' services. Holding technology constant, the elasticities of demand with respect to income, price and insurance were all small relative to the direct effect of the number of physicians on demand, and physician location appeared to be influenced most by private advantage, price of services, facilities, and availability of educational and cultural opportunities.

121   D. Hewitt, J. Milner, 'Components of the demand for hospital care'
IJE, Spring, 1972, 1(1), pp. 61–8.

Data on utilisation are used in a model to study the demand for hospital care
for nine diagnostic categories. The model is based on the postulate that any
small increment in the supply of hospital care will be associated with some
change in the amount of care absorbed by each particular category of use; the
size of the ratio between these proportional changes is an indication of the
urgency of the category of the admission.

122   J. R. Lave, S. Leinhardt, 'The delivery of ambulatory care to the poor: a
literature review'
MS, December, 1972, 19(4), pp. 78–99.

Literature on the state of health and perceptions of health of the poor in the
U.S. is reviewed. The 'vicious cycle of poverty' model linking ill-health and
poverty is discussed, and it is concluded that improved medical care for the
poor will not alone improve income levels.
See 1243.

123   H. H. Liebhafsky, 'The rational consumer's demand for psychiatric help:
a preference function generating a perfectly price-inelastic demand
function'
JPE, July–August, 1972, 80(4), pp. 829–32.

A demonstration that a perfectly rational consumer, fulfilling all the requirements of demand theory, will have a perfectly inelastic demand for psychiatric
help. See also the comment by J. C. Koeune, *JPE*, September–October, 1974,
82(5), pp. 1049–52.

124   R. F. L. Logan, J. S. A. Ashley, R. E. Klein, D. M. Robson,
*Dynamics of Medical Care – The Liverpool Study into Use of Hospital
Resources*
London: London School of Hygiene and Tropical Medicine, 1972, p.
152.

A thorough exploration of the problems of definition and measurement of need
for medical care were a major part of this study of the Liverpool hospital
services.
See 484.

125   S. W. Moore, H. B. Bock, 'Estimating the demand for medical care'
Inquiry, December, 1972, 9(4), pp. 64–7.

An outline is provided of the health services simulator in the Health Resources

Planning Unit of the Texas Hospital Association. The simulator is essentially a combination of multivariate regression equations to predict the demand of a population and a simulator model for measuring the requirements of medical care that processes the transition of patients between levels of care, recovery and death.

R. L. PARKER, A. K. MURTHY, J. C. BHATIA, 'Relating health services to community health needs'
Indian J.Med.Res., December 12th, 1972, 60(12), pp, 1835–48.

A study of the Punjab to estimate the needs for health care, the resources available for health care, and the resources that would be required to meet the needs. The approach used involved the relation of multiple health needs and diverse service activities to a relatively few functions. The information collected will provide a basis for cost-effectiveness studies of alternative health-care delivery patterns.

M. SILVER, 'An econometric analysis of spatial variations in mortality rates by race and sex'
In V. R. Fuchs (ed.) *Essays in the Economics of Health and Medical Care*, pp. 161–227 (27).

A large-scale regression study examining the relationship between age-adjusted mortality by race and sex and over 30 socio-economic, geographical and environmental variables. The regressions are run using data by state and by metropolitan area in the United States for the period 1959–61. Both ordinary least squares and two stage least squares methods are used.

J.-E. SPEK, 'On the economic analysis of health and medical care in a Swedish Health district'
In M. M. Hauser (ed.) *The Economics of Medical Care*, pp. 261–8 (28).

The processes of causation, medical and social, of ill-health are examined. Health and sickness and need and demand for medical care are discussed and a conceptual scheme is put forward that enables the identification of possible conflicts between society, medical experts and individuals over the existence of illness and the demand for and provision of medical treatment.

C. UPTON, W. SILVERMAN, 'The demand for dental services'
JHR, Spring, 1972, 7(2), pp. 250–61.

Estimates were made of the income elasticity of demand for a variety of dental services; for most types of treatment the income elasticity of demand was greater than one. The analysis also indicated that fluoridation of public water supplies would reduce demand for dental services by over 55 per cent.

130   K. L. WERTZ, 'Physicians and the demand for ethical drugs'
Amer.Econ., Spring, 1972, 16(1), pp. 120–5.

Demonstrates that the role of the physician interposed as a third party between drug companies and patients can explain two unexpected occurrences in the drug market, the first relating to price setting behaviour of profit-maximising drug producers, the second relating to the elasticities of demand of hospitalised and non-hospitalised patients for drugs.

1973

131   B. ABEL-SMITH, B. BENJAMIN, W. W. HOLLAND, J. W. PEARSON, D. F. PIACHAUD, O. GOLDSMITH, J. D. POLE, *Accounting for Health*
London: King Edward's Hospital Fund, 1973, p. 63.
See 32.

132   M. BERDIT, J. W. WILLIAMSON, 'Function limitation scale for measuring health outcomes'
In R. L. Berg (ed.) *Health Status Indexes*, pp. 59–65 (906).
See 904.

133   M. H. BRENNER, 'Fetal, infant, and maternal mortality during periods of economic instability'
IJHS, Spring, 1973, 3(2), pp. 145–59.

Evidence is found to suggest that fluctuations in the level of economic activity have played a significant role in fetal, infant and maternal mortality in the U.S.A. in the last 45 years. Economic instability may have been responsible for the lack of continuity of decline in infant mortality rates since 1950, despite continued growth of GNP.

134   A. DONABEDIAN, *Aspects of Medical Care Administration: Specifying Requirements for Health Care*
Cambridge, Massachusetts: Harvard University Press, 1973, p. 649.

The concept of need is examined, and a model presented to enable the assessment of need. The model considers client perspective, professional perspective and the interaction between them. The problems of measurement and evaluation are discussed extensively..
See 35.

R. G. EVANS, E. M. A. PARISH, F. SULLY, 'Medical productivity, scale effects and demand generation'
CJE, August, 1973, 6(3), pp. 376–93.
An econometric study using British Columbian data. A comparison of physician incomes in areas of very different physician density suggested substantial ability on the part of physicians to generate demand for their own services.
See 586.

M. S. FELDSTEIN, 'The welfare loss of excess health insurance'
JPE, March–April, 1973, 81(2 part 1), pp. 251–80.
See 1251.

P. J. FELDSTEIN, *Financing Dental Care: An Economic Analysis*
Lexington: D. C. Heath and Company, 1973, pp. xvii, 260.
See 36.

M. J. LEFCOWITZ, 'Poverty and health: a re-examination'
Inquiry, March, 1973, 10(1), pp. 3–13.
Casts doubt upon the conclusion that there is a direct causal relationship between poverty and low health care, and poverty and low health status. The relationship is complicated by the role of education. Present policies may be misdirected; a proper attack on the health poverty problem may involve only in part what is usually considered a health programme.

G. POVEY, D. UYENO, I. VERTINSKY, 'Social impact index for evaluation of regional resource allocation'
In R. L. Berg (ed.) *Health Status Indexes*, pp. 104–15 (906).
See 929.

A. REISMAN, B. V. DEAN, A. O. ESOGBUE, V. AGGARWAL, V. KAUJALGI, P. LEWY, J. S. GRAVENSTEIN, 'Physician supply and surgical demand forecasting: a regional manpower study'
MS, August, 1973, 19(12), pp. 1345–54.
See 306.

R. N. ROSETT, L. HUANG, 'The effect of health insurance on the demand for medical care'
JPE, March–April, 1973, 81(2 part 1), pp. 281–305.
See 1258.

142   I. VERTINSKY, D. UYENO, 'The demand for health services and the theory of time allocation'
AE, December, 1973, 5(4), pp. 249–60.

A theoretical model is constructed that recognises that a time input is an integral part of the act of consumption of many goods and services. The consumer must combine his resources (finances and time) so as to maximise his utility. Some implications for the quantity and type of medical services a consumer will choose, and some possible areas of application of the model, are outlined.

1974

143   J. G. ANDERSON, 'Effects of social and cultural processes on health'
Soc.-Econ.Plan.Sciences, January, 1974, 8(1), pp. 9–22.

A model is constructed linking infant mortality to the socio-demographic characteristics of a population. Data from 32 New Mexico counties were used to estimate parameters of the model. A significant relationship was found to exist between per capita income and infant mortality. Urbanisation and demographic composition of the population were also important.

144   J. R. ASHFORD, R. E. HUNT, 'The distribution of doctor–patient contacts in the NHS'
JRSS A, 1974, 137(3), pp. 347–83.

A sophisticated model of the distribution of doctor–patient contacts is constructed. Application to data from the Exeter study (J. R. Ashford, N. G. Pearson, *JRSS A*, 1970, 133(3), pp. 295–357) yielded a good fit for males and for female contacts excluding those connected with pregnancy.
See 91.

145   M. BLAXTER, 'Health "on the welfare" – a case study'
JSP, January, 1974, 3(1), pp. 39–51.

Examines the principles used in deciding need or entitlement to free or subsidised welfare services, and presents a case study of 237 individuals, half of whom were entitled to free prescriptions but were not receiving them.

146   M. H. COOPER, 'Economics of need: the experience of the British Health Service'

In M. Perlman (ed.) *The Economics of Health and Medical Care*, pp. 89–107 (44).
See 1137, 1141.

K. DAVIS, 'The role of technology, demand and labour markets in the determination of hospital cost'
In M. Perlman (ed.) *The Economics of Health and Medical Care*, pp. 283–301 (44).
See 445, 446, 468, 502, 503, 529.

R. G. EVANS, 'Supplier-induced demand: some empirical evidence and its implications'
In M. Perlman (ed.) *The Economics of Health and Medical Care*, pp. 162–73 (44).
The paper outlines two alternative specifications of physician behaviour that suggest that the demand for medical care will not be independent of the supply of physicians. Several pieces of empirical evidence from Canada are presented that are consistent with substantial demand influence by physicians.
See 318.

M. S. FELDSTEIN, 'Econometric studies of health economics'
In M. D. Intriligator, D. A. Kendrick (eds.) *Frontiers of Quantitative Economics*, Vol. 2, pp. 377–447, Amsterdam: North-Holland, 1974.
Discusses the problems associated with the role of the physician in determining household demand for medical care, and suggests that the relation between the patient and his physician is one of agency. The major studies to determine factors affecting demand for medical care and to estimate price and income elasticities are reviewed.
See 42.

B. FRIEDMAN, 'A test of alternative demand-shift responses to the Medicare programme'
In M. Perlman (ed.) *The Economics of Health and Medical Care*, pp. 234–47 (44).
The aggregate evidence on the effects of the Medicare programme on utilisation and costs is reviewed. The role of patient and physician in the increase in resource use is examined. A model in which professional preference plays a large role is developed. A study of possible changes in the early diagnosis and treatment of breast cancer, comparing years before and after the Medicare

programme began, gave support to the view that physicians make decisions reflecting their own preferences constrained by out-of-pocket costs to consumers.

151 J. GARRAD, 'Impairment and disability: their measurement, prevalence, and psychological cost'
In D. S. Lees, S. Shaw (eds.) *Impairment, Disability and Handicap*, pp. 141–56 (809).
See 937.

152 C. C. HAVIGHURST (ed.) *Regulating Health Facilities Construction*
Washington D.C.: American Enterprise Institute for Public Policy Research, 1974, p. 314.
See 1268.

153 C. E. PHELPS, J. P. NEWHOUSE, 'Coinsurance, the price of time, and the demand for medical services'
Rev.Econ.Stats., August, 1974, 56(3), pp. 334–42.
See 1245, 1247, 1277.

154 P. SAINSBURY, J. GRAD DE ALARCON, 'The cost of community care and the burden on the family of treating the mentally ill at home'
In D. S. Lees, S. Shaw (eds.) *Impairment, Disability and Handicap*, pp. 123–40 (809).
See 813.

155 A. WILLIAMS, '"Need" as a demand concept (with special reference to health)'
In A. J. Culyer (ed.) *Economic Policies and Social Goals*, pp. 60–76 (41).
An attempt to bridge the gap between economics and 'needology'. The paper explores need as a demand concept, need as a supply concept, and demand as a need concept. It is concluded that it would be wrong for economists to concentrate entirely on textbook notions of demand as the only proper way to determine the amount and distribution of goods such as medical care. If, on the other hand, they go further into the notions of merit goods and externalities they will come up against many of the problems 'needologists' have been grappling with.

D. E. YETT, L. DRABEK, M. D. INTRILIGATOR, L. J. KIMBELL, 'Econometric forecasts of health services and health manpower'
In M. Perlman (ed.) *The Economics of Health and Medical Care*, pp. 459–69 (44).
See 1424.

3 Supply of Health Services

The concern of this section is with the production aspects of health-care delivery. This divides conveniently into three groups of studies. The first group, titled Macro Productivity/Price Indices, is concerned essentially with general productivity questions: the relationships between resource inputs and 'health product' outputs at an aggregate level. The second group concentrates upon the characteristics of the supply of health service manpower, which is of particular importance both because of its special characteristics and because of its practical importance as a resource input. The third group relates to the organisational arrangements through which health service factors of production are co-ordinated. The counterpart of these studies in industrial economics would be, for example, the study of industry trends, of firm behaviour and of plant location decisions.

(a) Macro Productivity/Price Indices

The practical importance of questions of productivity in the delivery of health is unquestioned: its significance is matched only by the inherent difficulty of productivity studies in a field in which, in addition to the common problems of all such studies, researchers face obstacles such as the intangible nature of health output and the absence of markets or agreed value systems. The consequence of this has been that, while the number of studies that could be said to be concerned in some sense with productivity questions is quite large, the majority of these are directly concerned with a different objective; the light they throw on productivity questions is, so to speak, a by-product. Thus, this sub-section is relatively short, being restricted to studies directed explicitly at the measurement of input–output relationships, for the most part at an aggregated (general index, total health-care expenditure) rather than a unit (single hospital, medical unit) level.

Many of the studies in 3(b) and 3(c) have a bearing on productivity questions of this latter kind.

46

A good deal of the material included in this section is concerned with the deficiencies of the U.S. Bureau of Labor Statistics Medical-Care Price Index. The most important contributions are those of Scitovsky (158, 160), Barzel (164), Reder (165), Feldstein (166) and Klarman, Rice, Cooper and Stettler (167).

1964

S. E. HARRIS, *The Economics of American Medicine*
New York: The Macmillan Company, 1964, pp. xvi, 508.
See 6.

A. A. SCITOVSKY, 'An index of the cost of medical care – a proposed new approach'
In S. J. Mushkin (Chairman) *The Economics of Health and Medical Care*, pp. 128–41 (8).
The deficiencies of the Medical-Care Price Index in the U.S.A. are discussed. An index to supplement this showing changes in the average costs of treatment of individual illnesses is prepared, and the advantages of this type of index over the present Medical-Care Price Index outlined.

1965

H. E. KLARMAN, *The Economics of Health*
New York: Columbia University Press, 1965, pp. viii, 200.
See 11.

1967

A. A. SCITOVSKY, 'Changes in the costs of treatment of selected illnesses, 1951–65'
AER, December, 1967, 57(5), pp. 1182–95.
A study of the change in the cost of treating five illnesses (acute appendicitis, maternity care, otitis media in children, fracture of the forearm in children, and

cancer of the breast) in the U.S.A. between 1951–2 and 1964–5. The costs of treatment of all the illnesses increased by more than the BLS Medical-Care Price Index. The reasons for the differences are explored.

1968

161 W. F. BERRY, J. C. DAUGHERTY, 'A closer look at rising medical costs'
Mon.Lab.Rev., November, 1968, 91(11), pp. 1–8.

A review of the trends in medical care prices from 1946 as measured by the U.S. Bureau of Labor Statistics in the Consumer Price Index. The method of compiling the index and some of the conceptual problems faced are discussed. Some of the price rises are attributed to physicians using high rates for house calls to discourage them and to increasing specialisation.

162 V. R. FUCHS, 'The growing demand for medical care'
NEJM, July 25th, 1968, 279(192), pp. 190–5. Also in V. R. Fuchs (ed.)
Essays in the Economics of Health and Medical Care, pp. 61–8 (27).

A discussion of the factors contributing to the rise in medical care expenditures in the United States from 1947 to 1967.

163 A. A. SCITOVSKY, 'The higher cost of better medical care'
Trans-Action, December, 1968, 6(2), pp. 42–5.

A comparison of changes in the costs of treatment of five particular diagnoses with the Bureau of Labor Statistics Medical-Care Price Index, an index that considers price changes only on the costs of a fixed 'market basket' of goods. Costs of treatment have risen by considerably more than the BLS Index.

1969

164 Y. BARZEL, 'Productivity and the price of medical services'
JPE, November–December, 1969, 77(6), pp. 1014–27.

It is argued that the Consumer Price Index in the U.S.A. gives a misleading impression of productivity rise in medicine, and rather than lagging behind, the rate of increase of productivity in medicine has exceeded the overall rate of productivity increase in the economy. Support for this contention is provided by using data on insurance company expenses to provide estimates of the cost of maintaining health at a constant level, on the assumption that medical insurance will be used in such a way as to maintain the health level of the subscriber constant. These estimates of the cost of maintaining health at a constant level are then used to construct price indices of medical services.

M. W. REDER, 'Some problems in the measurement of productivity in the medical care industry'
In V. R. Fuchs (ed.) *Production and Productivity in the Service Industries*, New York: National Bureau of Economic Research, 1969, pp. 95–131.
The problems of measuring productivity are discussed and a proposal for a measure of output independent of service input is developed. The peculiar characteristics of the medical care industry, in particular consumer ignorance and price discrimination by producers, and the complications that they introduce, are discussed. Comments by H. E. Klarman, M. S. Feldstein, S. Fabricant, W. Z. Hirsch, and a reply by Reder, pp. 132–53.
See 864.

1970

M. S. FELDSTEIN, 'The rising price of physician services'
Rev.Econ.Stats., May, 1970, 52(2), pp. 121–33.
See 234.

H. E. KLARMAN, D. P. RICE, B. S. COOPER, H. L. STETTLER, 'Accounting for the rise in selected medical care expenditures, 1929–1969'
AJPH, June, 1970, 60(6), pp. 1023–39.
An accounting framework is established for analysing three categories of expenditures, for dental services, for physician services, and for short-term hospital care. The article provides basic data from 1929 to 1969, beginning with information on expenditures, price, per capita utilisation and population in 1929 and adding additional information for later years as it became available.

1971

C. P. McCLAUGHLIN, 'Technology and medical care costs: some basic evaluation problems'
EBB, Fall, 1971, 24(1), pp. 36–43.
See also H. A. Cohen, 'Technology and medical care costs: Comment', *JEB*, Fall, 1972, 25(1), pp. 68–89.

1972

169   V. R. Fuchs, M. J. Kramer, *Determinants of Expenditures for Physicians' Services in the United States 1948–68*
Washington D.C.: U.S. Department of Health, Education and Welfare, National Center for Health Services Research and Development, DHEW publication No. (HSM) 73–3013, December, 1972, p. 63.
See 120.

(b)   Manpower

The present state of manpower studies in the health-care field reflects the development of work of this kind in the general area of the economics of human resources and in particular the economics of education. Summarily, the insights provided by human resources studies have given new directions to the study of labour markets, and in particular have directed attention to the importance of 'human investment': the use of resources to enhance both the productive capacity of individuals and their ability simply to 'enjoy life' by improving, for example, their education/training or their health state. As a corollary, studies have been encouraged whose concern is with the implications for skilled labour requirements of plans for the development of the economy or for sectors thereof. There is a diversity of such studies, addressing themselves, for example, to the relation between the attainment of a given growth rate, the implied size and structure of the health sector, and the consequent requirements of skilled (health) manpower.

While this area of study has attracted considerable interest, however, it cannot be said that there is universal satisfaction with the end-product, in the sense that an agreed methodology for the study of manpower problems has emerged or is in immediate prospect. The essential problem is that of integration between two approaches. The first of these can be seen as a direct extension of the study of labour markets. It focuses upon the response of these markets to (e.g.) increases in the demand for 'better health', which in turn increase the 'yield' to individuals from investment in the acquisition of labour skills. Such studies are illuminating in providing understanding of the response of particular labour markets (e.g. the market for nurses) to specified changes in economic conditions. The second, 'manpower planning', approach attempts to discover the 'requirements' of skilled manpower implied by particular forecasts/extra-polations/projections of the state of an economy and/or its sectors.

The unsolved problem of the second approach is that of the translation of the results of an essentially technological exercise into a set of market processes, policies, prices, etc. Attempts have been made at integration, for example by relating the predicted shortages thrown up by manpower planning studies to the available data on labour markets, relative wages, manpower substitutabilities, etc. There have also been econometric studies attempting to bridge the gap. But there is continuing difference of opinion as to the actual or potential value of the manpower planning approach for practical policy decisions.

It is a consequence of this situation (an active research area, but an as yet untidy one) that no simple method of classifying the relevant works suggests itself. The reader will, we hope, be able to discern some general system in the commentary that follows; but this is an area in which the interested researcher has little option but to read our own annotations, and then work through the material guided simply by his own needs.

In addition to studies fitting the above general description, two special questions concerning medical manpower require mention. These are the nature and implications of restrictive labour practices and professional interest groups, and the geographical distribution of medical manpower between and within countries.

The best surveys of the field are provided by Butter (199), Fein (201), Klarman (221) and Rafferty (ed.) (329).

The major planning studies are those by Lee and Jones (170), Judek (182), Paige and Jones (196), Baker and Perlman (198), Fein (201), Taylor, Dirican and Deuschle (212) and Hall (220). Critical reviews of studies of the manpower planning type, including studies carried out by government commissions, are provided by Gales and Wright (191), Peacock and Shannon (209), Shannon (211) and Ahamad (291).

Studies of individual labour markets include: Friedman and Kuznets (171), Hansen (180), Sloan (243, 266, 331, 332), Fein and Weber (254), Lindsay (304) and Evans (318), dealing with doctor manpower; and Yett (189, 197, 214, 246, 247), Altman (228), Benham (249), Cohen (275), Bishop (292) and Hurd (303), dealing with nursing manpower.

The possibility of substitution of doctors by lower grade manpower is explored by Reinhardt (305, 330) and Zeckhauser and Eliastam (338).

Econometric studies by Yett, Drabek, and Intriligator (270) and Yett, Drabek, Intriligator and Kimbell (290) attempt to bridge the gap between the two approaches.

Restrictive labour practices and professional interest groups are the subject of the work of: Hyde and Wolff (172), Kessel (174, 239), Holen (184), Rayack (187, 205), Lees (193), Forgotson and Cook (202), Carlson (233), Newhouse (242), Hershey (257), Ruffin and Leigh (308) and Frech (322).

The geographical distribution of manpower within countries is the subject of the work of: Steele and Rimlinger (188), Last (204), Benham, Maurizi and Reder (207), Brown (230), Joroff and Navarro (259), Charles (274) and Butler (293). Movements of medical manpower between countries are dealt with by Abel-Smith and Gales (179), Margulies and Bloch (224), Butter (232, 251, 252), Kilgour (260) and Hambleton (280).

1933

170 R. I. LEE, L. W. JONES, *The Fundamentals of Good Medical Care*
Chicago: Publication of the Committee on the Costs of Medical Care, No. 22, University of Chicago Press, 1933, p. 302.

A study that estimated the requirements for United States medical manpower on the basis of expert assessment of the amount of care in terms of physician hours required to prevent, diagnose and treat specific diseases.

1945

171 M. FRIEDMAN, S. KUZNETS, *Income from Independent Professional Practice*
New York: Columbia University Press for the National Bureau of Economic Research, 1945.

A pioneering study of the professions in the U.S.A., discovering higher than market rates of return to physicians' training – particularly high in relation to those from dental training. It was concluded that the high returns could only be explained by limitations being placed on the numbers entering the profession, and not by differences in ability or rational choice by individuals of profession.

1954

2 D. R. HYDE, P. WOLFF, 'The American Medical Association: power, purpose and politics in organized medicine'
YLJ, May, 1954, 63(7), pp. 938–1022. A shortened version of the article appears in W. R. Scott, E. H. Volkart (eds.) *Medical Care*, New York: John Wiley and Sons, 1966, pp. 163–80.
A comprehensive study of the development of the A.M.A., the basis of its power, and the application of that power.

1956

3 O. L. PETERSON, L. P. ANDREWS, R. S. SPAIN, B. G. GREENBERG, 'An analytical study of North Carolina general practice 1953–1954'
JME, December, 1956, 31(12 part 2), pp. 1–165.
See 555.

1958

R. A. KESSEL, 'Price discrimination in medicine'
JLE, October, 1958, 1(2), pp. 20–53.
A lot of evidence is produced to support the discriminating monopoly hypothesis as an explanation of the pricing of doctors' services in the United States. The problem lies in demonstrating why competition among doctors has not established uniform prices. The majority of the evidence is concerned with the power of organised medicine to enforce price discipline on doctors. The major control has been the ability to cut off staff privileges at hospitals to price cutters, but rules of professional conduct, and discrimination in entry to medical school against groups thought likely to be price cutters, also help to maintain discipline.

1961

J. P. MEERMAN, 'Some comments on the predicted future shortage of physicians'
JAMA, September 16th, 1961, 177(11), pp. 793–9.

The deficiencies of planning the future number of doctors on the basis of doctor–population ratios is discussed. It is suggested that removing financial barriers to entry into medical education would allow better adjustment of doctor supply to patient demand.

176   M. I. ROEMER, 'Hospital utilization and the supply of physicians'
JAMA, December 9th, 1961, 178(10), pp. 989–93.
See 351.

1963

177   J. HOGARTH, *The Payment of the General Practitioner*
Oxford: Pergamon Press, 1963, pp. xii, 684.

A comprehensive study of the methods of paying general practitioners in Europe, the Soviet Union, Australia and New Zealand.

178   G. V. RIMLINGER, H. B. STEELE, 'An economic interpretation of the spatial distribution of physicians in the U.S.'
SEJ, July, 1963, 30(1), pp. 1–12.

A lot of United States data on the relationship between physician–population ratios and regional per capita incomes are brought together. High income areas are found to have substantially higher ratios. A variety of hypotheses on physician behaviour are tested: income maximisation, leisure preference and degree of mobility.

1964

179   B. ABEL-SMITH, K. GALES, *British Doctors at Home and Abroad*
London: G. Bell and Sons Ltd., Occasional Papers on Social Administration No. 8, 1964, p. 63.

A sample study to determine the nature and extent of medical emigration from the U.K. in the 1950s. The study came at the end of a debate on the volume of emigration, and the results indicated that while emigration was greater than that suggested in the official manpower planning document (Willink Report) it was substantially less than that suggested by some medical contributors to the debate.

0 W. Lee Hansen, '"Shortages" and investment in health manpower'
In S. J. Mushkin (Chairman) *The Economics of Health and Medical Care*, pp. 75–91 (8).

Estimates are made of the rates of return to physicians, dentists and male college graduates in the years 1939, 1949 and 1956 in the U.S.A. Evidence of declining relative rates of return suggests that the shortages of physicians and dentists have been diminishing quite rapidly since 1949.

1 S. E. Harris, *The Economics of American Medicine*
New York: The Macmillan Company, 1964, pp. xvi, 508.
See 6.

2 S. Judek, *Medical Manpower in Canada*
Ottawa: Royal Commission on Health Services, Queens Printer, 1964, pp. xx, 413.

A massive study containing a great deal of factual information. Chapters are included on the supply of physicians, Canadian medical graduates and students, the geographical distribution and professional characteristics of Canadian doctors, the demand for medical services, the economics of medical practice, an evaluation of supply and demand for physicians in Canada, and physician–population projections for the period 1961–91.
See 1169.

3 E. Rayack, 'The supply of physicians' services'
ILRR, January, 1964, 17(2), pp. 221–37.

Examination of data for the period 1939–60 on the relative income of physicians, and on the attempts by United States hospitals to find less costly substitutes for domestically trained physicians, both foreign medical graduates and paramedical personnel, suggests that the magnitude of the doctor shortage is even larger than that suggested by official manpower commissions.

1965

---

4 A. S. Holen, 'Effects of professional licensing arrangements on interstate labour mobility and resource allocation'
JPE, October, 1965, 73(5), pp. 492–8.

Considers the effect of state licensing arrangements on interstate mobility of physicians, dentists and lawyers. Data are presented to show that physicians were more mobile than the other two groups. A significant relationship was found between licensure exam failure rates and state incomes for lawyers and dentists but not for doctors. Dispersions of state average incomes of lawyers and dentists were consistent with the hypothesis that mobility restriction results in a geographic misallocation of these groups.

185   H. E. KLARMAN, *The Economics of Health*
New York: Columbia University Press, 1965, pp. viii, 200.
See 11.

186   R. PENCHANSKY, G. ROSENTHAL, 'Productivity, price and income in the physicians' services market – a tentative hypothesis'
MC, October–December, 1965, 3(4), pp. 240–4.
It is suggested that differences in physicians' incomes and prices reflect the different extent to which they are dependent on the use of hospital facilities. The more hospital-oriented the physician, the higher his income and the smaller the rise in his prices. There are two main sources for the differences: increased productivity, and the smaller time given free to the community in return for capital services provided free to physicians using hospital facilities.

187   E. RAYACK, 'The American Medical Association and the supply of physicians: a study of the internal contradictions in the concept of professionalism'
MC, January–March, 1965, 3(1), pp. 17–25.
The paper chronicles the actions of the A.M.A. in restricting the availability of medical school places by opposing government assistance to medical schools to expand enrolment in spite of increasing evidence of doctor shortage. This action was in marked contrast to their attitude in encouraging government sponsorship of research and hospital building.

188   H. B. STEELE, G. V. RIMLINGER, 'Income opportunities and physician location trends in the United States'
WEJ, Spring, 1965, 3(2), pp. 182–94.
A study to determine the change in the distribution of physicians in the U.S.A. between 1950 and 1959, and the factors producing the change. The most important factors over time were the degree of mobilisation and the increase in population. Income of the population was a less important factor than had been expected, although this may have been the result of using data on all physicians rather than for private physicians alone.

189   D. E. YETT, 'The supply of nurses: an economist's view'
HP, February, 1965, 96(2), pp. 88–102.
Looks at the problems in talking about shortage, in particular the problem in

talking about and estimating supply. The first part of the paper examines the view of a nursing administrator of the nurse shortage and finds it wanting. The second part of the paper discusses some projections, which indicate that even under favourable circumstances, i.e. nursing wages rising as fast as the general female wage level, a nursing shortage would still exist in 1970.

1966

T. D. BAKER, 'Dynamics of health manpower planning'
MC, October–December, 1966, 4(4), pp. 205–11.

A framework is provided for manpower planning. Problems encountered in dealing with the questions posed in the framework, and data sources, are discussed.

K. GALES, R. C. WRIGHT, *A Survey of Manpower Demand Forecasts for the Social Services*
London: National Council of Social Services, 1966, p. 96.

A critical review of manpower demand forecasts carried out in Great Britain for doctors, dental practitioners, nurses and medical auxiliaries.

D. L. HIESTAND, 'Research into manpower for health services'
MMFQ, October, 1966, 44(2), pp. 146–79.

Sets out priorities for research, noting a preoccupation in existing research with physicians and nurses, while in fact the other personnel groups are numerically larger and have expanded more rapidly in the post-war period. A catalogue of work that has been done (mainly empirical work) is provided, although not all the authors of the work reviewed are identified.

D. S. LEES, *Economic Consequences of the Professions*
London: The Institute of Economic Affairs, 1966, p. 48.

An examination of the nature of the professions and their consequences in the United Kingdom. It is concluded that while the professions contribute to the creation of valuable human skills, and to reducing the uncertainty facing consumers, they also impose restrictions on competition that produce mono-poly gains for members at the expense of consumers.

M. F. MCNULTY, 'Health manpower'
Hospitals, April 1st, 1966, 40(7), pp. 83–8.

A review of the United States manpower situation in the light of the 1965 literature; all types of health manpower are considered.

— **195**   OFFICE OF HEALTH ECONOMICS, *Medical Manpower*
London: Office of Health Economics, July, 1966, p. 32.

An examination of trends in the numbers of doctors in general practice and the
hospital service, and the problems of forecasting these numbers in the future.
See 4.

196   D. C. PAIGE, K. JONES, *Health and Welfare Services in Britain in 1975*
Cambridge: Cambridge University Press for the National Institute of
Economic and Social Research, Occasional Papers 22, 1966, p. 142.

Estimates are made of the requirements of manpower and facilities in the
different sectors of the British Health and Welfare Services up to 1975.
See 77, 1101.

197   D. E. YETT, 'The nursing shortage and the Nurse Training Act'
ILRR, January, 1966, 19(2), pp. 190–200.

An examination of the provisions of the 1964 Nurse Training Act, a five year
programme instituted in 1964 to increase the supply of nursing school
graduates in the U.S.A. by 75 per cent by 1970. While the Act is regarded as a
major step towards alleviating the nurse shortage, a basic cause of the shortage
is low salaries in nursing – a reflection of the often monopsony power of
hospitals – and the Act does not address itself to the demand side of the
problem.

1967

198   T. D. BAKER, M. PERLMAN, *Health Manpower in a Developing Economy*
Baltimore: Johns Hopkins Press, 1967, pp. xi, 203.

A comprehensive manpower planning study of Taiwan. The study includes a
census of health workers, a household survey to determine medical care
demands, an examination of medical training institutions, and an attitude
survey of students studying to become health professionals. A shortfall in the
supply of doctors but a surplus of nurses in 1973 and 1983 are predicted, but all
the deficiencies are seen to be correctable without serious difficulty.
See 212, 220.

199   I. BUTTER, 'Health manpower research: a survey'
Inquiry, December, 1967, 4(4), pp. 5–41.

An examination of the factors affecting the demand for, and supply of medical
manpower and the implications of various policy measures. The paper provides

a comprehensive survey of the United States literature including the work of government commissions.

0 CANADIAN MEDICAL ASSOCIATION, *Conference on Medical Manpower*
   CMAJ, December 23rd and 30th, 1967, 97(26), pp. 1555–609.

A collection of twelve short papers providing a good deal of information on the medical manpower situation in Canada.

J. H. Walters, 'The Canadian Medical Association manpower census: a preliminary report', pp. 1555–7.

T. C. Points, 'How to use a medical census', pp. 1557–61.

C. B. Stewart, 'The future availability of medical students', pp. 1562–8.

R. L. Perkin, 'Medical manpower in general practice', pp. 1569–72.

I. W. Bean, 'Future manpower needs in general practice', pp. 1573–7.

W. M. Goldberg, 'The present manpower situation with regard to specialists in Canada', pp. 1578–82.

R. B. Kerr, 'Future manpower needs in specialty practice', pp. 1583–6.

P. G. Fish, 'Medical manpower in teaching and research: the present situation', pp. 1587–91.

J. R. Evans, 'Future manpower needs in teaching and research', pp. 1592–6.

D. I. Rice, 'The future use of paramedical personnel in private medical practice', pp. 1597–602.

E. K. Lyon, 'Will group practice ease the physician's work load?' pp. 1602–5.

R. O. Jones, 'The responsibility of voluntary medical associations for future medical manpower', pp. 1605–9.

R. FEIN, *The Doctor Shortage: An Economic Diagnosis*
Washington D.C.: The Brookings Institution, 1967, pp. xi, 199.

An economic framework is outlined within which the problem of doctor shortage may be discussed, and a comprehensive study of the problem in the U.S.A. is presented. In the opening section of the book a variety of approaches that have been used to project requirements for health manpower are reviewed. The study of the U.S.A., which occupies the major part of the book, is an aggregative study with projections being made of the total demand for physicians' services, and of the total supply of physicians, but the problems of location patterns, and the shift to specialisation are discussed and the likely impact of such factors suggested. The analysis suggests that in the period 1965–75 total demand for services will grow by approximately 22–26 per cent, whereas the supply of physicians will increase by 19 per cent, and the balance of demand and supply in the period 1975–80 will if anything be rather worse. These results imply the need for productivity growth, and a discussion of methods of improving productivity, in particular group practice and new types of personnel, forms another major part of the book.

202   E. H. FORGOTSON, J. L. COOK, 'Innovations and experiments in uses of health manpower – the effect of licensure laws'
Law Contemp.Probl., Autumn, 1967, 32(4), pp. 731–50.

An examination of state licensure laws in the U.S.A., which regulate the tasks and responsibilities of various categories of health manpower. It is concluded that licensure does prevent optimal allocation of tasks between personnel, and acts as a barrier to training and utilisation of new kinds of manpower.

203   J. M. LAST, 'Objective measurement of quality in general practice'
AGP, June, 1967, 12(Supp. part 2), pp. 5–26.

See 566.

204   J. M. LAST, 'Regional distribution of general practitioners and consultants in the National Health Service'
BMJ, June, 1967, 2(5555), pp. 796–9.

The study revealed that general practitioners more often than consultants settle in the part of country where they spent their youth, rather than near the medical school they attended. Consultants tend to diffuse more widely throughout the country.

205   E. RAYACK, *Professional Power and American Medicine*
Cleveland: The World Publishing Company, 1967, pp. xvii, 298.

Sub-titled 'the economics of the American Medical Association', the book examines the areas of conflict between the A.M.A. and the social interest. The book discusses the growth and origins of the A.M.A.; its power and influences; the influence on medical education, on the supply of physicians, in the physician shortage debate, in jurisdictional disputes with related professions; and the Association's role in the development of private and social insurance.

206   H. M. STURM, *Technology and Manpower in the Health Services Industry 1965–75*
Washington D.C.: U.S. Department of Labor, Manpower Administration, Manpower Research Bulletin Number 14, May, 1967, pp. vii, 109.

A study based partly on published sources of information and partly on interviews with experts in various medical fields. The study has three main parts: the first analyses trends in health service employment and summarises major existing difficulties in meeting health manpower needs. The second part looks at technological developments and how these are likely to affect requirements for health manpower. The third part looks at the effects of the expected increase in the demand for health services and technological developments on the volume and structure of health services employment, and projections for 1975 of manpower requirements in the major health occupation groups are given. A summary of the main findings of the report can be found in H. M. Sturm, 'Technological developments and their effects upon health manpower', *Mon.Lab.Rev.*, January, 1967, 9(91), pp. 1–9.

1968

L. BENHAM, A. MAURIZI, M. W. REDER, 'Migration, location, and remuneration of medical personnel, physicians and dentists' *Rev.Econ.Stats.*, August, 1968, 50(3), pp. 332–47.

A study to determine how well the distribution of the national stock of physicians and dentists corresponds to the distribution of population across the states of the U.S.A., and to determine the influence exerted by effective demand, barriers to migration, and location preferences of the medics. Data from 1930, 1940, 1950 and 1960 were used in the study. The main results were that effective demand was found to have an impact on distribution; some secular correction of the inequality of distribution of 1930 was found; dentists however were impeded by state licensure arrangements; and the number of physicians per capita was found to increase with the volume of training facilities.

W. L. KISSICK, 'Health manpower in transition' *MMFQ*, January, 1968, 46(1 part 2), pp. 633–45.

A descriptive survey of the manpower field and its problems. The material covered is as follows: the difficulties of defining health manpower; determinants of need and demand; the methods used to forecast requirements; the resources on which we can draw for health manpower; and factors influencing the full utilisation of potentials – salaries, inflexibilities, restrictive practices. The paper then goes on to consider ways of improving utilisation and new approaches to manpower problems.

A. T. PEACOCK, J. R. SHANNON, 'The new doctors' dilemma' *LBR*, January, 1968, pp. 26–38.

Provides a criticism of manpower planning in the British National Health Service, taking the Paige and Jones study as an example of work that has been done. They suggest that an alternative approach is to make a realistic projection of public expenditure on the National Health Service, consistent with the development of other government services and the development of the economy as a whole, and then to try to maximise the output of 'health' subject to this budget constraint.

210   H. K. SCHONFELD, I. S. FALK, 'The development of standards for the audit and planning of medical care – good pediatric care – program content and methods of estimating needed personnel'
AJPH, November, 1968, 58(11), pp. 2097–110.

Standards of good care are established by interview of high quality pediatricians and dentists, and these standards are used to determine the scope of the programme. The time required to perform the procedures regarded as desirable is then calculated and from these calculations manpower requirements can be obtained.

211   J. R. SHANNON, 'Manpower planning in the National Health Service'
In G. McLachlan (ed.) *Problems and Progress in Medical Care, Essays on Current Research, Third Series*, pp. 51–62 (16).

A discussion of the weaknesses of the methods used by manpower planners in the United Kingdom, in particular their failure to take proper account of opportunity cost, and the fact that shortages are discussed as differences between projections of requirements and supply with no reference to costs or benefits of making up the shortfall.

212   C. E. TAYLOR, R. DIRICAN, K. W. DEUSCHLE, *Health Manpower in Turkey*
Baltimore: Johns Hopkins Press, 1968, pp. xi, 300.

One of a series of comprehensive manpower planning studies (other studies covered Taiwan, Peru and Nigeria), this study includes a survey of existing resources, manpower supply and demand projections, and a set of recommendations for policy. Evidence was produced suggesting poor utilisation and inadequate productivity of health manpower, and gross inequities in availability of health services.
See 198, 220.

213   A. J. WILLCOCKS, 'The staffing of the maternity services'
In G. McLachlan (ed.) *Problems and Progress in Medical Care, Essays on Current Research, Third Series*, pp. 63–89 (16).

The essay surveys the available data on the supply and distribution of midwives in England and Wales. The training, social and educational background, and employment of the midwives is discussed and topics for further research are suggested.

214   D. E. YETT, 'Lifetime earnings for nurses in comparison with college trained women'
Inquiry, December, 1968, 5(4), pp. 35–70.

Estimates are provided for the period 1939–66 of the internal rate of return, and rate of return over cost to nurse training. The rates are consistently low and sometimes negative, although this finding is not regarded as evidence of a surplus of nurses, but rather as evidence of monopsony power on the part of local hospitals being used to keep wages down.

1969

F. N. ARNHOFF, E. A. RUBINSTEIN, J. C. SPEISMAN, *Manpower for Mental Health*
Chicago: Aldine Publishing Company, 1969, pp. xii, 204.

A collection of nine papers plus a summary examining a wide variety of aspects of mental health manpower. Most of the papers have a theoretical orientation although the first paper by Arnhoff, Rubinstein, Shriver and Jones presents information on the growth in the numbers of various types of mental health manpower in the U.S.A. since 1945. A paper by Klarman reviews economic approaches to projecting health manpower requirements and develops a cost–benefit framework for looking at the mental health manpower problem. Several of the papers have substantial bibliographies.

D. C. E. CHEW, 'Wastage patterns in the nursing profession in Singapore: a study of manpower utilization'
ILR, December, 1969, 100(6), pp. 583–94.

A study to determine the causes of the high rate of attrition among qualified nurses, and in its light an evaluation of policies to increase the number of nurses. The major causes of resignations were found to be the desire to study abroad, coupled with limited admission to the post-basic midwifery course, and the universal difficulty of combining family obligations with nursing.

R. T. FLINT, K. C. SPENSLEY, 'Recent issues in nursing manpower: a review'
NR, May–June, 1969, 18(3), pp. 217–29.

398 books and articles appearing in the period 1956–68 are organised into ten sections: (1) overview: summaries and projection, (2) analytical studies; (3) sociological and psychological studies; (4) education; (5) refresher training; (6) recruitment; (7) utilisation; (8) suppertime personnel; (9) innovations; (10) attrition and turnover.

E. GINZBERG, M. OSTOW, *Men, Money and Medicine*
New York: Columbia University Press, 1969, pp. xii, 291.

The book presents an appraisal of what has been learned from studies in the

political economy of health, and assesses efforts to improve the United States health care system. Two of the book's four sections deal with manpower. The five chapters of section two deal with the medical profession and consider issues such as the market power of the physicians, physician shortage and women in the medical profession. The third section of the book concerns itself with problems relating to allied health manpower and includes chapters on nursing, clinical laboratory personnel and social workers.
See 1194.

219 H. I. GREENFIELD, *Allied Health Manpower: Trends and Prospects*
New York: Columbia University Press, 1969, pp. xvii, 195.

A study of the United States health manpower situation concentrating particularly on five categories of technicians (X-ray, medical records, occupational and physical therapy, medical and dental) and three categories of assistants (licensed practical nurses, nurses' aides and psychiatric aides). These groups together constitute 1.2 million of the 1.7 million persons classified as 'allied health manpower'. The study looks at the sources of supply, education and training, structure of labour markets, and federal programmes relating to these groups of health personnel.

220 T. L. HALL, *Health Manpower in Peru*
Baltimore: Johns Hopkins Press, 1969, pp. xvi, 281.

A manpower planning study for Peru considering all types of health manpower: doctors, dentists, pharmacists, nurses, midwives, technicians and auxiliaries. Demand projections up to 1984 are based on the achievement of particular staffing ratios for different health facilities. A second set of projections is made assuming a more moderate rate of growth of the health sector. Three sets of supply projections are made on the assumption of different staff retention rates. The costs of meeting the demand projections are calculated.
See 198, 212.

221 H. E. KLARMAN, 'Economic aspects of projecting requirements for health manpower'
JHR, Summer, 1969, 4(3), pp. 360–76.

A survey of methods used to project requirements for health manpower. A large bibliography is provided.

222 J. H. KNOWLES, 'The quantity and quality of medical manpower: a review of medicine's current efforts'
JME, February, 1969, 44(2), pp. 81–118.

A survey of the manpower situation in the U.S.A. Manpower shortages in the various specialty groups are examined. The medical needs of the poor are seen as the major requirement for the health-care system to meet in the future. A substantial bibliography is included.

J. H. KNOWLES, 'Radiology – a case study in technology and manpower' *NEJM*, June 5th, 1969, 280(23), pp. 1271–8, June 12th, 1969, 280(24), pp. 1323–9.

Brings together a lot of information on this specialty in the U.S.A. Restrictive practices, nature of the career, salaries, attitudes of medical students to the specialty, are discussed. Evidence of a shortage of radiologists in the U.S.A. is adduced from a large number of unfilled vacancies, and from evidence that the number of radiological examinations and treatments has grown faster than the supply of radiologists.

H. MARGULIES, L. BLOCH, *Foreign Medical Graduates in the United States* Cambridge, Massachusetts: Harvard University Press, 1969, pp. xx, 169.

A compilation and analysis of information available about foreign medical graduates in the United States, including information on salaries, type of activity, country of origin and performance in state examinations. The impact of the foreign medical graduates on medicine in the United States is examined. A final chapter discusses some policy solutions to dilemmas, both within the U.S.A. and for international relations, created by the employment of foreign medical graduates.

M. PERLMAN, 'Rationing of medical resources: the complexities of the supply and demand problem' *Sociological Review Monographs*, September, 1969, 4, pp. 105–19.

A review of the factors governing the supply of physicians in the U.S.A.; with substitution of other factors for physicians appearing inappropriate, various methods that might be used to retain physician services are discussed.

J. WISEMAN, 'Some economic problems of medical care' *JRCGP*, February, 1969, Supplement No. 1., 17(79), pp. 2–7. *See* 1008.

E. YOST, *The U.S. Health Industry: The Costs of Acceptable Medical Care by 1975* New York: F. A. Praeger Publishers, 1969, pp. xv, 138.

Projections are made of manpower requirements for physicians, registered nurses, dentists and other health occupations in 1975, first on the assumption that medical care be provided at the present level, with existing variations, to the projected population for 1975, and second that care be provided equal to that available in middle-class geographical areas in 1966–7. Estimates are also made of the costs of these increases.

1970

228   S. H. ALTMAN, 'The structure of nursing education and its impact on supply'
In H. E. Klarman (ed.) *Empirical Studies in Health Economics*, pp. 335–52 (18).

An examination of the structure of the nursing educational system and the effects it has on the type of labour market in which nursing services are provided. The paper analyses the behaviour of the training establishment and the benefits it derives from training, and the costs and benefits to the student. The last section of the paper considers recent experience in the training and employment of nurses in the United States.

229   M. BLAUG, *An Introduction to the Economics of Education*
Harmondsworth, England: Penguin Books Ltd., 1970, pp. xx, 363.
See 17.

230   R. G. S. BROWN, 'The supply of general practitioners to East Yorkshire'
YB, November, 1970, 22(2), pp. 164–79.

A review of the factors affecting general practitioner recruitment to a particular area. Financial factors appeared to be weighted relatively low; family connections, experience of the region and proximity of a medical school were the most significant variables.

231   J. P. BUNKER, 'Surgical manpower: a comparison of operations and surgeons in the United States and England and Wales'
NEJM, January 15th, 1970, 282(2), pp. 135–44.

An examination of evidence on the differences, socio-economic, organisational, philosophical and geographical, between the United States and England and Wales to try and explain why there are twice as many surgeons and twice as many operations per head of population in the United States compared to England and Wales. It is concluded that differences in the method of payment are the most likely reason for the disparity. It is further concluded that, with a disproportionate number of surgeons in the United States compared to the general manpower pool, some unnecessary surgery takes place.

I. BUTTER, J. GRENZKE, 'Training and utilization of foreign medical graduates in the United States'
JME, August, 1970, 45(8), pp. 607–17.

The implications of large-scale doctor immigration, both for the United States and for the donor countries, are examined. A brief survey is provided of work carried out by the authors on the geographic distribution, specialty distribution, distribution of professional activities, longitudinal comparisons, utilisation of foreign medical graduates and the extent to which foreign medical graduates alleviate the doctor shortage.

R. J. CARLSON, 'Health manpower licensing and emerging institutional responsibility for the quality of care'
Law Contemp.Probl., Autumn, 1970, 35(4), pp. 849–78.

An examination of the rationale of health manpower licensing laws, and how they operate in conjunction with malpractice law to thwart innovation and efficient utilisation of health manpower. A proposal for change to a system of institutional rather than individual licensure is outlined.

M. S. FELDSTEIN, 'The rising price of physician services'
Rev.Econ.Stats., May, 1970, 52(2), pp. 121–33.

It is shown that price and quantity behaviour in the market for physicians' services cannot be explained by traditional economic models. Rather it is suggested physicians sheltering behind permanent excess demand are free to vary both prices and the quantity of services they supply. There appeared to be a tendency for prices to rise with improved insurance coverage and increased ability of patients to pay. There was also evidence of physicians reducing the supply of services when fees rose. The study also provides revised estimates of the rates of increase of physicians' fees, output and productivity.
See also the comment by D. M. Brown, H. E. Lapan, *Rev.Econ.Stats.*, February, 1972, 54(1), pp. 101–5, and the reply by Feldstein, pp. 105–7; and D. M. Brown, M. S. Feldstein, H. Lapan, 'The rising price of physicians' services: a clarification', *Rev.Econ.Stats.*, August, 1974, 56(3), pp. 396–8.

P. J. FELDSTEIN, S. KELMAN, 'A framework for an econometric model of the medical care sector'
In H. E. Klarman (ed.) *Empirical Studies in Health Economics*, pp. 171–90 (18).
See 1389.

236   W. H. FRANKE, I. SOBEL, *The Shortage of Skilled and Technical Workers*
Lexington: Lexington Books, D.C. Heath and Company, 1970, pp. 391.

A detailed study of labour market operation, the attraction, training, placement and retention of workers in shortage occupations (shortage being defined as a situation in which employers have been unable to hire sufficient numbers of qualified personnel at existing wage rates). The study looks at the labour markets of Chicago and St. Louis. Six occupations were studied, two in the medical field – licensed practical nurses and medical technologists.

237   W. A. GLASER, *Paying the Doctor: Systems of Remuneration and their Effects*
Baltimore: The Johns Hopkins Press, 1970, pp. xii, 323.

A study of methods of payment of medical practitioners in sixteen countries, the development of the systems and their effects on work effort and quality of work, doctor–patient relations, patterns of care and the treatment of various groups of patients.
See 1066.

238   W. LEE HANSEN, 'An appraisal of physician manpower projection'
Inquiry, March, 1970, 7(1), pp. 102–13.

Discusses the key issues surrounding physician manpower planning. Six U.S. studies projecting physician requirements for 1965–75 are examined. The need for a more thorough understanding of the physician manpower market and the possibilities of substitution are stressed as necessary developments for further progress in forecasting.

239   R. A. KESSEL, 'The A.M.A. and the supply of physicians'
Law Contemp.Probl., Spring, 1970, 35(2), pp. 267–83.

An examination of the role of the American Medical Association in determining the rate of output of physicians and in limiting the choice of contractual relationships between physicians and their patients. The problem of physician shortage is seen to stem from the Flexner report of 1910, which specified 'how physicians were to be produced instead of specifying what the product should be and allowing schools to compete in efficiently producing that product'.

240   W. J. MCNERNEY, 'Why does medical care cost so much?'
NEJM, June, 1970, 282(26), pp. 1458–65.

It is argued that a substantial expansion of doctor supply, given the present systems of health-care delivery and financing, will do little to lower price or improve the distribution of care in the U.S.A., as there is a greater excess of unmet need than even the largest visualised expansions in supply could meet.

G. N. MONSMA, 'Marginal revenue and the demand for physicians' services'

In H. E. Klarman (ed.) *Empirical Studies in Health Economics*, pp. 145–60 (18).

An examination of empirical evidence to see if there is any support for the hypothesis that in situations where the purchase of physicians' services results in a positive marginal revenue to the physician there is a higher demand for physicians' services than in situations where there is no such financial advantage to the physician. As a whole the data supported this proposition, and this effect was more pronounced in surgery than in home and office visits.

J. P. NEWHOUSE, 'A model of physician pricing'
SEJ, October, 1970, 37(2), pp. 174–83.

The hypothesis is put forward that the market for physicians' services is monopolistic, although no attempt is made to distinguish simple and discriminating monopoly. The hypothesis was tested on the basis of inferences from two alternative models of the market for physicians' services, a simple monopoly model and a competitive model. The models were tested using data on charges for physician office visits and a few well-defined procedures – obstetrical care, an appendectomy, a tonsillectomy and tooth filling. Although the tests were relatively weak they did suggest that the market for physicians' services was monopolistic rather than competitive, and the same was true of the market for dental services. There was, however, some evidence that physicians do not maximise short-run profits, as price did not vary with age, education or insurance variables.

See also the comment by H. E. Frech, P. B. Ginsburg, *SEJ*, April, 1972, 38(4), pp. 573–7, and the reply by J. P. Newhouse and F. Sloan, pp. 577–80.

F. SLOAN, 'Lifetime earnings and physicians' choice of specialty'
ILRR, October, 1970, 24(1), pp. 47–56.

Present values of earnings and internal rates of return were calculated for general practice and for several specialties in the United States for the years 1955, 1959 and 1965. No systematic relationship was found between income differences and career choice within the medical profession. Possible explanations for these findings and policy implications are discussed.

J. J. SPENGLER, 'Cost of specialization in a service economy'
SSQ, September, 1970, 51(2), pp. 237–62.

The arguments in favour of specialisation and the costs associated with it are discussed. In a perfectly competitive situation specialisation would approximate the degree that is optimal, but when services are no longer competitively supplied, as in medical care, this is no longer the case. Specialisation in

American medical care is examined. The co-operation of existing specialists is seen to be inadequate for dealing with many problems; the solution does not lie with the old type general practitioner but in combining a measure of specialisation with general practice. It is suggested that 85,000 general practitioners could meet 85–90 per cent of the United States ordinary health needs, leaving 160,000 specialists for other services.

245   U.S. DEPARTMENT OF HEALTH, EDUCATION AND WELFARE, *Proceedings and Report of Conference on a Health Manpower Simulation Model* Washington D.C.: USDHEW, 1970.

In particular D. E. Yett, L. Drabek, M. D. Intrilagator, L. J. Kimbell, 'The development of a micro-simulation model of health manpower demand and supply', pp. 9–173.
See 1424.

246   D. E. YETT, 'The chronic "shortage" of nurses: a public policy dilemma' In H. E. Klarman (ed.) *Empirical Studies in Health Economics*, pp. 357–89 (18). Also in M. H. Cooper, A. J. Culyer (eds.) *Health Economics*, pp. 172–209 (33).

Two models developed to consider the 'shortage of engineers' are applied to the nursing market in the United States. The Blank–Stigler (changing relative remuneration) and Arrow–Capron (dynamic shortage) models are critically examined. This examination is in many ways more central to the paper than the application to nursing data. Most of the evidence favours the dynamic shortage model, but the aggregate magnitude of the shortage cannot be measured from available data. The policy implications of the findings are discussed.

247   D. E. YETT, 'Causes and consequences of salary differentials in nursing' *Inquiry*, March, 1970, 7(1), pp. 78–99.

The paper has four main parts. The first part of the paper reviews trends in vacancy rates by field of nursing and hospital position, and for full-time nurses by region, hospital type, control and bed size. The second part of the paper considers salary differentials between nurses and other groups, and within the nursing profession. The third part of the paper reviews various models of labour shortage and applies them to the nursing profession. The final part of the paper considers the effect on nurse shortages of different types of policies to change supply or demand elasticity, or to shift supply or demand.

*   *   *

1971

S. H. ALTMAN, 'Alternative measures of the regional availability of nursing manpower'
EBB, Fall, 1971, 24(1), pp. 68–75.

L. BENHAM, 'The labour market for registered nurses: a three equation model'
Rev.Econ.Stats., August, 1971, 53(3), pp. 246–52.
A complete model of the labour market for registered nurses in the U.S.A., with equations for demand, labour force participation and geographical location, is estimated by three stage least squares. All the coefficients had the expected signs and were similar in magnitude for both 1950 and 1960.

R. G. S. BROWN, C. WALKER, 'The distribution of medical manpower'
In G. McLachlan (ed.) *Problems and Progress in Medical Care, Fifth Series*, pp. 1–44 (24).
A study to throw light on the changes in the sources from which doctors have come to work in three parts of Great Britain, changes in the mobility of settled doctors, and the reasons for their career decisions. A profile of the medical population was constructed for each area for 1935, 1945, 1955 and 1965. The study areas were Hull and the East Riding, Cardiff and part of the Vale of Glamorgan, and Southampton and adjacent parts of Hampshire.

I. BUTTER, 'Migratory flows of M.D.s to and from the U.S.A.'
MC, January–February, 1971, 9(1), pp. 17–31.
American Medical Association data were used to estimate the outflow and inflow of foreign-trained doctors to the United States, and to determine their country of origin. The 'brain gain' was found to total 9,000 for the years 1967 and 1968, 7,500 excluding United States citizens. 50 per cent of the incoming physicians had the option of permanent stay in the United States.

I. BUTTER, R. SCHAFFNER, 'Foreign medical graduates and equal access to medical care'
MC, March–April, 1971, 9(2), pp. 136–43.
A study of foreign medical graduates in the United States in 1968 revealed that foreign medical graduates have increased the disparity, as measured by doctor–population ratios, between states and between urban and rural areas in the provision of medical care. The calculation, however, is carried out on the basis that the distribution of U.S. medical graduates is unaffected by the location pattern of foreign doctors.

253   I. J. FAHS, T. CHOI, K. BARCHAS, P. ZAKARIASEN, 'Indicators of need for health care personnel: the concept of need, alternative measures employed to determine need, and a suggested model'
MC, March–April, 1971, 9(2), pp. 144–51.

A brief discussion of indicators commonly used to show need for health-care personnel, health personnel/population ratios, need based on economic factors, mainly income, and need as indicated by geographic distance from care. A model incorporating these measures with study of entry and exit from the health care professions is suggested as a means of health manpower planning.

254   R. FEIN, G. I. WEBER, *Financing Medical Education: An Analysis of Alternative Policies and Mechanisms*
New York: McGraw-Hill Book Company, 1971, p. 279.

A comprehensive study of the American medical school system. The major features of the medical schools, the evaluation of their financial structure, the background of medical students, the factors affecting the number of applicants to the schools, the rate of return to medical education, the role of state and federal finance in medical education, are examined in the opening six chapters. The final chapter argues a case for greater federal government involvement in financing medical education, with provision of subsidies to both students and medical schools.

255   M. S. FELDSTEIN, 'Hospital cost inflation: a study of non-profit price dynamics'
AER, December, 1971, 61(5), pp. 835–72.
See 447.

256   O. GISH, *Doctor Migration and World Health*
London: G. Bell and Sons Ltd., Occasional Papers on Social Administration No. 43, 1971, p. 151.

Draws together a great deal of material on the scale and effects of international medical migration. The monograph is in two parts: the first part reviews work, much of it by the author, on migratory movements to and from the British Isles; the second part looks at health and development in the Third World countries and the impact on their health programmes of large-scale doctor migration. Appendices are included on the migration of nurses and 'other' health manpower.
See 1069.

N. HERSHEY, 'New directions in licensure of health personnel'
EBB, Fall, 1971, 24(1), pp. 22–35.

A survey of developments since 1969 in the U.S.A. to try and overcome the problems of restrictive licensing legislation in the health field, which inhibits realignment of the functions of licensed personnel and recognition of scopes of practice for the unlicensed. The principal suggestion for change is a move from individual licensure to institutional licensure, malpractice actions alone being enough to prevent abuse by institutions.

J. E. JONISH, 'U.S. physician manpower and immigration'
NJEB, Summer, 1971, 10(3), pp. 12–26.

The importance of immigration to health services in the U.S.A. is evidenced. While the largest absolute flows from individual countries come from Europe and Canada, the greatest relative impact is borne by the developing nations of the world. Emigration flows among countries were positively related to the current stock of physicians and the physician–population ratio of the country of emigration, and negatively related to the income per capita of the country of emigration.

S. JOROFF, V. NAVARRO, 'Medical manpower: a multivariate analysis of the distribution of physicians in urban United States'
MC, September–October, 1971, 9(5), pp. 428–38.

An examination of the relationship between ten community characteristics in 299 Standard Metropolitan Statistical Areas and the supply of physicians by individual specialty (21 specialties).

J. L. KILGOUR, 'Migration of doctors and medical manpower planning'
HT, 1971, 3(2), pp. 34–6.

A brief survey of information on the inflow and outflow of doctors to and from the U.K., and the factors responsible for these movements.

J. L. KILGOUR, 'The urgent need for a new staff structure'
BJHM, July, 1971, 6(1), pp. 18–22.

An introduction to the problems of the staffing structure in the National Health Service. The main problem lies in the imbalance between the number of doctors in the training grades and the number of available established posts in the hospital service.

J. R. LAVE, L. B. LAVE, T. E. MORTON, 'The physician's assistant. Exploration of the concept'
Hospitals, June 1st, 1971, 45(11), pp. 42–51.

A review of the literature on physicians' assistants, their training programmes, cost of training, potential functions, quality of care, productivity, methods of payment and education and career mobility. An extensive bibliography is provided.

263   E. RAYACK, 'The physicians' service industry'
In W. Adams (ed.) *The Structure of America's Industry*, 4th Edition, New York: Macmillan Company, 1971, pp. 419–56.

A study of the physician service industry (as opposed to the hospital service industry), its structure, conduct and performance. The study centres around an examination of professional power represented by the American Medical Association, and operating principally through licensing arrangements.

264   M. I. ROEMER, J. W. FRIEDMAN, *Doctors in Hospitals: Medical Staff Organisation and Hospital Performance*
Baltimore: the Johns Hopkins Press, 1971, pp. xiv, 322.
See 456.

265   L. J. SHUMAN, J. P. YOUNG, E. NADDOR, 'Manpower mix for health services: a prescriptive regional planning model'
HSR, Summer, 1971, 6(2), pp. 103–19.

A linear programming model is constructed to determine the mix of manpower and technology needed to provide health services of acceptable quality at a minimum total cost to the community. The costs include the costs of shortages and the costs of not providing facilities. The model is illustrated with reference to a neighbourhood health centre, and the sensitivity of the model to alternative policies is investigated.

266   F. SLOAN, 'The demand for medical education: a study of medical school applicant behaviour'
JHR, Fall, 1971, 6(4), pp. 466–89.

A demand model for medical education was constructed. The results indicated that potential medical students were responsive to differences in expected returns between occupations, with direct medical education costs having a substantial impact on occupational choice, although 'A' record students were less influenced by education costs and earnings.

267   C. M. STEVENS, 'Physician supply and national health care goals'
IR, May, 1971, 10(2), pp. 119–44.

It is concluded on the basis of either physician output or patient utilisation rates achieved under the Kaiser prepaid medical care scheme that the existing supply of physicians in the United States is in excess of the number that would be required if the system of care was suitably reorganised.

C. M. STEVENS, G. D. BROWN, 'Market structure approach to health manpower planning'
AJPH, October, 1971, 61(10), pp. 1988–95.
The approach outlined involves essentially an examination of the supply side of the manpower market to see if its structure might reasonably be expected to respond to changes in demand. The approach is illustrated by examination of three occupations requiring at least one year of formal training: registered nurses, licensed practical nurses and medical secretaries.

P. WING, M. S. BLUMBERG, 'Operating expenditures and sponsored research at U.S. medical schools: an empirical study of cost patterns'
JHR, Winter, 1971, 6(1), pp. 75–102.
See 457.

D. E. YETT, L. DRABEK, M. D. INTRILIGATOR, 'A macro-econometric model for regional health planning'
EBB, Fall, 1971, 24(1), pp. 1–21.
Seven categories of health manpower are included in the model: medical specialists in private practice, surgical specialists in private practice, physicians employed by hospitals, hospital interns and residents, registered nurses, allied health professionals and technicians, non-medical labour. The problem of estimating aggregate demand and supply equations for the different types of manpower are discussed.
See 1403.

1972

B. ABEL-SMITH, L. EKHOLM, H. E. KLARMAN, V. ROJO-FERNANDEZ, 'Can we reduce the cost of medical education?'
WHO Chronicle, October, 1972, 26(10), pp. 441–9. Also in *DD*, April, 1974, 12(2), pp. 97–108.
An examination of the issues to consider before deciding to establish a new medical school in a developing country: the health-care requirements, the available additional resources, the problems of using and keeping the newly trained doctors, and the alternatives to a new school.

272   R. F. Boaz, 'Manpower utilization by subsidized family planning clinics: an economic criterion for determining the professional skill mix'
JHR, Spring, 1972, 7(2), pp. 191–207.
See 576.

273   I. Butter, G. T. Moore, R. L. Robertson, E. Hall, 'Effects of manpower utilization on cost and productivity of a neighbourhood health centre'
MMFQ, October, 1972, 50(4 part 1), pp. 421–52.
See 577.

274   E. Charles, 'Policies to increase the supply of physicians in rural communities'
Amer.Econ., Fall, 1972, 16(2), pp. 36–42.
It is suggested that no foreseeable increase in the number of physicians, family practice specialities, drafts or incentives is likely to encourage a significantly larger number of physicians to locate in rural communities. Physicians' assistants may, however, provide some answer to the problem.
See also G. M. Scobie's comment, pp. 43–4.

275   H. A. Cohen, 'Monopsony and discriminating monopsony in the nursing market'
AE, 1972, 4(1), pp. 41–50.
An econometric study revealed that hospitals behave as monopsonists in the nursing market, but they did not appear to behave as discriminating monopsonists, nor could the wage pattern be explained by productivity differences. It is concluded that the explanation of the wage pattern must be sought in institutional factors such as the non-profit status of the hospitals, presence of a nursing school and the activities of nursing unions.

276   R. G. Evans, *Price Formation in the Market for Physician Services in Canada 1957–1969*
Ottawa: Queens Printer, 1972, pp. vi, 131.
A major study prepared for the Prices and Incomes Commission. The first chapter examines price and income trends and contains an appendix on the price indices used and their deficiencies. The second chapter explores various models of physician-pricing behaviour that have been suggested in the literature, and various of these elements are put together into a model 'whose most important feature is its demotion of the price variable from an equilibrating role'. The third chapter is an examination of the market behaviour of

physicians by province. The fourth chapter examines price changes within fee schedules as opposed to changes in the average overall level. A final chapter groups the conclusions of the study under three headings: the implications for data on medical prices, interpretations of medical market behaviour, and public policy towards medical care. An appendix is included on the future of the physician stock in Canada and in particular the development of domestic as opposed to the use of immigrant physicians.

N. R. E. FENDALL, *Auxiliaries in Health Care: Programs in Developing Countries*
Baltimore: Johns Hopkins Press, 1972, pp. xiii, 200.

Although not primarily an economic work, a great deal of information is provided on all aspects of the training and work of auxiliary medical personnel in the developing countries.

V. R. FUCHS, E. RAND, B. GARRETT, 'The distribution of earnings in health and other industries'
In V. R. Fuchs (ed.) *Essays in the Economics of Health and Medical Care*, pp. 119–31 (27).

The distributions of earnings of full-time year-round employed persons in health and nineteen other large industries in the United States are compared. The health industry was found to have a bimodal distribution; the distribution of earnings within hospitals alone was, however, more like that of a typical industry. An appendix is included on the distribution of earnings under prepaid group practice as opposed to the distribution in the health industry as a whole.

V. R. FUCHS, M. J. KRAMER, *Determinants of Expenditures for Physicians' Services in the United States 1948–68*
Washington D.C.: U.S. Department of Health, Education and Welfare, National Center for Health Services Research and Development, DHEW Publication No. (HSM)73–3013, December, 1972, p. 63.
See 120.

J. W. HAMBLETON, 'Foreign medical graduates and the doctor shortage'
Inquiry, December, 1972, 9(4), pp. 68–72.

It is argued that Schaffner and Butter (*Inquiry*, March, 1972, 9(1), pp. 24–33) may have been wrong to identify geographic maldistribution of physicians as an important aspect of the doctor shortage. Using data from postal zones it is demonstrated that poor neighbourhoods are not geographically disadvantaged

with respect to care, but they do not receive treatment from the nearby physicians. It is argued therefore that there must be institutional rather than geographic limitations to access to care.
See 286.

281   E. F. X. HUGHES, V. R. FUCHS, J. E. JACOBY, E. M. LEWIT, 'Surgical workloads in a community practice'
Surgery, March, 1972, 71(3), pp. 315–27.

A study of nineteen New York general surgeons indicated a mean weekly workload of 4.3 hernia equivalents, well below the 10 per week suggested by surgeons to be a realistic burden consistent with maintaining skills and continuing education. The study suggested a substantial underutilisation of highly specialised skills.

282   R. A. KESSEL, 'Higher education and the nation's health: a review of the Carnegie Commission report on medical education'
JLE, April, 1972, 15(1), pp. 115–27.

An examination of the findings and recommendations of the Carnegie Commission on medical education. The principal conclusion is that the commission failed to analyse why there is a shortage of doctors. Kessel holds that the shortage is a product of Flexner and A.M.A. restrictions; the former reduced the need for medical schools to rely on students for funds, removing the influence of market pressures. Some of the Carnegie recommendations go further in the same direction, reducing not increasing the financial incentives to expand medical school places.

283   R. J. LAVERS, M. REES, 'The distinction award system in England and Wales'
In G. McLachlan (ed.) *Problems and Progress in Medical Care, Essays on Current Research, Seventh Series*, pp. 33–68 (30).

A study of the distinction award system, a system whereby a third of consultants within the National Health Service receive additional payments of up to 100 per cent of salary, revealed that there were wide variations between specialities and regions in the expected value of award per consultant. Furthermore, it was found that these variations were not accounted for by any of a number of equity and efficiency criteria which were considered.

284   M. LYNCH, 'The physician "shortage": the economists' mirror'
AAAPSS, January, 1972, 399, pp. 82–8.

A survey of some of the literature on the physician shortage. It is concluded that by almost any criteria there was a shortage of physicians in the U.S.A. by the mid-1960s.

U. E. REINHARDT, 'A production function for physicians' services'
Rev.Econ.Stats., February, 1972, 54(1), pp. 55–66.
See 580.

R. SCHAFFNER, I. BUTTER, 'Geographic mobility of foreign medical
graduates and the doctor shortage. A longitudinal analysis'
Inquiry, March, 1972, 9(1), pp. 24–33.

A study to determine whether the interstate mobility of foreign medical
graduates does anything to relieve the disparity in the geographic distribution
of physicians in the United States. Evidence was found of a moderate trend
towards reducing relative shortages, but this was not sufficient to counteract
the geographic disparity that results from the initial choice of location.
See 280.

H. K. SCHONFELD, J. F. HESTON, I. S. FALK, 'Numbers of physicians
required for primary medical care'
NEJM, March 16th, 1972, 286(11), pp. 571–6.

Estimates of numbers of physicians required to provide good primary care are
developed on the basis of professional opinion of the services needed for such
care. Considering primary care providers to be internists and paediatricians, a
figure of 133 per 100,000 population in this type of practice in the United States
was thought desirable, or rather more than double the numbers available in
1966.

K. R. SMITH, M. MILLER, F. L. GOLLADAY, 'An analysis of the optimal use
of inputs in the production of medical services'
JHR, Spring, 1972, 7(2), pp. 208–25.

The possibilities and implications of using paramedical personnel in medical
practice are explored – the effects of efficient delegation of physician tasks on
physician productivity, leisure and costs of care. The implications of efficient
patterns of delegation are examined using data on primary care practices in
three states of the United States. The data are analysed in an activity analysis
model of primary care practice. Considerable potential for delegation was
revealed, although more and better data would be necessary for formulating
manpower policy.

A. YANKAUER, J. SCHNEIDER, S. H. JONES, L. M. HELLMAN, J. J. FELDMAN,
'Physician output, productivity and task delegation in obstetric-
gynecologic practices in the U.S.'
OG, January, 1972, 39(1), pp. 151–61.

Data from a survey of 90 per cent of the qualified practitioners in this specialty are examined. Information is provided on the number of visits and operations performed per week or per year and the number of hours worked by specialists of different ages and in different practice settings. The nature of tasks delegated and the frequency with which they are delegated to non-physician manpower are also discussed.

290   D. E. YETT, L. DRABEK, M. D. INTRILIGATOR, L. J. KIMBELL, 'Health manpower planning: an econometric approach'
HSR, Summer, 1972, 7(2), pp. 134–47.

The use of two econometric models of the entire health service system (a macro-econometric model and a micro-simulation model) in the analysis of health manpower policies for the U.S.A. is discussed. The great advantage of the models is that they treat explicitly many of the variables left out of account in the widely used ratio method of planning (e.g. doctor–population ratios).
See 1403, 1411.

1973

291   B. AHAMAD, 'Doctors in Britain, Canada, and the United States'
In B. Ahamad, M. Blaug (eds.) *The Practice of Manpower Forecasting*, Amsterdam: Elsevier Scientific Publishing Company, 1973, pp. 285–309.

A review of the doctor manpower forecasts and the techniques used to make them by the Goodenough Committee, the Willink Committee, the Royal Commission on Medical Education in Great Britain, the study by Judek carried out for the Royal Commission on the Health Services in Canada and the work of Fein in the United States.

292   C. E. BISHOP, 'Manpower policy and the supply of nurses'
IR, February, 1973, 12(1), pp. 86–94.

The possibility of increasing the supply of nurses in the short run by attracting back nurses no longer working was considered. The most encouraging result was that the participation of married nurses appears to be substantially influenced by salary increases, the supply elasticity with respect to wages being 0.54, a higher elasticity than that found by D. E. Yett in H. E. Klarman (ed.) *Empirical Studies in Health Economics*.
See 246.

293   J. R. BUTLER in collaboration with J. M. BEVAN, R. C. TAYLOR, *Family Doctors and Public Policy: A Study of Manpower Distribution*
London: Routledge and Kegan Paul, 1973, pp. x, 198.

A comprehensive study of the distribution of general practitioners in England. Historical aspects are investigated, and current policy to correct the maldistribution is assessed.

P. W. Cobb, D. M. Warner, 'Task substitution among skill classes of nursing personnel'
NR, March–April, 1973, 22(2), pp. 130–7.

An industrial engineering approach to measuring substitution, relying on accurate job descriptions and measuring the number of tasks performed by persons with skill levels not considered appropriate for the task.

E. A. Confrey, 'The logic of a "shortage of health manpower"'
IJHS, Spring, 1973, 3(2), pp. 253–9.

The difficulties associated with the concept and measurement of a 'shortage of health manpower' are discussed and a number of ways in which shortage may be more usefully depicted are suggested.

A. Donabedian, *Aspects of Medical Care Administration: Specifying Requirements for Health Care*
Cambridge, Massachusetts: Harvard University Press, 1973, p. 649.

The problems of measuring physicians' output are discussed (pp. 257–64), and the final chapter considers methods of estimating requirements for services and resources and reviews attempts in the United States at manpower forecasting. There are excellent bibliographies. In particular the bibliography at the end of chapter four (pp. 485–508) contains a lot of material on United States health manpower including official reports and commissions and the main statistical sources.
See 35.

R. G. Evans, E. M. A. Parish, F. Sully, 'Medical productivity, scale effects and demand generation'
CJE, August, 1973, 6(3), pp. 376–93.
See 586.

R. Fein, 'The Greater Medical Profession, economic consequences in the United States'
In Royal Society of Medicine, Josiah Macy Jr. Foundation, *The Greater Medical Profession*, pp. 168–79 (307).

Two different types of new health occupations are identified: the first is a product of a demand for personnel created by advances in science and technology, the second of a deliberate attempt to help rationalise labour inputs by making possible a subdivision of existing tasks. Development of the first type of manpower is not seen as a problem; the pressure for scientific progress from the medical profession will ensure demand for their services. Fein therefore concentrates on examining the obstacles and rigidities that might prevent utilisation of manpower of the second type.

299 P. J. FELDSTEIN, *Financing Dental Care: An Economic Analysis*
Lexington: D.C. Heath and Company, 1973, pp. xvii, 260.
See 36.

300 F. L. GOLLADAY, M. MILLER, K. R. SMITH, 'Allied health manpower strategies: estimates of the potential gains from efficient task delegation'
MC, November–December, 1973, 11(6), pp. 457–69.
See 587, *593.*

301 J. N. HAUG, R. STEVENS, 'Foreign medical graduates in the United States in 1963 and 1971: a cohort study'
Inquiry, March, 1973, 10(1), pp. 26–32.
An eight year follow-up study of the activities of all foreign medical graduates known to be in the U.S.A. in 1963 revealed that 83.6 per cent were still resident in 1971, and 73.7 per cent of those ostensibly in the U.S.A. for training in 1963 were still there in 1971.

302 C. R. HEARN, 'Evaluation of patients' nursing needs: prediction of staffing'
In G. McLachlan (ed.) *The Future – and Present Indicatives, Problems and Progress in Medical Care, Essays on Current Research, Ninth Series*, pp. 157–93 (38).
Patients' nursing needs are used to calculate the nursing workload generated and hence to determine staff required. Successful applications in the Birmingham hospital group are described.

303 R. W. HURD, 'Equilibrium vacancies in a labour market dominated by non-profit firms: the shortage of nurses'
Rev.Econ.Stats., May, 1973, 55(2), pp. 234–40.
Demonstrates that the hypothesis that vacancies may be advertised at prevailing wages by monopsonists in equilibrium is consistent with a wide variety of behavioural assumptions appropriate for non-profit organisations as well as

profit maximisers. An empirical test suggests that monopsony power in the labour market for nurses is used in the U.S.A. to keep wages down.

C. M. LINDSAY, 'Real returns to medical education'
JHR, Summer, 1973, 8(3), pp. 331–48.
Correction for a bias in the measurement of human capital returns (developed in C. M. Lindsay, 'Measuring human capital returns', *JPE*, November–December, 1971, 79(6), pp. 1195–215) eliminates the alleged monopoly rents earned by United States doctors on their training, evidenced in studies by Fein and Weber, Sloan, and Friedman and Kuznets.
See 171, 243, 254.

U. E. REINHARDT, 'Manpower substitution and productivity in medical practice: review of research'
HSR, Fall, 1973, 8(3), pp. 200–27.
A survey of empirical research on manpower substitution in health. Both continuous production functions and activity analysis are examined, and the problems of estimation and the likely biases are discussed. Almost all existing work indicates the potential for productivity gains from substitution of paramedical for medical personnel.

A. REISMAN, B. V. DEAN, A. O. ESOGBUE, V. AGGARWAL, V. KAUJALGI, P. LEWY, J. S. GRAVENSTEIN, 'Physician supply and surgical demand forecasting: a regional manpower study'
MS, August, 1973, 19(12), pp. 1345–54.
Regression models were used to predict demand for and supply of anaesthesiologists in an Ohio county in 1980. The results from these models were rather below those obtained by canvassing experts (DELPHI exercise) as to the likely demand for anaesthesiologists. The projection models were however based on the current state of health-care delivery.

ROYAL SOCIETY OF MEDICINE, JOSIAH MACY JR. FOUNDATION, *The Greater Medical Profession*
New York: Josiah Macy Jr. Foundation, 1973, pp. x, 253.
A report of a symposium that considered some of the implications and the problems produced by the dramatic growth in the numbers of auxiliary health personnel in relation to the number of physicians in the twentieth century. Representatives from Britain and the U.S.A., from the fields of medical education and practice, public health, nursing, dentistry, economics and sociology discussed the issues as they related to the experience of the two countries.
See 298, 311.

308   R. J. Ruffin, D. E. Leigh, 'Charity, competition, and the pricing of doctors' services'
JHR, Spring, 1973, 8(2), pp. 212–22.

A charity-competition model is posed as alternative to Kessel's profit-maximising monopoly model to explain price discrimination by physicians. The model has price discrimination emerging as a consequence of utility maximisation by the individual doctor and the necessity of market equilibrium. Several implications of the model are shown to be consistent with observed tendencies in the medical profession.

309   C. T. Stewart, C. M. Siddayao, *Increasing the Supply of Medical Personnel: Needs and Alternatives*
Washington D. C.: American Enterprise Institute for Public Policy Research, 1973, p. 81.

A concise study of medical personnel, principally doctor, shortage in the U.S.A.; causes of the shortage, estimates of the shortage, federal policy to eliminate the shortage, the scope for more efficient utilisation of resources and alternative ways to improve health are all examined. It is concluded that federal policy has been to offer long-term solutions to what are short-term problems, and that there is a possibility of excess capacity in medical schools and a surplus of physicians by the late 1970s.

310   G. L. Stoddart, 'Effort reporting and cost analysis of medical education'
JME, September, 1973, 48(9), pp. 814–23.

An examination of the problem of allocating salary expenses between patient care and teaching. The effort reporting technique and previous applications of the technique are discussed. An activity reporting technique used in a family practice teaching unit to determine the costs of education and patient-care functions is outlined.

311   J. Wiseman, 'The Greater Medical Profession, economic consequences in Great Britain'
In Royal Society of Medicine, Josiah Macy Jr. Foundation, *The Greater Medical Profession*, pp. 160–8 (307).

A number of issues relating to the general theme of the volume, the implications of co-operation between doctors and other groups in providing care, are examined. The major issues discussed are the possibilities for gains from specialisation and division of labour, how professional motivations may prevent or inhibit the realisation of these gains, and finally why the NHS, at least in its present form, may not lead to efficient groupings of professionals or at least of professional activities.

1974

D. F. BERGWALL, P. N. REEVES, N. B. WOODSIDE, *Introduction to Health Planning*
Washington D.C.: Information Resources Press, 1974, pp. vii, 231.
A chapter of the book is devoted to the problems of providing and maintaining a growing and properly distributed supply of health manpower. A variety of studies and projections of health manpower in the United States is outlined. *See* 1418.

E. A. BLACKSTONE, 'Misallocation of medical resources: the problem of excessive surgery'
PP, Summer, 1974, 22(3), pp. 329–52.
Evidence is produced that suggests the existence of excess surgical capacity and unnecessary surgery in the United States. It is suggested that 10 per cent or 9,000 surgeons could be reallocated without serious effect on health; shifting 9,000 surgeons into general practice would alleviate between 30 and 50 per cent of projected overall doctor shortages.

M. F. BOGNANNO, J. S. HIXSON, J. R. JEFFERS, 'The short-run supply of nurses' time'
JHR, Winter, 1974, 11(1), pp. 80–94.
The participation of married nurses in the labour market was found to be most affected by husbands' earnings, and not significantly affected by the nurses' wage rate. The supply of services offered by the employed nurse was responsive to both variation in wage rate and the husband's earnings.

J. R. BUTLER, R. KNIGHT, 'General practice manpower and health service reorganisation'
JSP, July, 1974, 3(3), pp. 235–50.
Looks at the three major strategies employed since 1948 to correct the imbalance in the distribution of general practitioner manpower in the United Kingdom. The reorganisation it is feared, by setting up new machinery alongside the old, will lead to a fragmentation of authority and to a worsening of the imbalance.

H. S. COHEN, W. J. DEAN, 'To practice or not to practice: developing state law and policy on physicians' assistants'
MMFQ, Fall, 1974, 52(4), pp. 349–76.
An analysis is provided of the regulations governing the role, degree of

supervision and training of physicians' assistants in the U.S.A. A considerable variability in approaches to regulation in different states is evidenced; recommendations are made that would encourage greater uniformity in regulations.

317   R. G. EHRENBERG, 'Organisational control and the economic efficiency of hospitals: the production of nursing services'
JHR, Winter, 1974, 9(1), pp. 21–32.
See 532.

318   R. G. EVANS, 'Supplier-induced demand: some empirical evidence and implications'
In M. Perlman (ed.) *The Economics of Health and Medical Care*, pp. 162–73 (44).

The paper outlines two alternative specifications of physician behaviour that suggest the possibility of perverse response of price to increases in the supply of physicians or of the quantity of health care demanded to price. The first model involves a maximising framework, physicians having a broad objective function including exercise of discretion in treatment by the physician and his income or workload. The second is a general target model, the physician having rough targets for income and leisure, and adjusting price or discretionary behaviour so as to approach the moving targets.
See 148.

319   M. S. FELDSTEIN, 'Econometric studies of health economics'
In M. D. Intriligator, D. A. Kendrick (eds.) *Frontiers of Quantitative Economics*, Vol. 2, pp. 377–447, Amsterdam: North-Holland, 1974.

Discusses studies that deal with the supply of doctors, their distribution, choice of specialty, and the effect of price and other variables on the supply of doctors' and nurses' services.
See 42.

320   P. J. FELDSTEIN, 'A preliminary evaluation of federal dental manpower subsidy programs'
Inquiry, September, 1974, 11(3), pp. 196–206.

321   P. J. FELDSTEIN, 'A review of productivity in dentistry'
In J. Rafferty (ed.) *Health Manpower and Productivity*, pp. 107–18 (329).

Reviews work on the potential for increasing productivity in dentistry by use of auxiliary personnel.

H. E. FRECH, 'Occupational licensure and health care productivity: the issues and the literature'
In J. Rafferty (ed.) *Health Manpower and Productivity*, pp. 119–39 (329).

A survey of the literature on occupational licensing in the health professions in the U.S.A., the forms that restrictions on entry have taken, and their effects. Directions for future research on licensing are suggested.

V. R. FUCHS, *Who Shall Live? Health, Economics, and Social Choice*
New York: Basic Books Inc., 1974, pp. vii, 168.
See 43.

J. HADLEY, 'Research on health manpower productivity: a general overview'
In J. Rafferty (ed.) *Health and Productivity*, pp. 143–203 (329).

A survey paper that draws together the material of the previous six papers in the book, and adds material on such topics as capital substitution, the effect of different reimbursement schemes on physician productivity, and the role of technical change in increasing manpower productivity.

J. L. HARRISON, K. D. NASH, 'The income redistribution effects of publicly supported medical education'
Miss.Val.J.Bus.Econ., Spring, 1974, 9(3), pp. 1–16.

A study of four states of the U.S.A. is presented, comparing the proportion of total tax revenue paid by different income groups with the distribution of medical students by income group. It is concluded that public support of medical education involves a significant redistribution from relatively low to relatively high income groups. Alternative methods of financing medical education that have been canvassed are discussed.

B. H. KEHRER, M. D. INTRILIGATOR, 'Task delegation in physician office practice'
Inquiry, December, 1974, 11(4), pp. 292–9.
See 594, 595.

E. LIEFMANN-KEIL, 'Consumer protection, incentives and externalities in the drug market'
In M. Perlman (ed.) *The Economics of Health and Medical Care*, pp. 117–29 (44).
See 1047.

328 R. T. MASSON, S. WU, 'Price discrimination for physicians' services'
JHR, Winter, 1974, 9(1), pp. 63–79.
See 597.

329 J. RAFFERTY (ed.) *Health Manpower and Productivity*
Lexington, Massachusetts: Lexington Books, D.C. Heath and Company, 1974, pp. xxiv, 228.
A collection of seven survey papers reviewing the problems of measuring and improving productivity in the health services industry:
1   U. E. Reinhardt, K. R. Smith, 'Manpower substitution in ambulatory care'
2   R. M. Scheffler, 'Productivity and economies of scale in medical practice'
3   F. A. Sloan, 'Effects of incentives on physician performance'
4   F. L. Golladay 'Patient participation and productivity in the medical care sector'
5   P. J. Feldstein, 'A review of productivity in dentistry'
6   H. E. Frech, 'Occupational licensure and health care productivity'
7   J. Hadley, 'Research on health manpower productivity: a general overview'
All the papers have extensive bibliographies; all contain suggestions for future research.
See 321, 322, 324, 330, 332, 600, 807

330 U. E. REINHARDT, K. R. SMITH, 'Manpower substitution in ambulatory care'
In J. Rafferty (ed.) *Health Manpower and Productivity*, pp. 3–37 (329).
Surveys the literature on health manpower substitution, the problems of specifying and estimating production functions, activity analyses and descriptive studies. An illustration with the case of paediatric care is provided to show how information from various sources may be synthesised into an overall production function for that type of service.

331 F. A. SLOAN, 'A microanalysis of physicians' hours of work decisions'
In M. Perlman (ed.) *The Economics of Health and Medical Care*, pp. 302–25 (44).
Separate estimations were made of physician supply response to weekly and hourly wage rate changes. A positive supply response to the weekly rate, but negative response to the hourly rate were found. The physician–population ratio in the area in which the physician works was found to affect individual physician supply negatively.

332 F. A. SLOAN, 'Effects of incentives on physician performance'
In J. Rafferty (ed.) *Health Manpower and Productivity*, pp. 53–84 (329).

Develops models to examine the impact of group practice on physician output, price and input purchase decisions under a variety of cost and revenue sharing arrangements and with fee and non-fee for service methods of physician compensation. Reviews empirical evidence on costs and productivity of different types of practice and physician choice of mode of practice.

R. A. STEVENS, L. W. GOODMAN, S. S. MICK, 'What happens to foreign trained doctors who came to the United States?'
Inquiry, June, 1974, 11(2), pp. 112–24.
Reports a follow-up study of graduates of foreign medical schools who were appointed to graduate training positions in Connecticut hospitals in 1964. The study attempted to determine which graduates left the U.S.A., which remained, and their experiences in the U.S.A. Graduates from the poorest countries remained in larger numbers than those from higher income Western European countries.

K. N. WILLIAMS, B. A. LOCKETT, 'Migration of foreign physicians to the United States: the perspective of health manpower planning'
IJHS, Spring, 1974, 4(2), pp. 213–43.
A discussion of the difficulties in interpreting the data concerning migration of foreign medical graduates into the U.S.A. Includes a review of immigration and professional regulations and presents many useful data for the period 1950–72.

S. WOLFE, R. F. BADGLEY, 'How much is enough? The payment of doctors – implications for health policy in Canada'
IJHS, Spring, 1974, 4(2), pp. 245–64.
Argues that the medical profession has successfully influenced Canadian policy as regards both physician payment and manpower planning, to its substantial pecuniary advantage. Principal recommendations include: immigration restrictions; provincial medical manpower quotas; the establishment of health centres.

D. E. YETT, L. DRABEK, M. D. INTRILIGATOR, L. J. KIMBELL, 'Econometric forecasts of health services and health manpower'
In M. Perlman (ed.) *The Economics of Health and Medical Care*, pp. 459–69 (44).
See 1424.

337   D. E. Yett, F. A. Sloan, 'Migration patterns of recent medical school graduates'
Inquiry, June, 1974, 11(2), pp. 125–42.

A statistical examination of the location patterns of recent medical school graduates revealed that they had a higher propensity to establish practices in states where their previous level of attachment is strongest and most recent. General environmental conditions and growth in per capita personal income of the population of a state also had a significant effect on physician inflows.

338   R. Zeckhauser, M. Eliastam, 'The productivity potential of the physician assistant'
JHR, Winter, 1974, 9(1), pp. 95–116.

The paper discusses the possibilities for delegation of medical tasks to physicians' assistants. A CES production function is estimated for physicians and physicians' assistants working together. With optimal factor mix and efficient assignment of tasks a physician's assistant achieves half the productivity of a physician.

(c)   Supply Institutions

The relevant works are divided into three groups. The first two relate to the two major types of 'production unit': hospitals and general practice. The third group is concerned with locational questions: it might be described by analogy as the health economics equivalent of the economics of industrial location.

(i)   Hospitals

The economics of hospitals is probably the most thoroughly researched single area within health economics. Even in the U.S.A. the literature has concentrated less on price–output–investment decisions than might be expected by those seeing it primarily as an extension of the theory of the firm, and more on the estimation of cost functions (together with the analysis of hospital outputs). Nevertheless, the burgeoning of behavioural models of hospital decision-making, particularly since concern developed over hospital cost inflation and the nature of the incentives for efficiency confronting administrators, has recently brought the analysis of hospitals as economic decision-making units into the mainstream of economic theories of the firm.

On the cost side the standard reference continues to be Feldstein (392). Useful reviews are in Mann and Yett (403), Berki (462) and Feldstein (534). Other major innovating recent contributions have been Lave and Lave (432), Feldstein (448) and Evans and Walker (472).

Behavioural models are reviewed in Davis (467), Jacobs (540) and Pauly (548).

Around these central issues other important specific questions have also been addressed, including queues (e.g. Bailey, 341), 'adequacy' of bed stocks (e.g. Forsyth and Logan, 346), patient outcomes as output (e.g. Rosser and Watts, 490), costs of specific diseases (e.g. Babson 499), the interaction of demand and supply (e.g. Roemer, 351) and the differences between not-for-profit and for-profit hospitals (e.g. Stewart, 520).

1914

E. A. CODMAN, 'The product of a hospital'
SGO, January–June, 1914, 18, pp. 491–6.

An early paper recognising the distinction between inputs and outputs and discussing the problems of output measurement. It is argued that a type of hospital report showing as nearly as possible the results of treatment obtained at different institutions would be a good basis on which to begin asking questions about management and efficiency.

1951

H. B. MAKOVER, 'The quality of medical care'
AJPH, July, 1951, 41(7), pp. 824–32.

A classification of hospitals covered by a health insurance plan into four categories of quality based on a rating of clinical performance rather than conformance to standards. The lower quality hospitals had less-trained physicians and older physicians on average, and fewer laboratories and centralised facilities.

1954

341   N. T. J. BAILEY, 'Queuing for medical care'
AS, 1954, pp. 137–45.

An early illustration of the use of queuing theory to consider the problems of how many inpatient beds to provide in a given specialty, to determine the number or size of clinic sessions required in an outpatient department, and finally to design an appointment system to reduce waiting time for outpatients.

1955

342   M. C. SHEPS, 'Approaches to the quality of hospital care'
PHR, September, 1955, 70(9), pp. 877–86.
See 841.

1956

343   N. T. J. BAILEY, 'Statistics in hospital planning and design'
AS, November, 1956, 5(3), pp. 146–57.

A brief survey of a number of areas of hospital planning in which the discipline of statistics has proved useful. The problems for which statistics has proved useful are the determination of the amount of hospital accommodation, the construction of appointment systems, the internal design of hospitals, and keeping check on the performance of existing facilities.

1957

344   L. S. ROSENFELD, 'Quality of medical care in hospitals'
AJPH, July, 1957, 47(7), pp. 856–65.

Evaluation of quality of care is carried out on the basis of the judgement by specialists of the way the hospitals manage a particular set of illnesses and operations.

1959

J. D. LYTTON, 'Recent productivity trends in the Federal Government: an exploratory study'
Rev.Econ.Stats., November, 1959, 41(4), pp. 341–59.
A study of eight agencies in the federal government of which only the Veterans Administration hospitals had experienced no productivity increase (productivity had in fact declined). The measure of output used in the study is inpatient daily load.

1960

G. FORSYTH, R. F. L. LOGAN, *The Demand for Medical Care*
London: Oxford University Press, 1960, p. 153.
Sub-titled, 'A study of the case-load in the Barrow and Furness group of hospitals', it is one of the studies commissioned by the Nuffield Provincial Hospitals Trust to aid hospital bed planning. A figure of 2.5 acute beds per 1,000 population is suggested as appropriate for Barrow, about half the figure suggested as appropriate on the founding of the National Health Service, and less than the existing national average of 3.1 for acute specialties.

1961

B. BENJAMIN, T. A. PERKINS, 'The measurement of bed use and demand'
The Hospital, January, 1961, 57(1), pp. 31–3.
Clarifies a number of issues relating to the measurement of bed use and demand. The relationship between average duration of stay and average occupied beds, the relationship between turnover interval, average beds available and average beds occupied, and the measurement of occupancy rate and pressure on beds, are among the issues explored.

P. J. FELDSTEIN, *An Empirical Investigation of the Marginal Cost of Hospital Services*
Chicago: Graduate Programme in Hospital Administration, University of Chicago, 1961, p. 77.

349   C. E. RICE, 'Measuring social restoration performance of public psychiatric hospitals'
PHR, May, 1961, 76(5), pp. 437–46.
See 847.

350   M. I. ROEMER, 'Bed supply and hospitalization: a natural experiment'
Hospitals, November 1st, 1961, pp. 35–42.
Examination of data from a New York county revealed that bed supply determined utilisation; admissions rose and length of stay increased as a result of increasing bed supply. The major conclusion is that controlling bed supply is essential in any attempt to control utilisation effectively.

351   M. I. ROEMER, 'Hospital utilization and the supply of physicians'
JAMA, December 9th, 1961, 178(10), pp. 989–93.
A study of admissions to hospitals in the 48 states of the United States revealed, after standardisation for available bed supply and insurance coverage of the population, that when the supply of doctors was less than 110 per 100,000 population the number of admissions tended to rise. It is hypothesised that hospitalisation is a method that allows the overworked physician to save time.

1962

352   A. D. AIRTH, D. J. NEWELL, *The Demand for Hospital Beds, Results of an Enquiry on Tees-side*
Newcastle upon Tyne: University of Durham, Kings College, 1962, p. 91.
One of a series of studies commissioned in the 1950s by the Nuffield Provincial Hospitals Trust to aid hospital bed planning (the other studies are referenced in this volume). This study examines the current demand for non-mental hospital care and on this basis assesses the adequacy of existing provision. The method used involves the calculation of the number of patients recommended for admission in each specialty (admissions plus increases in the waiting list) and then calculating the number of beds required at 85 per cent occupancy to meet this demand.

353   P. A. BRINKER, B. WALKER, 'The Hill–Burton Act: 1948–1954'
Rev.Econ.Stats., May, 1962, 44(2), pp. 208–12.
The Hill–Burton formula for allocating funds between states for the construction of hospital facilities is explained, and illustrative examples of the

working of the formula provided. The operation of the programme in its first seven years is then evaluated. It is concluded that the Act has reduced the gap between bed need and supply nationally, and that more hospital facilities have been constructed in low income than in high income states.

W. J. MCNERNEY and Study Staff, *Hospital and Medical Economics: A Study of Population, Services, Costs, Methods of Payment, and Controls* Chicago: Hospital Research and Educational Trust, 1962, p. 1492 (2 vols.).
See 1160.

OFFICE OF HEALTH ECONOMICS, *Studies on Current Health Problems* London: Office of Health Economics, 1962–
See 4.

1963

J. H. F. BROTHERSTON, 'The use of the hospital: review of research in the United Kingdom'
MC, July–September, 1963, 1(3), pp. 142–50, and *MC*, October–December, 1963, 1(4), pp. 225–31.
A review of early work (operations research, work study, sociological, economic, statistical) on planning the availability of hospital services, the efficiency of their use and the role of the hospital in the wider health services system.

P. COWAN, 'The size of hospitals'
MC, January–March, 1963, 1(1), pp. 1–9.
Examines the size distribution of hospitals in England and Wales, and the effect that the Hospital Plan for England and Wales will have; mental and non-mental hospitals are separated. Comparisons are also made with the size distributions in Sweden, Denmark, United States, Portugal, Greece, Israel and India.

H. E. KLARMAN, *Hospital Care in New York City, the Roles of Voluntary and Municipal Hospitals*
New York: Columbia University Press, 1963, pp. xxxii, 573.
The report of a major study, the book has twenty-one chapters in three

sections: four chapters on the background (the population, patterns of hospital use, characteristics of patients in short-term hospitals), seven chapters on personnel, plant and organisation, and ten chapters on the financing of hospital care (sources of income, costs of care, comparisons with other areas and proposals for improvement).

359   J. D. THOMPSON, R. B. FETTER, 'The economics of the maternity service'
YJBM, August, 1963, pp. 91–103.

It is demonstrated that the larger an obstetrical service the higher is its average occupancy, even when correction is made for differences in the length of stay. A simulation model is used to predict the occupancy that can be expected from any set of population characteristics and any number of beds. The maternity services in smaller hospitals are also found to cost more.

1964

---

360   E. M. BROOKE, J. H. MABRY, 'Problems in determining the needs for mental health facilities in Britain'
JCD, September, 1964, 17(9), pp. 773–8.

A review of the problems in planning mental health facility needs in Britain. It is argued that planning can be based on short period experience but that there is a need for frequent review. It is pointed out that the output of the service since the Mental Health Act is not directly comparable with the output before the Act. Legislation having viewed rehabilitation as the primary goal has led to greater strain being placed on the community.

361   R. L. CARDWELL, 'How to measure hospital bed needs'
MH, August, 1964, 103(2), pp. 107–11, 181.

Illustrates the calculation of regional hospital bed needs within metropolitan Chicago. A bed–population ratio is used, adjusted for differences in length of stay and average occupancy levels, with a further adjustment for flows of patients across regional boundaries.

362   M. S. FELDSTEIN, 'Effects of differences in hospital bed scarcity on type of use'
BMJ, August 29th, 1964, 5408, pp. 561–6.

Regional data are used to investigate the effects of bed scarcity on a large number of different types of patient. Bed scarcity was found to have a 50 per cent greater effect on the number of cases treated than on average stay per case. Environmental explanations of this situation were found to be unsatisfactory, but a number of possible behavioural explanations are suggested. It is concluded that medical staff may be making choices implicitly, not realising that they are choosing to leave cases untreated rather than shorten length of stay, a choice that they may not be prepared to make explicitly. Responsiveness to bed scarcity according to age, sex and diagnosis of the patient is also examined in the study.

3   M. S. FELDSTEIN, 'Hospital planning and the demand for care'
    BOUIES, November, 1964, 26(4), pp. 361–8.
    It is demonstrated empirically that in Great Britain observed demand for hospital beds cannot serve as an adequate basis for planning the future provision of hospital beds, as the demand in any region reflects supply too closely for it to be considered an independent measure of 'need' or ability to benefit from additional beds. Waiting lists do not provide a suitable basis, as the effect of a larger bed supply on waiting lists is small.

4   T. B. FITZPATRICK, D. C. RIEDEL, 'Some general comments on methods of studying hospital use'
    Inquiry, January, 1964, 1(2), pp. 49–68.

5   S. E. HARRIS, *The Economics of American Medicine*
    New York: The Macmillan Company, 1964, pp. xvi, 508.
    See 6.

6   H. E. KLARMAN, 'The increased cost of hospital care'
    In S. J. Mushkin (Chairman) *The Economics of Health and Medical Care*, pp. 227–54 (8).
    An examination of the trend in hospital costs in the 1950s, and suggested explanations of these trends with particular reference to New York City. The evidence for most of the 1950s was consistent with the view that hospital wages and working conditions had lagged behind those in other industries, and were simply catching up in the 1950s.

7   H. E. KLARMAN, 'Some technical problems in area-wide planning for hospital care'
    JCD, September, 1964, 17(9), pp. 735–47.
    An outline of some of the problems encountered by the Hospital Council of New York in providing hospital care, and methods that have been used or suggested to overcome them. The major problems were connected with delineating areas served by different facilities, determining medical needs,

projecting population changes and determining hospital size. The most effective immediate action was felt to be the development of a better data base.

368   M. F. LONG, 'Efficient use of hospitals'
In S. J. Mushkin (Chairman) *The Economics of Health and Medical Care*, pp. 211–26 (8).

A discussion of possible responses to fluctuations over time in the demand for hospital services, which at present cause unnecessary duplication and waste of facilities.

369   D. J. NEWELL, 'Statistical aspects of the demand for maternity beds'
JRSS, 1964, 127(1), pp. 1–40.

370   D. J. NEWELL, 'The demand for hospital beds'
BISI, 1964, pp. 1085–102.

A survey of the early British work attempting to assess the demand for hospital care on the basis of bed use. Despite the deficiencies of the approach, the data collection involved threw up many interesting facts and questions, including confirmation that in the British setting demand for hospital care is modified by the existing supply of beds.

371   D. J. NEWELL, 'Problems in estimating the demand for hospital beds'
JCD, September, 1964, 17(9), pp. 749–59.

The results of a number of studies on the use of hospital facilities in Great Britain are discussed. A Nuffield survey of the Teesside area is considered at some length. The major finding of this study was that the supply of beds itself modifies the demand for beds.

372   G. D. ROSENTHAL, *The Demand for General Hospital Facilities*
Chicago: American Hospital Association, Hospital Monograph Series No. 14, 1964, p. 101.
See 66

1965

373   J. S. DEEBLE, 'An economic analysis of hospital costs'
MC, July–September, 1965, 3(3), pp. 138–46.

A study of general hospitals in Victoria to determine the effects on the cost of treatment of changes in the length of patient stay. It is suggested that fixed costs, and therefore high bed occupancy, are less important than is often thought, and that the cost of treating a patient is very little affected by reduction in length of stay because of the increased intensity of treatment necessary.

M. S. FELDSTEIN, 'Improving the use of hospital maternity beds'
ORQ, March, 1965, 16(1), pp. 65–76.

Two studies are described dealing with the problem of hospital admission and duration of stay for maternity care. In the first study bed supply is shown to have a significant effect on maternity admissions and deliveries, but not on length of stay. As only one woman in three delivers in a fully equipped hospital in Great Britain, the problem of selection for such care is important, and a model to assist such selection is outlined.

M. S. FELDSTEIN, 'Hospital cost variations and case-mix differences'
MC, April–June, 1965, 3(2), pp. 95–103. Also in M. H. Cooper, A. J. Culyer (eds.) *Health Economics*, pp. 260–75 (33).

The study examines the extent to which differences in the cost between British acute hospitals can be explained by differences between them in the proportions they treat of eight types of case. The study found that ward costs per case and, to a lesser extent, per patient week, were substantially influenced by the case-mix composition of hospital workload.

M. S. FELDSTEIN, 'Hospital bed scarcity: an analysis of the effects of inter-regional differences'
EC, November, 1965, 32(128), pp. 393–409.
See 362.

M. S. FELDSTEIN, 'Studying hospital costliness'
HSF, 1965, pp. 3–20.

It is argued that crude cost per case comparisons of hospitals are inadequate, and that adjustments for differences in case-mix are necessary. A method of adjustment for case-mix is outlined, which involves regression analysis to derive a set of weights, one for each type of case, 'with which to predict what every hospital's cost would be if its cost for each type of case were the same as the national average for that case type'. The results of applying the adjustment to 177 acute non-teaching hospitals are set out.

P. J. FELDSTEIN, J. J. GERMAN, 'Predicting hospital utilization: an evaluation of three approaches'
Inquiry, June, 1965, 2(1), pp. 13–36.

379   R. B. FETTER, J. D. THOMPSON, 'The simulation of hospital systems'
OR, September–October, 1965, 13(5), pp. 689–711.

A description of a project concerned with the design and utilisation of hospital facilities. Three models of hospital sub-systems are described: a maternity suite model, a model of a surgical position and a model of an outpatient clinic. Further models under development are also discussed.

380   H. E. KLARMAN, *The Economics of Health*
New York: Columbia University Press, 1965, pp. viii, 200.
See 11.

381   R. PENCHANSKY, G. ROSENTHAL, 'Productivity, price and income in the physicians' services market – a tentative hypothesis'
MC, October–December, 1965, 3(4), pp. 240–4.
See 186.

382   M. W. REDER, 'Economic theory and non-profit enterprise, some problems in the economics of hospitals'
AER, May, 1965, 55(2), pp. 472–80.

The paper considers some of the obstacles to efficient utilisation of resources associated with the private non-profit public service corporation. The problems concern the achievement of a socially optimal stock and utilisation of hospital facilities, the pricing policy of hospitals, and the tendency to duplicate facilities thus generating excess capacity.

383   B. A. WEISBROD, 'Some problems of pricing and resource allocation in a non-profit industry – the hospitals'
JB, 1965, 38(1), pp. 18–28.

It is argued that a number of inefficiencies arise in the U.S. hospital system as a result of an absence of market pressures on hospitals and a lack of incentive to consumers, because of insurance, to be influenced by relative prices. Two problems are examined in this light, the structure of hospital room prices and the range of accommodation available, and the instability of hospital utilisation.

1966

384   J. C. G. BURNHAM, 'Estimation of hospital bed requirements'
W. Hosp., 1966, 2, pp. 110–18.

A discussion of demand and need for health care. It is argued that in the short term planning must use statistics available on demand (utilisation), but longer term discussions should be based on need determined by detailed morbidity studies.

M. L. INGBAR, B. J. WHITNEY, L. D. TAYLOR, 'Differences in the costs of nursing service: a statistical study of community hospitals in Massachusetts'
AJPH, October, 1966, 56(10), pp. 1699–715.
A study of a large group of Massachusetts hospitals with a wide range of nursing costs – the nursing service cost in some hospitals was more than twice that in others. Two factors, number of students and total number of nursing personnel per available bed-day, explained over 40 per cent of the variance in unit cost of nursing service. Available bed-days and percentage of occupancy did not explain differences in cost, nor did differences in relative proportions of different types of nursing staff.

J. R. LAVE, 'A review of the methods used to study hospital costs'
Inquiry, May, 1966, 3(2), pp. 57–81.

D. C. PAIGE, K. JONES, *Health and Welfare Services in Britain in 1975*   —
Cambridge: Cambridge University Press for the National Institute of Economic and Social Research, Occasional Papers 22, 1966, p. 142.
See 77, 1101.

R. G. RICE, 'Analysis of the hospital as an economic organism'
MH, April, 1966, 106(4), pp. 87–91.
A model of the behaviour of a hospital similar to Baumol's model of the firm (sales maximisation subject to a profit constraint) is developed. Output maximisation is the goal, and a variety of possible financial constraints on voluntary hospitals are suggested.

1967

R. E. BERRY, 'Returns to scale in the production of hospital services'
HSR, Summer, 1967, 2(2), pp. 123–39.
The a priori case for the existence of economies of scale in the production of hospital services and the results of empirical work are reviewed. The main part of the paper is an attempt to overcome the problem of product heterogeneity, which bedevils attempts to discover the nature of the long-run average cost

function of hospitals. Using American Hospital Association data, which reports on the existence or non-existence of 28 separate facilities in over 5,000 hospitals, 40 groups containing hospitals of different size but similar facilities are constructed. Within most of these groups there is evidence of economies of scale.

390   W. J. CARR, P. J. FELDSTEIN, 'The relationship of cost to hospital size' *Inquiry*, June, 1967, 4(2), pp. 45–65.

Multiple regression analysis was used to examine the relationship between hospital costs and size. Controlling for number of services, outpatient visits, presence of a nursing school, number of student nurses, number and types of interns and residents and affiliation to a medical school, the study looked at 3,147 voluntary short-term hospitals in the United States. Average cost declined up to sizes of 200 beds, and then rose at larger sizes, although the authors were doubtful of the existence of diseconomies because of the unsatisfactoriness of adjustments for case-mix. Further analysis, by division of the hospitals into five categories according to number of facilities and services, confirmed the presence of falling average costs. Only for the very largest hospitals was there any indication of diseconomies of scale.

391   H. A. COHEN, 'Variations in cost among hospitals of different sizes' *SEJ*, January, 1967, 33(3), pp. 355–66.

Adjustments for salary and wage differentials between hospital staff in different communities, and a measure of output more sophisticated than crude patient-days (although still based upon service inputs) are used in estimating a long-run average cost curve for hospitals. The findings suggested that hospitals of between 150 and 350 beds were most efficient for ordinary patient care in areas of fairly dense population.

—   **392**   M. S. FELDSTEIN, *Economic Analysis for Health Service Efficiency* Amsterdam: North-Holland Publishing Company, 1967, pp. xii, 322.

A massive econometric study of the British National Health Service with particular attention to the hospital system. The objective of the study is stated on the first page: it is concerned with 'identifying and estimating relevant decision-making information and with applying optimizing methods to improve the efficiency of the British National Health Service'. The book is divided into two parts: the first is concerned with the hospital as a producing unit; the second deals with planning the supply and use of health-care resources. The first part of the book contains extensive analyses of cost and productivity of non-teaching acute hospitals. It includes a chapter on estimating a production function for acute hospitals, and a chapter applying linear programming to hospital production. The second part of the book contains a chapter examining approaches to planning bed supply, a chapter on improving the planning of maternity services and a chapter on an aggregate planning model of the health care sector. The book has been the starting point for a great deal of work on the economics of hospitals. An article length review of this important book is provided by J. R. Lave, L. B. Lave, *AE*, January, 1970, 1(4), pp. 293–305. *See* 82, 1381.

M. S. FELDSTEIN, 'An aggregate planning model of the health care sector' *MC*, November–December, 1967, 5(6), pp. 369–81. Also in M. H. Cooper, A. J. Culyer (eds.) *Health Economics*, pp. 210–29 (33). *See* 1380.

E. A. JOHNSON, 'Cost calculations show where Medicare reimbursement formula fails' *Hospitals*, March 1st, 1967, 41, pp. 42–7. *See* 1282.

H. E. KLARMAN, 'Economic factors in hospital planning in urban areas' *PHR*, August, 1967, 82(8), pp. 721–8. The original basis for the establishment by the United States Government of area-wide hospital planning agencies is outlined, and further reasons why economic intervention may be desirable in this area are provided. The need for recommendations by planners to be geared to flexibility of future use, because of the difficulties of accurately forecasting hospital use in localities, is stressed.

M. F. LONG, P. J. FELDSTEIN, 'Economics of hospital systems, peak loads, and regional co-ordination' *AER*, May, 1967, 57(2), pp. 119–29. A study to determine the optimal number of obstetrical units and the number of beds, taking account of the costs of hospital care, travel and inconvenience. A hypothetical system of scale in terms of births, similar to that of the Chicago region, is constructed to illustrate the use of the method. A study of the actual Chicago region showed that because of shifts in population the existing beds are far from optimally distributed.

H. M. SOMERS, A. R. SOMERS, *Medicare and the Hospitals, Issues and Prospects* Washington D.C.: The Brookings Institution, 1967, pp. xvi, 303. A large number of issues relating to the United States hospital system and the interaction between that system and Medicare are examined: the adequacy of facilities when Medicare was established, the development of hospital quality controls, staffing shortages, the method of paying the hospital, the development of hospital planning and methods of containing costs.

398 J. L. STAMBAUGH, 'A study of the sources of capital funds for hospital construction in the United States'
Inquiry, June, 1967, 4(2), pp. 3–22.

A survey is carried out to determine the sources of capital funds for 143 projects under construction in July/August of 1965. Six types of U.S. hospitals were included in the study, and fund sources were classified into six different categories. Private contributors were found to provide a larger proportion of capital funds for hospital construction than any other source.

1968

399 C. COOPER, 'Improved baselines for cost comparisons'
The Hospitals, April, 1968, 64(4), pp. 115–19.

Outlines the difficulties associated with calculating national average costs for groups of hospitals that are very diverse in nature. As a first step towards more meaningful cost comparisons, an attempt is made to see if there is any correlation between existing cost headings and hospital size (staffed beds), and between individual cost headings and degree of clinical activity (as measured by medical staff salaries).

400 M. L. INGBAR, L. D. TAYLOR, *Hospital Costs in Massachusetts*
Cambridge, Massachusetts: Harvard University Press, 1968, pp. xv, 237.

Regression analysis and factor analysis are used to estimate a hospital cost structure from data on a group of Massachusetts hospitals for the years 1958 and 1959, and 1962 and 1963. The structure is tested by using the 1962 and 1963 data to test the cost relationships estimated from 1958 and 1959 data, and by comparison with the results obtained from applying the techniques to data on other hospital groups. One of the results of the study was the suggestion that the average cost curve was an inverted U with a peak at about 150 beds and economies of scale thereafter. The results also suggested that when the occupancy rate increases, costs per patient-day are definitely lowered. Comparisons are made with the results of other studies. An extensive bibliography is provided.

401 E. M. KAITZ, *Pricing Policy and Cost Behaviour in the Hospital Industry*
New York: F.A. Praeger Publishers, 1968, pp. xiii, 192.

An investigation of management behaviour in short-term general hospitals. A study is made of pricing policy, costing, the role of competition and capital budgeting policies. It is concluded that no adequate notion of administrative efficiency has evolved in the hospital industry. The implications for third party payment for care are examined, and it is argued that Blue Cross should no longer be allowed to purchase hospital care on a 'wholesale' basis.

I. LEVESON, 'Medical care cost incentives: some questions and approaches for research'
Inquiry, December, 1968, 5(4), pp. 3–13.
A survey of the types of incentives that might be used to control costs. The need to identify objectives, the choice of stage in the production process at which they are to operate and the likely effects over time, are stressed. The sorts of information needed to operate the incentives are discussed.

J. K. MANN, D. E. YETT, 'The analysis of hospital costs: a review article'
JB, April, 1968, 4(2), pp. 191–202. Also in M. H. Cooper, A. J. Culyer (eds.) *Health Economics*, pp. 276–92 (33).
The work of W. J. Carr and P. J. Feldstein, M. S. Feldstein, and L. D. Taylor on hospital costs (on optimum size and utilisation) is reviewed in an effort to determine the reasons for their apparently conflicting results. The reason for the difference between their results is their differing interpretation of the relation between 'output' and 'scale'. An alternative theoretical formulation of the cost/output relationship based on the work of Alchian and Hirshleifer (rate–volume theory) is suggested as a way forward in the study of cost behaviour.

R. L. MORRILL, R. EARICKSON, 'Variation in the character and use of Chicago area hospitals'
HSR, Fall, 1968, 3(3), pp. 224–38.
Three related studies are reported. The first involves the estimation of the hierarchy of hospital services – the level of services offered by different hospitals. The major differentiating characteristics are size, facilities and presence of medical and intern programmes. The second study uses a principal components analysis to reduce 99 variables to nine major components, to allow a classification of hospitals on the basis of characteristics. The third study uses regression analysis of flows between communities and hospitals to predict the use of general hospitals.

K-K. RO, 'Determinants of hospital costs'
YEE, Fall, 1968, pp. 185–257.
Examines the impact on hospital costs of capacity utilisation, scope of services,

technology and size. Multiple regression analysis of cross-section and time series data for 68 hospitals over an eleven-year period is carried out. Evidence of economies of scale in hospital operations was found – lower unit costs were associated with higher capacity utilisation. There was no statistically significant difference in unit costs between hospitals with approved intern or residency programmes and those without. These and other results are compared to results obtained by other researchers in the field.

406 M. ROEMER, A. T. MOUSTAFA, C. E. HOPKINS, 'A proposed hospital quality index: hospital death rates adjusted for case severity'
HSR, Summer, 1968, 3(2), pp. 96–118.

A quality index based on the crude death rate adjusted for case severity by average length of stay, corrected in turn by the occupancy rate to compensate for differences in pressure for hospital use, is proposed. Empirical work based on a sample of hospitals in Southern California is used to illustrate the efficacy of the technique.
See 539

407 U.S. DEPARTMENT OF HEALTH, EDUCATION AND WELFARE, *Reimbursement Incentives for Hospital and Medical Care: Objectives and Alternatives* Washington D.C.: USDHEW, Research Report No. 26, U.S. Govt. Printing Office, 1968, pp. vii, 103.
See 1190.

1969

408 R. ANDERSEN, J. T. HULL, 'Hospital utilisation and cost trends in Canada, and the United States'
HSR, Fall, 1969, 4(3), pp. 198–222.

A descriptive study looking at the reasons for rising costs and hospital utilisation in the period 1950–67. It is argued that differences in systems of financing and reimbursement for medical care have little effect on relative cost increases. Other industrialised nations experienced similar cost trends.

409 H. H. BALIGH, D. J. LAUGHHUNN, 'An economic and linear model of the hospital'
HSR, Winter, 1969, 4(4), pp. 293–303.

The main feature of the model is the use of patient equivalence classes, defined by average requirements for goods and services of different cases. Output of the hospital is measured as a weighted sum of all patients in all equivalence classes, the weights being attached to the equivalence class by the hospital policy-making group.

T. R. HEFTY, 'Returns to scale in hospitals: a critical review of recent research'
HSR, Winter, 1969, 4(4), pp. 267–80.

A survey of empirical research on hospital cost curves, discussing the problems and limitations of the approaches that have been used. See also the comment by J. Kushner (*HSR*, Winter, 1970, 5(4), pp. 370–3).

R. C. JELINEK, 'An operational analysis of the patient care function'
Inquiry, June, 1969, 6(2), pp. 53–61.

A model of the patient-care function of a general care community hospital is described, and the sort of information on quantity and quality of output required for a performance measure is discussed.

H. E. KLARMAN, 'Approaches to moderating the increases in medical care costs'
MC, May–June, 1969, 7(3), pp. 175–90.

Reviews current knowledge on the effects of the supply of hospital beds on use, the advantages of prepaid group practice and the problems of reimbursing providers of care, with a view to making policy proposals. Only a move to curtail the supply of beds to limit use is seen as reasonable in the light of current knowledge. Current reimbursement mechanisms are seen to be deficient, but more research is needed before it is possible to propose constructive alternatives with assurance.

H. E. KLARMAN, 'Reimbursing the hospital – the differences the third party makes'
JRI, December, 1969, 36(5), pp. 553–66.
See 1195.

C. E. MULLER, P. WORTHINGTON, 'The time structure of capital formation: design and construction of municipal hospital projects'
Inquiry, June, 1969, 6(2), pp. 42–52.

An examination of data on 21 New York City hospital projects to discover the time lags between budget allocations and actual expenditures. The length of time before expenditures actually equalled allocations was found to have been increasing, design of a project was found to take as long as building and larger projects were found to economise on time per dollar spent.

415   P. J. PHILLIP, 'Some considerations involved in determining the optimum size of specialized hospital facilities'
Inquiry, December, 1969, 6(4), pp. 44–8.

Optimum size is defined as the size that strikes an acceptable balance between excess capacity and unmet demand. Choosing the size of a hospital emergency department in the light of these objectives is used as an illustrative example.

416   M. W. REDER, 'Some problems in the measurement of productivity in the medical care industry'
In V. R. Fuchs (ed.) *Production and Productivity in the Service Industries*, New York: National Bureau of Economic Research, 1969, pp. 95–131.
See 165, 864.

417   K-K. RO, 'Incremental pricing would increase efficiency in hospitals'
Inquiry, March, 1969, 6(1), pp. 28–36.

The case is presented for a price policy based solely on economic considerations to increase efficiency. This policy would allow more even spreading of the patient load over a seven- instead of five-day week. Incremental pricing requires the identification of different hospital activities so that prices can be based on equal charge for equal cost.

414   K-K. RO, 'Patient characteristics, hospital characteristics, and hospital use'
MC, July–August, 1969, 7(4), pp. 295–312. Also in V. R. Fuchs (ed.) *Essays in the Economics of Health and Medical Care*, pp. 69–96 (27).

The consumption of hospital services is viewed as resulting from interaction among physicians, patients and hospitals. The direct interaction takes place between physicians and patients; hospital characteristics enter as a factor influencing this interaction. Medical condition and socio-economic class shape the patient's expectations concerning hospital use; the doctor is conditioned by his personal and medical background. A simplified and formalised version of the model (four equations) is tested in the paper. The results indicate systematic variation in hospital use according to some variables representing patient characteristics and some of those representing hospital characteristics. The data also support the view that hospital and patient characteristics are significantly interrelated.

419   K-K. RO, R. AUSTER, 'An output approach to incentive reimbursement for hospitals'
HSR, Fall, 1969, 4(3), pp. 177–87.
See 1197.

E. YOST, *The U.S. Health Industry: The Costs of Acceptable Medical Care by 1975*
New York: F.A. Praeger Publishers, 1969, pp. xv, 138.

Projections are made of health facility requirements for general hospital beds, mental hospital beds, long-term-care beds, diagnostic and treatment centres, rehabilitations facilities and public health centres in 1975, first on the assumption that care be provided at the present level to the projected population for 1975, and second that care be provided equal to that available in middle-class geographical areas in 1966–7. Estimates are also made of the costs of these increases.

1970

S. H. ALTMAN, 'The structure of nursing education and its impact on supply'
In H. E. Klarman (ed.) *Empirical Studies in Health Economics*, pp. 335–52 (18).
See 228.

J. C. BERESFORD, D. A. T. GRIFFITHS, 'Hospital costing for planning and development'
The Hospital, February, 1970, 66(2), pp. 48–53.

The fallacy of using cost per inpatient week as an indicator of hospital efficiency is demonstrated by examining the relationship between cost per week, cost per case and throughput. The case is developed for high tempo hospitals offering more intensive treatment during a shorter stay. Allied with this is the need for a more precise definition of the type of care a particular hospital, of whatever type, is meant to provide.

R. E. BERRY, 'Product heterogeneity and hospital cost analysis'
Inquiry, March, 1970, 7(1), pp. 67–75.

Seven dummy variables representing accreditation and approval, and twenty-seven dummy variables representing availability of facilities or services, average length of stay, proportion of outpatient activity, proportion of births and number of students and trainees per patient, are used to adjust for case-mix differences in attempting to estimate hospital cost functions. These variables added significantly to the explanatory power of the cost estimating equations. Factor analysis was then used to generate eight factors which explained 60 per cent of the variation in these variables.

424   M. Brown, 'An economic analysis of hospital operation'
HA, Spring, 1970, 15(2), pp. 60–74.

Attempts to clarify the idea of a production function for hospitals. The problems of defining inputs and outputs and measuring them, and the source of economies of scale are discussed.

425   J. M. Buchanan, C. M. Lindsay, 'The organisation and financing of medical care in the United States'
Appendix Q of British Medical Association, *Health Services Financing*, pp. 535–85 (1065).
See 1012, 1207.

426   W. J. Carr, 'Economic efficiency in the allocation of hospital resources: central planning versus evolutionary development'
In H. E. Klarman (ed.) *Empirical Studies in Health Economics*, pp. 195–221 (18).

Simulation analysis is used to compare the efficiency of the allocation of hospital resources under a perfect planning system and a pure market system. In the planning system, decisions about hospital size and location are made on the basis of parameters measured with error. In the market system, a trial and error process of evolution is assumed. At what appear to be attainable levels of error the planning system has potential for attainment of lower levels of cost. Comment by J. Rothenberg, pp. 222–8.

427   H. A. Cohen, 'Hospital cost curves with emphasis on measuring patient care output'
In H. E. Klarman (ed.) *Empirical Studies in Health Economics*, pp. 279–93 (18).

A measure of hospital size based upon weighted units of intermediate services is developed. The weighting is based upon the average cost of the service in a group of hospitals. The relationship between cost and weighted units of service is estimated for hospitals that are members of the United Hospital Fund of New York.

428   M. H. Cooper, A. J. Culyer, 'An economic assessment of some aspects of the operation of the National Health Service'
Appendix A of British Medical Association, *Health Services Financing*, pp. 187–250 (1065).

Information is examined on the regional variations in hospital and staff salary expenditures, and regional percentage deviations from national average length of stay and national average unit cost per patient-week are calculated. *See* 1112.

E. W. FRANCISCO, 'Analysis of cost variations among short-term general hospitals'
In H. E. Klarman (ed.) *Empirical Studies in Health Economics*, pp. 321–32 (18).

Three methods of analysis are used to examine the relationship between costs and output. Linear and curvilinear regression analysis is undertaken for each sizeable group of hospitals homogeneous with regard to the number of facilities and services available. Regression analysis with dummy variables is used to represent each of the facility and service combinations studied. Finally, multiple regression analysis is used, including an unweighted index of facilities and services. The results with all methods were similar: significant economies of scale were absent in the overall analysis; separation of large and small hospitals suggested economies of scale for small hospitals and constant returns for large hospitals.

C. P. HARDWICK, H. WOLFE, 'Incentive reimbursement'
Hospitals, September 16th, 1970, 44(18), pp. 45–8.
See 1205.

I. HESS, K. S. SRIKANTAN, 'Recommended variables for the multiple stratification of general hospitals'
HSR, Spring, 1970, 5(1), pp. 12–24.

Variables available for stratification are investigated to determine the most useful numbers and combinations of these variables (e.g. number of size classes, number of geographic divisions) for multiple stratification of hospitals. Illustrative tabulations of data on 5,078 hospitals are provided.

J. R. LAVE, L. B. LAVE, 'Hospital cost functions'
AER, June, 1970, 60(3), pp. 379–95.

Time series data are used in estimating cost functions that attempt to deal with the multi-product nature of hospital output. Two different procedures are used to deal with the problem of multiple products. The first involves the estimation of the relationship between cost, utilisation, size and time for each hospital; an explanation is then sought for differences in parameters between the hospitals. The second procedure relies on the assumption that all hospitals have the same cost function; the data are pooled and a single cost function estimated. The results suggest an L-shaped short-run average cost function, and if scale economies exist in the hospital industry they are very weak. The results also suggest an accelerating rate of cost increase for the period 1961–7.

433   J. R. LAVE, L. B. LAVE, 'Estimated cost functions for Pennsylvania hospitals'
Inquiry, June, 1970, 7(2), pp. 3–14.

A cross-section, time series model is developed to examine the nature of the average cost curve of hospitals, and to examine changes in hospital costs over time. The model is constructed on the assumption that, while there are output differences between hospitals, within a single hospital output is constant over a short period of time.

434   C. E. MULLER, P. WORTHINGTON, 'Factors entering into capital decisions of hospitals'
In H. E. Klarman (ed.) *Empirical Studies in Health Economics*, pp. 399–415 (18).

The paper examines the hypothesis that the rate of investment in voluntary hospitals is influenced by anticipated changes in future demand. The hypothesis is tested in three different forms using data on forty voluntary hospitals in New York. The hypothesis is confirmed in two of the three forms.
See also the comment by J. R. Lave, R. M. Sigmond, pp. 416–19.

435   J. P. NEWHOUSE, 'Toward a theory of non-profit institutions: an economic model of a hospital'
AER, May, 1970, 60(2), pp. 64–74. Also in M. H. Cooper, A. J. Culyer (eds.) *Health Economics*, pp. 243–59 (33).

A utility maximising model for the hospital is developed. The maximand for the hospital decision-maker contains two elements: the quantity of services and the quality of services. The implications of the model for economic efficiency are examined. A bias is found against the production of lower quality products, products that would be demanded by certain sections of the population and produced by profit-maximising firms. Movement to a socially optimal outcome is thought unlikely because the non-profit status of voluntary hospitals raises barriers to entry for potential competitors.

436   M. V. PAULY, 'Efficiency, incentives and reimbursement for health care'
Inquiry, March, 1970, 7(1), pp. 114–31.

A demonstration of how incentives affect the three major actors in the medical care field, the physician, the hospital and the consumer, with respect to economic efficiency. The effects of different remuneration and reimbursement systems on output, scale of organisation, locus of patient care and combination of inputs, are discussed.

M. V. PAULY, D. F. DRAKE, 'Effect of third-party methods of reimbursement on hospital performance'
In H. E. Klarman (ed.) *Empirical Studies in Health Economics*, pp.
297–314 (18).

The study attempts to determine whether differences in the method of payment
of hospitals can alter the hospital's operating behaviour. Four different
reimbursement methods that have been used by Blue Cross are examined in the
study. The evidence suggested that the incentive schemes differed little in their
impact on hospital behaviour and had practically no effect on short-run
production efficiency, nor did the presence of direct controls affect short-run
efficiency. It was found, however, that direct controls did affect the pattern of
capital allocation to hospitals, causing large hospitals to grow more than
proportionately. See also the comment by H. E. Klarman, pp. 315–19.

G. D. ROSENTHAL, 'Price elasticity of demand for short-term general
hospital services'
In H. E. Klarman (ed.) *Empirical Studies in Health Economics*, pp.
101–17 (18).
See 97.

D. S. SALKEVER, 'Hospital cost studies and planning under uncertainty:
analysis of a simple model'
SEJ, January, 1970, 36(3), pp. 263–7.

It is shown that the long-run average cost curve is not a useful planning tool
when output is uncertain; knowledge of both long- and short-run cost
behaviour is required. It is then shown that a marginal increase in uncertainty
would increase optimal size if the derivative of the rate of increase of marginal
cost with respect to size was negative. Illustrative calculations of change in
optimal size under different degrees of uncertainty are presented.

W. SHONICK, 'A stochastic model for occupancy–related random variables
in general–acute hospitals'
JASA, December, 1970, 65(332), pp. 1474–1500.

A model for the behaviour of the daily census in general-acute hospitals is
presented. The model allows computation of expected overfill rate, percentage
occupancy, waiting time for admission, waiting list length and loss of emergency patients.

B. STEINWALD, D. NEUHAUSER, 'The role of the proprietary hospital'
Law Contemp.Probl., Autumn, 1970, 35(4), pp. 817–38.

A review of the history, the current characteristics and some of the arguments levelled against proprietary hospitals in the United States. It is concluded that these hospitals play a useful but limited role and should be allowed to continue to do so. They are not, however, a panacea for the problems besetting the health field.

442 C. M. STEVENS, 'Hospital market efficiency: the anatomy of the supply response'
In H. E. Klarman (ed.) *Empirical Studies in Health Economics*, pp. 229–48 (18).

The paper is concerned with the determinants of hospital capacity. The findings of a study of a sample of hospitals in the Portland area suggested that the supply of hospital services is systematically related to market demand. The process is viewed as a chain reaction of increasing demand for services associated with an increasing supply of physicians, resulting in pressure on hospitals to expand capacity. A measure of demand pressure is constructed, based on the concepts of required occupancy and maximum occupancy (required occupancy is estimated by observed occupancy). See also the comment by E. S. Mills, pp. 249–51.

443 W. WORTHINGTON, L. H. SILVER, 'Regulation of quality of care in hospitals: the need for change'
Law Contemp.Probl., Spring, 1970, 35(2), pp. 305–33.

A review of hospital regulation at state level and certification and accreditation at national level in the U.S.A. Suggestions for improvement include the greater involvement of the Department of Health, Education and Welfare (through the Medicare programme) in the certification of hospitals.

1971

444 C. W. BAIRD, 'On profits and hospitals'
JEI, March, 1971, 5(1), pp. 57–66.
See 1014.

445 K. DAVIS, 'Relationship of hospital prices to costs'
AE, 1971, 3, pp. 115–25.

Three hypotheses about hospital pricing policies are tested using data for a ten-year period from the 50 states of the U.S.A. The hypotheses tested are: the price-average cost ratio is a constant; the price-average cost ratio is a function of the need for additional investment; the price-average cost ratio is a function of demand and supply conditions. The first two hypotheses were not substantiated, but price-average cost ratios were found to be sensitive to certain demand and supply conditions; in particular they are higher in states with higher per capita incomes.

R. G. EVANS, ' "Behavioural" cost functions for hospitals'
CJE, May, 1971, 4(2), pp. 198–215.

The functions that are estimated are not technical cost functions, they are cost–output relations descriptive of the way the Ontario hospital industry behaves subject to the process of budgetary review, which is part of the process of reimbursement. The major innovation in the paper is the correction for case-mix differences using data on age, sex and discharge diagnosis of patients. The empirical analysis suggested that diagnostic mix was an extremely important determinant of hospital costs. It was found that cost per case was constant or slowly rising with hospital size; but cost per day fell to a minimum at 300–400 beds and then rose.
See 472.

M. S. FELDSTEIN, 'Hospital cost inflation: a study of non-profit price dynamics'
AER, December, 1971, 61(5), pp. 835–72.

An econometric model of the economic behaviour of hospitals is constructed, which consists of twelve equations divided into four groups: demand relations price adjustment, components of cost and expansion of capacity. The demand and price adjustment equations are estimated using a mixed cross-section of time-series sample of ten annual observations for each state. The major conclusions are that: there are substantial price and income elasticities of demand for care; the source of inflation is the pressure of demand induced by increases in insurance coverage, income and the availability of hospital-oriented specialists; increases in the components of cost are the result not the cause of higher prices.
See 448, 491.

M. S. FELDSTEIN, *The Rising Cost of Hospital Care*
Washington D.C.: National Center for Health Services Research and Development, Information Resources Press, 1971, p. 88.

A study of the rise in the cost of hospital care over the period 1950–69. The study examines the role of the growth of insurance coverage, government subsidies, changing technology and the increase in wages of hospital employees as factors contributing to the rise in the cost of hospital care. The work emphasises the importance of health insurance as an explanatory variable.
See 447, 491.

449   B. FERBER, 'An analysis of chain-operated for-profit hospitals'
HSR, Spring, 1971, 6(1), pp. 49–60.

A descriptive survey using 1969 data to present statistics comparing chain-operated for-profit hospitals with other for-profit hospitals and non-profit hospitals on a wide variety of details: size, types of services offered, regional distribution, length of stay, occupancy, staffing levels and cost per case.

450   R. D. FRASER, *Canadian Hospital Costs and Efficiency*
Ottawa: Economic Council for Canada, Special Study No. 13, 1971, pp. v, 159.

A study using 1966 data to estimate hospital cost and production functions. Hospital output is measured as services provided by the hospital weighted by their average cost. No evidence was found to support the existence of a U-shaped average cost curve. The evidence suggested continually declining, though not sharply declining, average costs. A number of policy recommendations and recommendations for further study are made.

451   T. HU, 'Hospital costs and pricing behaviour: the maternity ward'
Inquiry, December, 1971, 8(4), pp. 19–26.

Estimation of a cost function using data from 30 non-profit hospitals suggested that hospital maternity wards were of sizes in the range of economies of scale, and that existing wards were underutilised. A comparison of point estimates of average cost of delivery and average charges suggested that hospitals were pricing maternity services at average cost.

452   J. R. LAVE, L. B. LAVE, 'The extent of role differentiation among hospitals'
HSR, Spring, 1971, 6(1), pp. 15–38.

A study of case-mix variation among hospitals in an area of Western Pennsylvania. A crude case-mix measure was constructed based upon a percentage of patients in each of 17 ICDA groupings. This measure was supplemented with measures of the incidence of surgery and of secondary diagnoses, estimates of the extent of common diagnosis and surgical procedures and an index of surgical complexity. The variations in these measures across the study hospitals were measured. Among the findings were that a small subset of diagnoses and surgical procedures was found to account for a large proportion of all cases, case-mix within a hospital was stable over short periods, and institutional characteristics only explain 25–45 per cent of the variation in the case-mix measures, indicating that facilities were not a good surrogate for case-mix.

M. L. LEE, 'A conspicuous production theory of hospital behaviour'
SEJ, July, 1971, 38(1), pp. 48–58.

A theory of hospital behaviour is developed on the basis of the proposition that the preferences of hospitals are interdependent and certain inputs are acquired for purposes other than efficient production. Each hospital is assumed to have a desired status and an actual status, and decision-takers act to minimise the gap between the two.

L. McCOY, 'The nursing home as a public utility'
JEI, March, 1971, 5(1), pp. 67–76.
See 1024.

J. A. RAFFERTY, 'Patterns of hospital use: an analysis of short-run variations'
JPE, January–February, 1971, 79(1), pp. 154–65.

Study of hospital use in thirty-five diagnoses over a period of four years revealed predictable variations in case-mix patterns. Admissions in seven categories increased and in six categories decreased in months in which occupancy rose above the normal levels. Illnesses of the latter group were those for which hospital admission might reasonably be regarded as postponeable or discretionary.

M. I. ROEMER, J. W. FRIEDMAN, *Doctors in Hospitals: Medical Staff Organisation and Hospital Performance*
Baltimore: The Johns Hopkins Press, 1971, pp. xiv, 322.

A comprehensive study of the organisational patterns by which physicians work in hospitals in the U.S.A. A chapter is included on doctor–hospital relations in the rest of the world, and comparisons are made between American and European forms of organisation.

P. WING, M. S. BLUMBERG, 'Operating expenditures and sponsored research at U.S. medical schools: an empirical study of cost patterns'
JHR, Winter, 1971, 6(1), pp. 75–102.

An estimate was made of the operating cost of undergraduate medical education for the entire group of four-year medical schools and for four sub-groups of the schools. The costs to medical schools of interns, residents and basic science students were also estimated. No conclusive evidence was found of economies of scale in medical education, although there were indications of a U-shaped cost curve. A high correlation was found between sponsored and non-sponsored research expenditures. A marked positive correlation was found between sponsored research expenditures and the number of students who became researchers at the same establishment.

458   D. E. YETT, L. DRABEK, M. D. INTRILIGATOR, 'A macro-econometric model for regional health planning.
EBB, Fall, 1971, 24(1), pp. 1–21.

Six categories of supply institutions are included in the model: voluntary and proprietary short-term hospitals, state and local governmental hospitals, skilled nursing homes, outpatient clinics of non-federal hospitals, offices of medical specialists in private practice, and offices of surgical specialists in private practice.
See 1403.

1972

459   R. ANDERSEN, J. J. MAY, 'Factors associated with the increasing cost of hospital care'
AAAPSS, January, 1972, 399, pp. 62–72.

The increase in the total cost of hospital care is split into the increase caused by increases in use and the increase caused by increases in the price per unit of service. The former accounts for a much smaller proportion of the increase than the latter. No single factor, increases in numbers of staff, in wages of staff, in amount or price of capital, appeared to be primarily responsible for the increase in cost per unit of service.

460   J. H. BABSON, *Health Care Delivery Systems: A Multinational Survey*
London: Pitman and Sons Ltd., 1972, pp. vii, 128.

A study of hospital financing mechanisms, patterns of hospital ownership, and procedures for accreditation and licensing of hospitals.
See 1073.

461   J. C. BERESFORD, 'Use of hospital costs in planning'
In M. M. Hauser (ed.) *The Economics of Medical Care*, pp. 165–76 (28).

A demonstration of the usefulness of a calculation relating costs per inpatient-week and cost per case to hospital throughput. It is found that cost per inpatient-week increases linearly with throughput, but cost per patient-week decreases with rising throughput up to a throughput of 0.75 or an average stay of 9 days. It is suggested that if two unselective hospitals (general hospitals) were replaced by a high throughput and a low throughput hospital offering different intensities of treatment, there would be a worthwhile reduction in hospital costs.

S. E. BERKI, *Hospital Economics*
Lexington, Massachusetts: Lexington Books, D.C. Heath and Company, 1972, pp. xxi, 270.

The book is an extended critical survey of mainly American literature on hospital economics. Chapters are included on hospital objectives, hospital outputs, productivity and efficiency, hospital costs, the demand for and utilisation of hospital services, pricing and reimbursement strategies and on the special problems facing the municipal hospital. Four problems are identified as being in particular need of greater analytical and empirical attention: the development of a satisfactory behavioural model of a hospital, both as an entity in itself and as one interacting with other entities within a health care system; the development of satisfactory measures of output and quality; the identification of production functions, especially disaggregated ones; and the collection of a better statistical base for the testing of models and for planning. *See* 113, 1233, 1484.

S. E. BERKI, 'The pricing of hospital services'
In S. J. Mushkin (ed.) *Public Prices for Public Products*, Washington: The Urban Institute, 1972, pp. 351–69.

A review of many of the major issues in hospital economics: output and productivity measurement, hospital cost curve estimation, hospital pricing policies, and incentives for efficiency.

K. W. CLARKSON, 'Some implications of property rights in hospital management'
JLE, October, 1972, 15(2), pp. 363–84.

The paper derives and tests some implications about differences in behaviour resulting from differences in managerial property rights between proprietary and non-proprietary hospitals. Evidence is presented to support the implications that non-proprietary hospitals will have different and more explicit internal rules than proprietary hospitals, that there is a different distribution of work effort in the two types of institutions, that non-proprietary hospital managers use market value information less than their proprietary counterparts, and that there is a greater variance in input combinations to produce similar products in non-proprietary hospitals.

H. A. COHEN, 'Monopsony and discriminating monopsony in the nursing market'
AE, 1972, 4(1), pp. 41–50.
See 275.

466   K. DAVIS, 'Community hospital expenses and revenues: pre-Medicare inflation'
SSB, October, 1972, 35(10), pp. 3–19.

Support was found for the demand-pull view of hospital inflation and for views emphasising changes in technology and expansion of the community hospitals role as explanations of hospital inflation in the period 1962–6. The labour cost-push model was found to be inadequate; hospital costs per patient day would have increased at an annual rate of 4 per cent even if wages had remained constant.

467   K. DAVIS, 'Economic theories of behaviour in non-profit, private hospitals'
EBB, Winter, 1972, 24(2), pp. 1–13.

A survey of the literature. Some evidence is presented to assess the validity of five alternative hypotheses about the behaviour of non-profit hospitals. The models considered are: recovery of costs, output maximisation, output and quality maximisation, utility maximisation and cash flow maximisation. It is tentatively suggested on the basis of the evidence that more dynamic models of behaviour are required.

468   K. DAVIS, 'Rising hospital costs: possible causes and cures'
Bull.N.Y.Acad.Med., December, 1972, 48(11), pp. 1354–71.

A survey of different theories of hospital cost inflation and the policy prescriptions that they imply. The empirical evidence in support of the various theories is also reviewed, and although no single theory has been decisively confirmed in the U.S. context, a number of results support a demand-pull hypothesis, raising concern about the possible inflationary impact of proposed increases in insurance coverage.

469   K. DAVIS, L. B. RUSSELL, 'The substitution of hospital outpatient care for inpatient care'
Rev.Econ.Stats., May, 1972, 54(2), pp. 109–20.
See 118.

470   H. G. DOVE, C. G. RICHIE, 'Predicting hospital admissions by state'
Inquiry, September, 1972, 9(3), pp. 51–6.
See 119.

471   R. A. ELNICKI, 'Effect of phase II price controls on hospital services'
HSR, Summer, 1972, 7(2), pp. 106–17.

A study of three Connecticut hospitals over the period 1960–9 to determine the contributions to total costs per discharge made by increases in cost per unit of service and by increases in units of service. It was found that the growth in total costs allowed under the Economic Stabilization Act was likely to be more than taken up by increases in costs of current services without any increase in the total number of services.

R. G. EVANS, H. D. WALKER, 'Information theory and the analysis of hospital cost structure'
CJE, August, 1972, 5(3), pp. 398–418.
The paper extends the approach of an earlier paper (by Evans) to British Columbia hospitals, with similar results. The paper introduces a measure drawn from information theory, defined on diagnostic proportions as an alternative method of adjusting for diagnostic mix.
See 446.

V. R. FUCHS, E. RAND, B. GARRETT, 'The distribution of earnings in health and other industries'
In V. R. Fuchs (ed.) *Essays in the Economics of Health and Medical Care*, pp. 119–31 (27).
See 278.

P. GEDLING, D. J. NEWELL, 'Hospital beds for the elderly'
In G. McLachlan (ed.) *Problems and Progress in Medical Care, Essays on Current Research, Seventh Series*, pp. 131–45 (30).
An examination of the factors determining the demand for hospital care for the elderly. The results of a study of hospitalisation of the elderly in three areas are presented, and likely future demands for care are projected.

P. B. GINSBURG, 'Resource allocation in the hospital industry: the role of capital financing'
SSB, October, 1972, 35(10), pp. 20–30.
A behavioural model of the non-profit private hospital is outlined. In the model, hospital decision-takers try to maximise the output of the various services produced, subject to the constraints of current income and the availability of capital funds. In the United States those institutions with the greatest access to capital funds are not necessarily those with the greatest demands for their services. This produces differences in the output-mix and capital intensity of services produced by hospitals. The final section of the paper presents a summary of an extensive analysis of the determinants of hospital investment and flows of capital financing as they relate to the model of hospital behaviour.

476   P. F. GROSS, 'Urban health disorders, spatial analysis, and the economics of health facility location'
IJHS, February, 1972, 2(1), pp. 63–84.

A critical review of existing bed planning methodologies. A major deficiency is the frequent failure to take account of the link between optimal facility size and the size of the service area. Four areas at present developed largely in isolation are identified as a natural base for future health planning: identifying urban health disorder and the patterns of interaction between particular disorder and patterns of socio-economic, demographic and environmental conditions; discovering the determinants of utilisation of existing health services; work on the determinants of supply and costs of health services; and finally work on the location of new health services and facilities.

477   M. A. HEASMAN, 'Increasing the efficiency of inpatient treatment'
In M. M. Hauser (ed.) *The Economics of Medical Care*, pp. 212–20 (28).

The need for data on the total cost of sickness in attempts to improve hospital efficiency is outlined. Some problems connected with the provision of incentives to consultants to adopt more efficient treatments are discussed.

478   D. HEWITT, J. MILNER, 'Components of the demand for hospital care'
IJE, Spring, 1972, 1(1), pp. 61–8.
See 121.

479   H. JOSEPH, S. FOLLAND, 'Uncertainty and hospital costs'
SEJ, October, 1972, 39(2), pp. 267–73.

The issue examined is whether the balance struck between the costs of excess capacity and the hazards of insufficient capacity has been an appropriate one. On the assumption that the daily census of patients is Poisson distributed, results from Iowa suggest that the costs incurred to avoid turning away patients were very high. The paper highlights the whole issue of option demand and who should bear the burden of the costs of additional capacity.

480   J. R. LAVE, L. B. LAVE, L. P. SILVERMAN, 'Hospital cost estimation, controlling for case-mix'
AE, September, 1972, 4(3), pp. 165–80.

A hospital cost function with case-mix variables included is estimated. Three techniques are used to reduce the problem of collinearity resulting from the introduction of the case-mix variables: principal component analysis, cluster analysis and another technique that reduces the number of explanatory variables by aggregating variables with similar estimated marginal costs. The cost function estimated by these techniques revealed that marginal cost was approximately 70 per cent of average cost, that there were no significant economies of scale, and that teaching hospitals, hospitals in metropolitan areas, hospitals performing complex surgery and hospitals treating difficult cases have higher costs.

R. J. LAVERS, 'The implicit valuation of forms of hospital treatment'
In M. M. Hauser (ed.) *The Economics of Medical Care*, 1972, pp. 190–205 (28).

The paper examines the possibility of making inferences about the relative value placed on the treatment of patients for particular disorders from a knowledge of the decisions actually made in the hospital system. Two approaches to the problem are explored. The first approach involves positing that decision-makers attempt to maximise an objective function that depends on the numbers and diagnostic categories of patients treated in a given time period, constrained by the fact that a certain number of bed-days must be occupied. The second approach is inverse programming: hospital authorities aim to maximise some objective function subject to maximum available levels of beds, doctors and nurses. See also the comment by R. Morley, pp. 206–11.

M. L. LEE, 'Interdependent behaviour and resource misallocation in hospital care production'
RSE, March, 1972, 30(1), pp. 84–95.

A conspicuous production theory of hospital behaviour is presented, in which a difference between the desired status of a hospital and its actual status drives hospital decision-takers to acquire inputs that will be underutilised or inappropriate for many types of care. This process is held to increase patient costs by more than any corresponding increase in quality.

M. L. LEE, R. L. WALLACE, 'Classification of diseases for hospital cost analysis'
Inquiry, June, 1972, 9(2), pp. 69–72.

Five different classification schemes for hospital cases are considered. The statistical results obtained by relating average cost per patient-day to the five classification schemes are compared to the results of simply relating average cost per patient-day to the aggregate number of patient-days produced.

R. F. L. LOGAN, J. S. A. ASHLEY, R. E. KLEIN, D. M. ROBSON, *Dynamics of Medical Care – The Liverpool Study into Use of Hospital Resources*
London: London School of Hygiene and Tropical Medicine, 1972, p. 152.

A report of a five-year study into resource allocation in the hospital services. The study considers need, demand, availability and utilisation of resources and costs in the Liverpool area. For surgery, the study found an absence of unmet need, long lengths of stay and low waiting lists; the study recommended closing beds. In the medical sphere, some acute beds were functioning as chronic beds; reclassification of these beds improved the performance of the Liverpool hospitals substantially.

485   G. M. Luck, 'Decision-making within hospitals'
In M. M. Hauser (ed.) *The Economics of Medical Care*, pp. 179–86 (28).

The paper looks at the role of operational research in providing information for decision-taking on two hospital projects – the commissioning of a new 600-bed hospital in the Birmingham hospital group, and a short-term re-organisation of a hospital group involving the closure of a casualty ward and provision of 65 new beds.

486   D. Neuhauser, F. Turcotte, 'Costs and quality of care in different types of hospitals'
AAAPSS, January, 1972, 399, pp. 50–61.

A review of some of the evidence on differences in cost and quality of care in different types of hospitals in the United States. It is concluded that the major potential for cost saving lies in the field of mental care.

487   J. Rafferty, 'Measurement of hospital case-mix: a note on alternative patient classifications'
AE, 1972, 4, pp. 301–5.

A case-mix adjustment index (developed more fully in Rafferty, 'Hospital output indices', *EBB*, 1972, 24(2), pp. 21–7) was calculated using the utilisation data of a small hospital system. The calculations were carried out for a variety of case-type specifications: fifty leading diagnoses, forty-four groups of diagnoses, seventeen clinical departments, medical versus surgical cases, and age groups of patients. The specific diagnostic categories were better for identifying short-run variations in case-mix.
See 488.

488   J. Rafferty, 'Hospital output indices'
EBB, 1972, 24(2), pp. 21–7.

An index measuring case-mix variation is constructed. The index is composed of two elements – the number of patients with a particular diagnosis, and the average length of stay for that diagnosis across hospitals.
See 487.

H. ROSE, B. ABEL-SMITH, *Doctors, Patients, and Pathology*
London: G. Bell and Sons Ltd., Occasional Papers on Social
Administration No. 49, 1972, p. 79.
A study of the demand for pathology services within one group of hospitals,
and the implications for resource allocation.

R. M. ROSSER, V. C. WATTS, 'The measurement of hospital output'
IJE, December, 1972, 1(4), pp. 361–7.
See 897.

D. S. SALKEVER, 'A microeconometric study of hospital cost inflation'
JPE, November–December, 1972, 80(6), pp. 1144–66.
A behavioural model of hospital cost inflation is constructed in which average
cost per day is a multiplicative function of factors affecting demand for hospital
services, the supply functions of factors, hospital decision-takers' preferences,
and the previous year's average cost per day. The model has the advantage that
potential causes of inflation are incorporated as parameters in the model. The
model is estimated using data from federal non-profit hospitals in south-eastern
New York State. The results indicate that a variety of factors contribute to cost
inflation but that average cost per day responds only slowly to these changes; a
considerable amount of inflation is therefore already in the pipeline.
See 447, 448.

W. SHONICK, 'Understanding the nature of the random fluctuations of the
hospital daily census'
MC, March–April, 1972, 10(2), pp. 118–42.
The deficiencies of the Hill–Burton hospital bed allocation formula are
analysed, and an alternative methodology based upon probability distributions
of the daily census and various waiting times is suggested.

L. J. SHUMAN, H. WOLFE, C. P. HARDWICK, 'Predictive hospital reimbursement and evaluation model'
Inquiry, June, 1972, 9(2), pp. 17–33.
Three regression models, one linear, two non-linear, are developed to predict
hospital costs. The models have a potential use in evaluating hospital performance and as a basis for incentive reimbursement. The independent variables
used in the model are six indices representing services, education, location,
medical staff/case-mix, outpatient activity and size classes; the dependent
variable is the total audited cost of the hospital.

494   R. A. TAYLOR, 'Principles of the economic behaviour of hospitals'
NJEB, Spring, 1972, 11(2), pp. 45–53.

An explanation of the alleged quality bias, i.e. quality higher than would exist under competitive market conditions, in American hospital treatment is provided in terms of the price discriminating behaviour of physicians and the availability of a variety of quantity/quality combinations of care needed to provide a cure. The mode of hospital organisation is held to be an important factor in the quality bias, and prepaid group practice and proprietary hospitals are seen as being less likely to have this bias.

1973

495   B. ABEL-SMITH, B. BENJAMIN, W. W. HOLLAND, J. W. PEARSON, D. F. J. PIACHAUD, O. GOLDSMITH, J. D. POLE, *Accounting for Health*
London: King Edward's Hospital Fund, 1973, p. 63.
See 32.

496   J. G. ANDERSON, 'Demographic factors affecting health services utilization: a causal model'
MC, March–April, 1973, 11(2), pp. 104–20.

In those areas where alternative health services are lacking it was found that an increase in the supply of beds significantly alters both the admission rate and the average length of stay. The usual economic factors – income, ethnic group and educational level – appeared to have little effect on length of stay.

497   J. R. ASHFORD, G. FERSTER, D. M. MAKUC, 'An approach to resource allocation in the reorganised National Health Service'
In G. McLachlan (ed.) *The Future — and Present Indicatives, Problems and Progress in Medical Care, Essays on Current Research, Ninth Series*, pp. 57–90 (38).
See 1412.

498   J. R. ASHFORD, K. L. O. READ, V. C. RILEY, 'An analysis of variations in perinatal mortality amongst local authorities in England and Wales'
IJE, Spring, 1973, 2(1), pp. 31–46.

An attempt to determine the relationship between the output of the maternity care system and the inputs of resources in the different local authorities of England and Wales. Information on perinatal mortality was used to measure

output; inputs were measured by the proportions of institutional confinements for different birthweight groups. In addition, the characteristics and general environment of each local authority were represented by a set of 88 descriptive variables representing features not directly related to the maternity services. Although a large proportion of the variation in mortality remained unexplained, the techniques used appeared to be a fruitful base for future research.
See 902.

J. H. BABSON, *Disease Costing*
Manchester: University Press, 1973, pp. viii, 151.
See 762.

R. E. BERRY, 'On grouping hospitals for economic analysis'
Inquiry, December, 1973, 10(4), pp. 5–12.
There are significant differences between short-term hospitals, but it is possible to identify distinct groups of hospitals on the basis of numbers of distinct facilities or services provided, and these groupings provide a satisfactory basis for further analysis. Four basic types of hospitals are identified in this study. The hospitals within these groups are different in major respects (costs, size, patient stay) from hospitals outside the group. This sort of analysis shifts emphasis from the question of optimal hospital size to the question of optimal mix of types of hospitals.

H. A. COHEN, 'Cost functions of hospital diagnostic procedures: a possible argument for diagnostic centres'
JEB, Winter, 1973, 25(2), pp. 83–8.
Long-run total cost schedules are estimated for a variety of diagnostic services. The results lend support to the proposal for large diagnostic centres. Unfortunately the elimination of heteroscedasticity greatly reduced the exploratory power of the functions estimated.

K. DAVIS, 'Theories of hospital inflation: some empirical evidence'
JHR, Spring, 1973 8(2), pp. 181–201.
Two theories of hospital cost inflation, the cost-reimbursement hypothesis and the labour cost-push theory, were examined. Theoretical reasons were found that suggested the cost reimbursement theory may be inapplicable at present. No empirical support was found for the hypothesis that costs varied with the extent of reimbursement, nor for the hypothesis that the growth of cost reimbursement was significant in explaining wage rates. Both hospital average costs and wages, suitably adjusted for other changes, were however significantly higher in the Medicare than in the pre-Medicare period.

503   K. Davis, 'Hospital costs and the Medicare programme'
SSB, August, 1973, 36(8), pp. 18–36.

Information is provided on overall trends in hospital revenues and expenses, labour and capital components of cost inflation, trends in revenues and expenses of individual hospital services, and the sources of hospital revenues in the first two years of Medicare. Regression analysis of hospital costs using individual non-profit hospital data for the period 1962–8 was also carried out. The findings of the study tended to support demand-pull theories of hospital cost inflation and theories emphasising changes in technology and an expanded role for the hospital, rather than labour cost-push models. Medicare did not appear to have changed the nature of hospital cost inflation, rather having accelerated trends already produced by the growth of private insurance in the pre-Medicare period.

504   A. Donabedian, *Aspects of Medical Care Administration: Specifying Requirements for Health Care*
Cambridge, Massachusetts: Harvard University Press, 1973, p. 649.

Sections are included on methods of planning hospital bed supply, measuring hospital output, the relationship between hospital and ambulatory care, and hospital productivity trends.
See 35.

505   C. Driver, 'Blood collection policies: towards a cost minimum'
SEA, January, 1973, 7(1), pp. 20–9.

A model for the overall planning of blood collection is developed that enables the determination of the required size of donor population and the number of calls to each donor to attend a session to meet the required level of blood demand. Estimates are provided of some of the parameters of the model using regional data.

506   G. Ferster, R. J. Pethybridge, 'The costs of a local maternity care system'
The Hospital, July, 1973, 69(7), pp. 243–7.

Estimates are made of the current costs of care by subdividing total costs according to case-mix and corresponding lengths of stay or items of service. Estimates of average costs are provided for eight different places of confinement with separate estimates for cases involving intervention during delivery.

507   H. I. Greenfield, *Hospital Efficiency and Public Policy*
New York: Praeger Publishers Ltd., 1973, pp. x, 82.

An examination of the hospital as a decision-taking unit, a critical review of recent empirical research on hospitals, and the problem of influencing hospitals to produce an efficient allocation of resources are dealt with in chapters 1, 2, 4 and 5. The third chapter examines the problem of hospital output measurement; a proposal to measure output by quality adjusted patient days is put forward, and illustrative calculations carried out for New York hospitals.

D. B. HILL, D. A. STEWART, 'Proprietary hospitals versus non-profit hospitals: a matched sample analysis in California'
BCRRS, March, 1973, 9, pp. 10–16.

Profit and non-profit hospitals comparable in size and geographical location were studied to shed light on the similarities and differences between the two types. Data comparing several aspects of performance are presented (e.g. occupancy, length of stay), though no attempt is made to compare the quality of care or the types of patient treated.

W. C. HILLES, 'Program cost allocation and the validation of faculty activity involvement'
JME, September, 1973, 48, pp. 805–13.

Reviews the use of effort reporting in cost allocation studies. The deficiencies of the approach and attempts to achieve a more valid measure of faculty activities are discussed.

R. W. HURD, 'Equilibrium vacancies in a labour market dominated by non-profit firms: the shortage of nurses'
Rev.Econ.Stats., May, 1973, 55(2), pp. 234–40.
See 303.

J. R. LAVE, L. B. LAVE, L. P. SILVERMAN, 'A proposal for incentive reimbursement for hospitals'
MC, March–April, 1973, 11(2), pp. 79–90.

Incentive reimbursement schemes are discussed briefly. A scheme is analysed in which reimbursement is based upon incurred costs, with a ceiling rate related to average costs in a hospital group. Evidence suggested a tendency for hospital costs to converge, and the authors saw no reason to expect that average cost increase across hospitals had decreased.

M. L. LEE, R. L. WALLACE, 'Problems in estimating multiproduct cost functions: an application to hospitals'
WEJ, September, 1973, pp. 350–63.

A hospital model is constructed in which the multiproduct nature of hospital output is recognised. The model also takes account of the effects of market structure and case-mix on the average cost of providing general hospital care. To illustrate the model's usefulness, calculations showing the influence of case-mix on hospital costs are carried out.

513 S. M. LEE, 'An aggregative resource allocation model for hospital administration'
Soc.-Econ.Plan. Sciences, 1973, 7(4), pp. 381–95.

An application of the goal programming approach to the problem of budget planning of a hospital. The approach requires that the administrator be capable of defining, quantifying and ordering objectives.

514 L. J. OPIT, K. W. CROSS, 'Comparing hospital costs'
The Hospital, February, 1973, 69(2), pp. 44–9.

An alternative framework for comparison of hospital costs is suggested. The framework involves comparison of expenditures on individual inputs as fractions of total medical salary expenditure on general clinical services (medical salary costs were a constant proportion of total expenditure in six acute hospitals considered). See also the comment by J. G. Cullis, P. A. West, August, 1973, 69(8), pp. 282–6.

515 M. V. PAULY, M. REDISCH, 'The not-for-profit hospital as a physicians' co-operative'
AER, March, 1973, 63(1), pp. 87–99.

A model of the hospital is developed in which physicians are the decision-takers and act to maximise net income per member of the physician staff. Among the implications of the model are that less than perfect co-operation among physician staff will tend to keep the physician staff small, and third-party payment for services will increase physician prices and incomes.

516 H. S. RUCHLIN, D. C. ROGERS, *Economics and Health Care*
Springfield, Illinois: Charles C. Thomas Publisher, 1973, pp. xvii, 317.
See 39.

517 H. S. RUCHLIN, D. D. POINTER, L. L. CANNEDY, 'A comparison of for-profit investor-owned chain and non-profit hospitals'
Inquiry, December, 1973, 10(4), pp. 13–23.

A report of the findings of a study using a matched sample of 56 hospital pairs, each pair consisting of one investor-owned chain and one non-profit voluntary or state and local government hospital. Findings comparing patient demographic characteristics, medical characteristics, medical education and financial characteristics, are presented. Some evidence was found to support the claim that proprietary hospitals attract easier, more profitable cases, although a great many similarities were found between the two types of hospital.

R. I. SCHULZ, J. ROSE, 'Can hospitals be expected to control costs?' *Inquiry*, June, 1973, 10(2), pp. 3–8.

It is suggested that the criteria of managerial success in the hospital industry contribute to the rapid rise in costs, there being few incentives and no rewards to reduce unnecessary admission, length of stay or overutilisation of ancillary services. It is argued that it would be easier for hospitals to contain costs if controls are established externally by regulatory agencies, or by the market through prepaid plans.

D. E. SKINNER, D. E. YETT, 'Debility index for long-term-care patients' In R. L. Berg (ed.) *Health Status Indexes*, pp. 69–82 (906). *See* 931.

D. A. STEWART, 'The history and status of proprietary hospitals' *BCRRS*, March, 1973, 9, pp. 2–9.

Reviews the history and the current status of for-profit hospitals in the U.S.A. The charges of lower quality care and 'cream skimming' in choice of patient and type of case treated are examined, as is the counter-argument that proprietary hospitals are more efficient. It is concluded that insufficient information is available to substantiate any of these claims.

G. L. STODDART, 'Effort reporting and cost analysis of medical education' *JME*, September, 1973, 48(9), pp. 814–23. *See* 310.

P. A. WEST, 'Allocation and equity in the public sector: the hospital revenue allocation formula' *AE*, September, 1973, 5(3), pp. 153–66. *See* 1140.

1974

523　R. C. AUGER, V. P. GOLDBERG, 'Prepaid health plans and moral hazard'
PP, Summer, 1974, 22(3), pp. 353–97.
See 1262.

524　D. P. BARON, 'A study of hospital cost inflation'
JHR, Winter, 1974, 9(1), pp. 33–49.

An attempt to estimate the amount of hospital cost inflation (per patient-day, and per admission cost) associated with increases in factor prices, technological and case-mix change and growth in demand for hospital services. Increases in factor prices were the main element in the increase (responsible for 60–80 per cent of the per day increase, and 75–100 per cent of the per case increase); changes in technology and case-mix were also significant factors.

525　R. E. BERRY, 'Cost and efficiency in the production of hospital services'
MMFQ, Summer, 1974, 52(3), pp. 291–313.

An econometric investigation to attempt to identify the factors affecting short-term general hospital costs in the U.S.A. Data from 6,000 hospitals for 1965, 1966 and 1967 are used. Input and throughput data are used as a proxy for output variables. Common characteristics of high and low average cost hospitals are identified.

526　J. CROMWELL, 'Hospital productivity trends in short-term general non-teaching hospitals'
Inquiry, September, 1974, 11(3), pp. 181–7.

527　A. J. CULYER, J. G. CULLIS, 'Private patients in NHS hospitals: waiting lists and subsidies'
In M. Perlman (ed.) *The Economics of Health and Medical Care*, pp. 108–16 (44).
See 1142.

528　P. D. CUMMING, E. L. WALLACE, D. M. SURGENOR, B. D. MIERZWA, F. A. SMITH, 'Public interest pricing of blood services'
MC, September, 1974, 12(9), pp. 743–53.

A study of blood service cost and pricing policy, partly by interview of blood centre managers, and partly by analysis of financial data of several blood centres. Most of the large price variations that characterise blood service in the

U.S.A. are shown to depend upon pricing policy rather than differential efficiency. Various policies for blood pricing are examined.

9 K. DAVIS, 'The role of technology, demand and labour markets in the determination of hospital cost'
In M. Perlman (ed.) *The Economics of Health and Medical Care*, pp. 283–301 (44).

Estimates a reduced form equation of hospital costs to sort out the roles of demand factors, labour market conditions and changing technology in the determination of hospital costs in the U.S.A. Of the predicted increase in expenses per hospital admission, demand variables counted for 45 per cent of the increase, case-mix variables 7 per cent, and increases in the earnings of hospital employees a further 10 per cent.

W. L. DOWLING, 'Prospective reimbursement of hospitals'
Inquiry, September, 1974, 11(3), pp. 163–80.
See 1264.

R. DUSANSKY, P. J. KALMAN, 'Toward an economic model of the teaching hospital'
JET, February, 1974, 7(2), pp. 210–23.

A dual objective model of the teaching hospital is constructed. The objectives are cost-efficient quality patient care, and determination of optimal case-mix overtime from the point of view of physician training.

R. G. EHRENBERG, 'Organisational control and the economic efficiency of hospitals: the production of nursing services'
JHR, Winter, 1974, 9(1), pp. 21–32.

Wage elasticities of demand for registered and licensed practical nurses are estimated. An attempt is then made to ascertain if these elasticities, and the extent to which hospitals substitute across classes of nurses, vary across types and size of hospital. First results suggested substitution of LPNs for RNs occurred as their relative wages change, in both public non-profit and private for-profit hospitals, but the extent of the substitution varies with the size of the hospital, and each category's (LPN, RN) employment level is more sensitive to its own wage level than to the wage level of the other category. In the main, the publicly operated hospitals' nursing employment levels seemed relatively insensitive to the wages of different categories of nurses.

M. S. FELDSTEIN, 'The quality of hospital services: an analysis of geographic variation and intertemporal change'

In M. Perlman (ed.) *The Economics of Health and Medical Care*, pp. 402–19 (44).

Discusses the conceptual problems involved in defining an index for aggregative analyses of the quality of hospital services. A quality measure is calculated using a price index for hospitals' non-labour inputs. The rest of the paper is devoted to an analysis of the geographic variation in the overall price of inputs, and to an examination of the intertemporal change and geographic variation in the quality of hospital services in the U.S.A.

534   M. S. FELDSTEIN, 'Econometric studies of health economics'
In M. D. Intriligator, D. A. Kendrick (eds.) *Frontiers of Quantitative Economics*, Vol. 2, pp. 377–447, Amsterdam: North-Holland, 1974.

Reviews work on models of hospital behaviour, economies of scale in the provision of hospital care, the causes of hospital cost inflation and input price determination.
See 42.

535   G. FERSTER, R. J. PETHYBRIDGE, 'Comparative costs of maternity care in three H.M.C. areas'
The Hospital, March, 1974, 70(3), pp. 82–6.

Cost estimates are presented for maternity care in consultant units, general practitioner units and by local authority domiciliary midwife services. The costing methods used involve the identification of resource use measured in physical units by different classes of patients, and then costing these resources. Information is also provided on perinatal mortality per 1,000 births in the different places of confinement.

536   M. D. FOTTLER, W. K. ROCK, 'Some correlates of hospital costs in public and private hospital systems: New York City'
QREB, Spring, 1974, 14(1), pp. 39–53.

A study to determine the relative effects of a variety of factors on the costs of voluntary and municipal hospitals in New York City in 1965 and 1970. The only major difference in hospital cost determinants in the two hospital systems was the effect of size on costs; the voluntary system exhibited diseconomies of scale, the municipal system showed no relationship between hospital size and cost.

537   B. FRIEDMAN, 'A test of alternative demand-shift responses to the Medicare programme'

In M. Perlman (ed.) *The Economics of Health and Medical Care*, pp. 234–47 (44).
See 150.

V. R. FUCHS, *Who Shall Live? Health, Economics, and Social Choice*
New York: Basic Books Inc., 1974, pp. vii, 168.
See 43.

M. E. W. GOSS, J. I. REED, 'Evaluating the quality of hospital care through severity-adjusted death rates: some pitfalls'
MC, March, 1974, 12(3), pp. 202–13.

A study to examine the validity of the hospital quality index suggested by Roemer, Moustafa and Hopkins (*HSR*, 1968, 3(2), pp. 96–118). Examination of data from New York City suggested that occupancy-connected length of stay was not such a good indicator of case severity as Roemer *et al.* had suggested; furthermore, severity-adjusted death rates were found to be essentially unrelated to the technological adequacy of the New York hospitals.
See 406.

P. JACOBS, 'A survey of economic models of hospitals'
Inquiry, June, 1974, 11(2), pp. 83–97.

A survey of the literature on models of hospitals. The models fall into two types, 'organism' models where the hospital is the acting body, and 'exchange' models, with the emphasis on the individuals who use the hospital as an institution to further their own aims.

J. KRIZAY, A. WILSON, *The Patient as Consumer: Health Care Financing in the United States*
Lexington, Mass.: Lexington Books, D. C. Heath, 1974, pp. xxii, 229.
See 1272.

J. K. KWON, 'On the relative efficiency of health care systems' *Kyklos*, 1974, 27(4), pp. 821–39.

Compares four types of hospital – the physician controlled non-profit hospital, the proprietary hospital, the consumer controlled co-operative hospital and the government controlled hospital – with regard to pricing policy, output and employment of resources. The implications of a zero user cost are also examined, and it is concluded that the waste of resources is likely to be larger under proposed U.S. plans than under the NHS in Britain, largely because of the inelastic supply response of the existing U.S. health care industry.

543 J. R. LAVE, L. B. LAVE, *The Hospital Construction Act: An Evaluation of the Hill–Burton Program, 1948–1973*
Washington D.C.: American Enterprise Institute for Public Policy Research, 1974, p. 71.

544 M. L. LEE, 'Theoretical foundations of hospital planning'
Inquiry, December, 1974, 11(4), pp. 276–81.

It is argued that the attempt by hospitals to provide treatment for all types of disease results in their having a large number of underutilised facilities. To eliminate this inefficiency, specialisation of hospitals by type of case treated is held to be necessary.

545 E. V. MORSE, G. GORDON, M. MOCH, 'Hospital costs and quality of care: an organisational perspective'
MMFQ, Summer, 1974, 52(3), pp. 315–46.

An examination of data from 388 government non-federal and voluntary general service hospitals to assess the impact of organisational structure (centralisation/decentralisation) on hospital efficiency (total expenses) and quality (level of adoption of new technology).

546 D. NEUHAUSER, 'The future of proprietaries in American health services'
In C. C. Havighurst (ed.) *Regulating Health Facilities Construction*, pp. 233–47 (1268).

The paper examines the future of for-profit hospitals and for-profit health maintenance organisations. This is done by examining society's goals for the health services industry, the working of the industry, the nature of the proprietaries, and the ideology underlying the support for them.
See 1268.

547 M. V. PAULY, 'Hospital capital investment: the roles of demand, profits, and physicians'
JHR, Winter, 1974, 9(1), pp. 7–20.

Sets out to test the Pauly/Redisch model of physician income maximisation as an explanation of hospital behaviour. Analysis of hospital investment with reference to this model yielded a positive relationship between physician income and hospital capital investment (i.e. hospitals operated to augment physician income). An accelerator model did receive some confirmation, but not as strongly as in the case of for-profit firms. Hospital profits were not important in determining total investment.
See 515.

M. V. PAULY, 'The behaviour of non-profit hospital monopolies: alternative models of the hospital'
In C. C. Havighurst (ed.) *Regulating Health Facilities Construction*, pp. 143–61 (1268).

A review of alternative models of the hospital. Models that explicitly consider physician behaviour and, within that group, models in which there is not perfect co-operation, are considered to be the most appropriate. The implications for hospital regulation are discussed.
See 1268.

J. RAFFERTY, S. O. SCHWEITZER, 'Comparison of for-profit and non-profit hospitals: a re-evaluation'
Inquiry, December, 1974, 11(4), pp. 304–9.

A comment on Ruchlin, Pointer, Cannedy (*Inquiry*, December, 1973, 10(4), pp. 13–24). It is suggested that these authors underestimate the extent to which proprietary hospitals 'skim off' easier to treat, more profitable cases. They go on to point out that a more interesting question is why the proprietary hospitals are able to skim, the answer to which must lie in the pricing policies or the efficiency of non-profit hospitals.
See 517.

N. P. ROOS, 'Influencing the health care system: policy alternatives'
PP, Spring, 1974, 22(2), pp. 139–67.

The differences between rational maximising models of health institutions and behavioural models are outlined. The different policy implications of the models are demonstrated, and it is shown how policy based on an inappropriate model can lead to results far removed from the original intentions of the policy makers. A case study of a laboratory merger decision by hospitals is examined.

R. M. ROSSER, V. C. WATTS, 'The development of a classification of the symptoms of sickness and its use to measure the output of a hospital'
In D. S. Lees, S. Shaw (eds.) *Impairment, Disability and Handicap*, pp. 157–70 (809).
See 897.

R. N. ROSETT, 'Proprietary hospitals in the United States'
In M. Perlman (ed.) *The Economics of Health and Medical Care*, pp. 57–65 (44).

The hypothesis is put forward that non-profit hospitals are preferred to profit hospitals by physicians because in larger institutions with diminished incentive for each doctor to cut costs it is more profitable to accept the tax and legal advantages of non-profit status, and to take a profit in the form of services provided by the hospital.

553   L. H. SILVER, 'The legal accountability of non-profit hospitals'
In C. C. Havighurst (ed.) *Regulating Health Facilities Construction*, pp. 183–200.
See 1268.

554   P. N. WORTHINGTON, 'Capital–labour ratios in short-term voluntary hospitals'
Inquiry, June, 1974, 11(2), pp. 98–111.
Empirical analysis revealed a high and systematic responsiveness of capital–labour ratios to variations in hospital wage (unit payroll cost). A wage elasticity (the responsiveness of the capital–labour ratio to changes in the wage) of 2.0 for non-teaching and 1.0 for teaching hospitals was found.

(ii)   *General Practice, Physician Practice, Community Care*

This field has been less thoroughly investigated than have hospitals (see preceding section), perhaps because general/physician practice presents less obvious analogies with the theory of the firm, and perhaps because the growing claims of hospitals on community resources have been the more obvious. It is also true that, in the nature of things, data are more difficult to come by in this field. At one level there are several detailed investigations of the workload of G.P.s, but the genuinely *economic* contribution has been made by those studies that have attempted cost-effectiveness assessments of group practice (e.g. Evans *et al.* 586) and input substitution in community practice (e.g. Reinhardt 580, 589).

1956

555   O. L. PETERSON, L. P. ANDREWS, R. S. SPAIN, B. G. GREENBERG, 'An analytical study of North Carolina general practice 1953–1954'
JME, December, 1956, 31(12 part 2), pp. 1–165.
A great deal of information is provided on the background and education of general practitioners, the type of patients they deal with and the type of care they give, the organisation of practice and the choice of practice location.

1962

OFFICE OF HEALTH ECONOMICS, *Studies on Current Health Problems*
London: Office of Health Economics, 1962–
See 4.

1963

H. E. KLARMAN, 'Effect of prepaid group practice on hospital use'
PHR, November, 1963, 78(11), pp. 955–65.
See 1162.

D. S. LEES, M. H. COOPER, 'Research into general practice'
JCGP, 1963, 6(3), pp. 233–41.
A paper indicating the scope and context of thirty-seven studies of general practice carried out since 1945 in the United Kingdom.

D. S. LEES, M. H. COOPER, 'The work of the general practitioner: an analytical survey of studies of general practice'
JCGP, 1963, 6(4), pp. 408–35.
After considering the problems of defining such entities as population at risk, consultation and the fact that different age groupings and classifications of disease are used in different studies, a survey of general practice is carried out. Aspects of practice considered in the paper include percentage of list seen, consultation rates, the proportion of home visits and types of illness; clear age and sex patterns existed for all of these aspects of practice, but variations between practices meant that meaningful generalisations about a doctor's work were difficult to make.

1964

J. FRY, 'Operations research in general clinical practice'
JCD, September, 1964, 17(9), pp. 803–13.
A review of work that has been done on a number of aspects of general practice, the G.P.'s work, his techniques, the organisation of his practice, his premises, and his relationship with other branches of medical care.

561   S. JUDEK, *Medical Manpower in Canada*
Ottawa: Royal Commission on Health Services, Queens Printer, 1964,
pp. xx, 413.
See 182.

1966

562   J. A. BOAN, *Group Practice*
Ottawa: Royal Commission on Health Services, Queens Printer, 1966.
On the basis of a survey of Canadian physicians carried out by the Royal
Commission on Health Services, which indicated a higher net income for
physicians with a higher per physician employment of supporting staff and a
lower value of medical equipment per physician in group practice, it is
concluded that group practice is more productive than solo practice.
See 1169.

563   R. B. FETTER, J. D. THOMPSON, 'Patients' waiting time and doctor's idle
time in the outpatient setting'
HSR, Summer, 1966, 1(1), pp. 66–90.
A simulation model is constructed to examine the effect on physicians' and
patients' idle time of appointment interval, service time, patients' arrival
pattern, number of no-shows, number of walk-ins, physicians' arrival pattern
and interruptions in patient services.

564   E. R. WEINERMAN, 'Research into the organisation of medical practice'
MMFQ, October, 1966, pp. 104–35.
A review of research in the U.S.A. and U.K. since 1950 on forms of medical
practice, the social role of the physician and the evaluation of different types of
medical practice organisation. The research methods used in the studies are
discussed and further needed research outlined.

1967

565   M. S. FELDSTEIN, *Economic Analysis for Health Service Efficiency*
Amsterdam: North-Holland Publishing Company, 1967, pp. xii, 322.
See 392.

J. M. LAST, 'Objective measurement of quality in general practice'
AGP, June, 1967, 12(Supp. part 2), pp. 5–26.

A survey of work on general practice: mainly social medicine work on the prerequisites for adequate care (numbers of doctors, distribution, organisation, equipment, hospital access, ability of doctors, doctor–patient relationship and quality control), on aspects of performance (diagnosis, referral, methods used, continuity of care), on the effects of care, and attempts to evaluate clinical performance are reviewed. The paper also includes the results from a prescribing study, covering a number of aspects of general practice: training, previous experience, methods of keeping up to date and prescribing habits.

D. E. YETT, 'An evaluation of alternative methods of estimating physicians' expenses relative to output'
Inquiry, March, 1967, 4(1), pp. 3–27.

Both clinical and rate-volume cost functions are estimated to examine the relationship between physician practice output and expenses for a sample of 1262 physicians in the U.S.A. Although the empirical results were such that neither type of function could be decisively preferred, both suggested the presence of economies of scale in expenses. Output was measured as the number of patient visits per year.

1969

A. DONABEDIAN, 'An evaluation of prepaid group practice'
Inquiry, September, 1969, 6(3), pp. 3–27.
See 1193, *1257*.

M. I. ROEMER, D. M. DUBOIS, 'Medical costs in relation to the organisation of ambulatory care'
NEJM, May 1st, 1969, pp. 988–93.
Group practice and individual practice costs are compared.

1970

R. M. BAILEY, 'Philosophy, faith, and facts(?) in the production of medical services'
Inquiry, March, 1970, 7(1), pp. 37–53.
Doubt is expressed about the existence of economies of scale in group practice.

The evidence cited in support of such economies comes from analysis of financial data showing increased income in group practice. Bailey suggests that the increased income comes from the sale of additional services, which are not an essential part of the physician's production function, and which can often be produced by outside organisations. It is argued that there is a tendency to presume that economies of scale exist in physician practice because there are known to be economies of scale in other industries.

571   R. M. Bailey, 'Economies of scale in medical practice'
In H. E. Klarman (ed.) *Empirical studies in Health Economics*, pp. 255–273 (18).

The view that there are economies of scale in physician group practice is disputed, supported by empirical evidence suggesting constant returns to scale. See also the comment by M. Reder pp. 274–7.
See 570.

572   R. Fein, 'An economist's view of the neighbourhood health centre as a new social institution'
MC, March–April, 1970, 8(2), pp. 104–7.

One of a series of papers in this issue of the journal by social scientists and doctors on the goals and potentials of neighbourhood health centres. Fein contends that while the centres go some way to providing care for the poor they are only a second best solution. Universal health insurance would enable the poor to choose the type of care they wanted, which may, or may not, be from neighbourhood health centres.

573   J. P. Newhouse, 'A model of physician pricing'
SEJ, October, 1970, 37(2), pp. 174–83.
See 242.

1971

574   I. G. Greenberg, M. L. Rodburg, 'The role of prepaid group practice in relieving the medical care crisis'
HLR, February, 1971, 84(4), pp. 887–1001.
See 1219.

575   L. J. Shuman, J. P. Young, E. Naddor, 'Manpower mix for health services: a prescriptive regional planning model'
HSR, Summer, 1971, 6(2), pp. 103–19.
See 265.

1972

R. F. BOAZ, 'Manpower utilization by subsidized family planning clinics: an economic criterion for determining the professional skill mix'
JHR, Spring, 1972, 7(2), pp. 191–207.
A study to determine the efficiency of manpower resource use. Two production functions, a Cobb-Douglas and a modified exponential, were estimated from data on nineteen clinics. The results indicated that the marginal cost of physicians' services was much lower than the cost of services rendered by the other clinic personnel, suggesting that a relative increase in the use of physician services was necessary to obtain an optimal skill mix.

I. BUTTER, G. T. MOORE, R. L. ROBERTSON, E. HALL, 'Effects of manpower utilization on cost and productivity of a neighbourhood health centre'
MMFQ, October, 1972, 50(4 part 1), pp. 421–52.
A study of a community health centre. Manpower input was measured by time study, and patient visits were used as a measure of output. The study considered the efficiency of manpower utilisation in the departments of paediatrics, internal medicine, nursing, nutrition, community mental health and social services.

D. L. CROMBIE, 'A model of the medical care system: a general systems approach'
In M. M. Hauser (ed.) *The Economics of Medical Care*, pp. 61–98 (28).
See 1404.

J. M. GLASGOW, 'Prepaid group practice as a national health policy: problems and perspectives'
Inquiry, March, 1972, 9(1), pp. 3–15.
See 1319.

U. E. REINHARDT, 'A production function for physicians' services'
Rev.Econ.Stats., February, 1972, 54(1), pp. 55–66.
A production function for physicians' services was estimated with data from two nationwide surveys of self-employed American physicians. Three output measures were used: the weekly rate of office visits, total patient visits and aggregate annual billings. The relationship between physician hours and output, and the effects of group practice and physician aides on output, were

examined. The study indicated that the average practice in the sample could have profitably employed nearly four aides per physician, or twice the observed sample average.

581   M. I. ROEMER, *Evaluation of Community Health Centres*
Geneva: World Health Organisation, Public Health Papers No. 48, 1972, p. 42.

582   K. R. SMITH, M. MILLER, F. L. GOLLADAY, 'An analysis of the optimal use of inputs in the production of medical services'
JHR, Spring, 1972, 7(2), pp. 208–25.
See 587, 593.

583   A. YANKAUER, J. SCHNEIDER, S. H. JONES, K. M. HELLMAN, J. J. FELDMAN, 'Physician output, productivity and task delegation in obstetric-gynecologic practices in the U.S.'
OG, January, 1972, 39(1), pp. 151–61.
See 289.

1973

---

584   R. F. BOAZ, 'Free standing subsidized planning clinics: the manpower cost of patient services'
Inquiry, March, 1973, 10(1), pp. 14–25.
A study to determine the factors that affect cost per unit of output to indicate appropriate policy when considering expansion. Two surrogate measures of output were used: the number of patients who receive pregnancy preventing services and the number of visits to the clinic.

585   A. DONABEDIAN, *Aspects of Medical Care Administration: Specifying Requirements for Health Care*
Cambridge, Massachusetts: Harvard University Press, 1973, p. 649.
See 35.

586   R. G. EVANS, E. M. A. PARISH, F. SULLY, 'Medical productivity, scale effects and demand generation'
CJE, August, 1973, 6(3), pp. 376–93.
An econometric study that uses British Columbian data. Some evidence is

found to support the hypothesis that group practices generate more output per physician, but the effect is substantially different between specialties and the gains for large groups appear to be small. A comparison of physician incomes in areas of very different physician density suggested substantial discretion on the part of physicians to generate demand for their own services.

F. L. GOLLADAY, M. MILLER, K. R. SMITH, 'Allied health manpower strategies: estimates of the potential gains from efficient task delegation'
MC, November–December, 1973, 11(6), pp. 457–69.

A simulation model of an efficient primary medical care practice is constructed that reveals that the productivity of a primary care practice could be increased by as much as 74 per cent by delegation of tasks to a physician's assistant.

J. P. NEWHOUSE, 'The economics of group practice'
JHR, Winter, 1973, 8(1), pp. 37–56.

A theoretical and empirical examination of the way in which the costs of medical services vary with the size of the group providing the services. It is suggested that the sharing of costs and revenues will tend to dilute the incentive to the physician to keep the cost of practice down and his work effort high. The evidence, comparing twenty single-specialty groups, three clinics and part of a hospital, tends to support the hypotheses that group practice reduces incentives to keep costs down and effort high.

U. E. REINHARDT, 'Manpower substitution and productivity in medical practice: review of research'
HSR, Fall, 1973, 8(3), pp. 200–27.
See 305.

M. I. ROEMER, W. SHONICK, 'HMO performance: the recent evidence'
MMFQ, Summer, 1973, 51(3), pp. 271–317.
See 1193, 1257.

1974

M. S. FELDSTEIN, 'Econometric studies of health economics'
In M. D. Intriligator, D. A. Kendrick (eds.) *Frontiers of Quantitative Economics*, Vol. 2, pp. 377–447, Amsterdam: North-Holland, 1974.
Reviews work on the economic behaviour of physicians – the extent of their

ability to set prices, the level at which they fix prices and the labour supply function of physicians.
See 42.

592   H. E. FRECH, P. B. GINSBURG, 'Optimal scale in medical practice: a survivor analysis'
JB, January, 1974, 47(1), pp. 23–36.

A survivor analysis is carried out using data on the size distribution of medical practice in the U.S.A. in 1965 and 1969. The underlying model rests upon the presumption that physicians will alter their size of practice when another size appears to be more profitable in terms of the physician's utility function, so that those practice sizes that are growing most rapidly can be identified as the most efficient at the margin. The evidence suggests that groups are more efficient than solo practice, with large and small groups more efficient than middle sized (7–25 physicians).

593   F. L. GOLLADAY, M. E. MANSER, K. R. SMITH, 'Scale economies in the delivery of medical care: a mixed integer programming analysis of efficient manpower utilization'
JHR, Winter, 1974, 9(1), pp. 50–62.

An extension of an earlier model (*JHR*, Spring, 1972, 7(2)), which looked at optimal use of inputs, to allow for the institutional constraint that labour inputs must be employed in discrete units; staffing patterns and optimal techniques thus depend on the scale of practice. Empirical investigation indicated that staffing and optimal techniques are sensitive to the scale of practice (measured by patient visits), and that sub-optimal practice scale results in substantially higher costs.
See 582, 587.

594   M. D. INTRILIGATOR, B. H. KEHRER, 'Allied health personnel in physicians' offices: an econometric approach'
In M. Perlman (ed.) *The Economics of Health and Medical Care*, pp. 442–58 (44).

A simultaneous equation model is developed to study the employment and utilisation of allied health personnel (nurses, technicians and secretaries) by solo practice physicians. The model is estimated separately for four specialties: general practice, internal medicine, paediatrics and obstetrics-gynaecology, using two stage least squares.

595   B. H. KEHRER, M. D. INTRILIGATOR, 'Task delegation in physician office practice'
Inquiry, December, 1974, 11(4), pp. 292–9.

A summary of the replies on the subject of task delegation obtained in the A.M.A. Seventh Periodic Survey of Physicians (1971). Various specialties were asked about the delegation of ten tasks, the percentage of times tasks were performed by allied health personnel and which allied health personnel most frequently performed the tasks.

J. D. E. KNOX, D. C. MORRELL, 'Studies of general practice (demand, need, quality)'
BMB, 1974, 30(3), pp. 209–13.
A brief review of studies of general practice in the U.K. – mostly non-economic. A useful bibliography is provided.

R. T. MASSON, S. WU, 'Price discrimination for physicians' services'
JHR, Winter, 1974, 9(1), pp. 63–79.
On the assumption that there are costs to obtaining information on price and quality of physician services, it is shown that profit-maximising physicians will practise price discrimination among income groups. Charity motives on the part of physicians are introduced to explain provision of some services to poor patients at zero prices or prices below marginal cost.

U. E. REINHARDT, K. R. SMITH, 'Manpower substitution in ambulatory care'
In J. Rafferty (ed.) *Health Manpower and Productivity*, pp. 3–37 (329).
See 330.

J. H. RICKARD, 'The costs of domiciliary nursing care'
JRCGP, December, 1974, pp. 839–45.
The study indicates that the costs of domiciliary nursing care are about half of those of hospital care (£13–16 compared with £32 for 1972), but excluded from the study are the costs that may have to be borne by family or friends of persons ill at home, and the benefits to the patient of being at home.

R. M. SCHEFFLER, 'Productivity and economies of scale in medical practice'
In J. Rafferty (ed.) *Health Manpower and Productivity*, pp. 39–51 (329).
Reviews work on economies of scale and on productivity differences between group and solo medical practice, and concludes that existing studies are confounded by data deficiencies and measurement problems, and that the problem of scale may be beyond existing methodology and priority should be given to research on productivity differences.

601   M. H. SHORTRIDGE, 'Quality of medical care in an outpatient setting'
MC, April, 1974, 12(4), pp. 283–300.

Reviews ten studies up to 1970 that examine the problem of defining and
measuring the quality of care in an ambulatory setting.

602   F. A. SLOAN, 'A microanalysis of physicians' hours of work decisions'
In M. Perlman (ed.) *The Economics of Health and Medical Care*, pp.
302–25 (44).
See 331.

603   F. A. SLOAN, 'Effects of incentives on physician performance'
In J. Rafferty (ed.) *Health Manpower and Productivity*, pp. 53–84 (329).
See 332.

604   R. ZECKHAUSER, M. ELIASTAM, 'The productivity potential of the physi-
cian assistant'
JHR, Winter, 1974, 9(1), pp. 95–116.
See 338.

(iii)   *Location of Health-Care Facilities*

The guiding principle in selecting items for classification in this section
rather than elsewhere is rather a narrow one: we have included items
whose main concern is with the consequences of locational decisions, but
excluded those whose concern is with other questions, even though these
are recognised as having significant locational consequences. The implications of this are best appreciated by some examples of the kind of
material that is excluded: the English allocation formula, concepts of
'territorial justice' in health service provision, regional morbidity as a
measure of need.

1967

605   M. F. LONG, P. J. FELDSTEIN, 'Economics of hospital systems, peak loads,
and regional co-ordination'
AER, May, 1967, 5 7(2), pp. 119–29.
See 396

J. B. SCHNEIDER, 'Measuring the locational efficiency of the urban hospital'
HSR, Summer, 1967, 2(2), pp. 154–69.

Locational efficiency is measured according to the degree of success in minimising the value of travel time of those who use the hospital. Examination of the behaviour of various groups of hospitals suggests that the locational efficiency of any hospital can be approximated by the success in minimising the value of travelling time of inpatients (hospital staff and doctors locate themselves to reduce their travel time). An examination of the location of Cincinatti hospitals on this criterion suggests that the hospitals are badly sited and the situation is likely to worsen as population moves out of the city.

1968

R. L. MORRILL, R. EARICKSON, 'Hospital variation and patient travel distances'
Inquiry, December, 1968, 5(4), pp. 26–34.

A principal components analysis was used to produce nine major components from 99 variables on which Chicago area hospitals showed meaningful variation. The scores of hospitals on the nine component dimensions were then used to group the hospitals. An analysis was then carried out of distances travelled by patients to hospitals in the different groups.

J. B. SCHNEIDER, 'Measuring, evaluating, and redesigning hospital–physician–patient spatial relationships in a metropolitan area'
Inquiry, June, 1968, 5(2), pp. 24–43.

An analysis is provided of locational patterns of short-term hospitals in relation to patients, and physician office and residence location (by specialty) in relation to patients and hospitals in Cincinatti. Two techniques are used: a locational inefficiency index based on linear distance measures, and a sectorgram involving measurement of size, shape and directional orientation of a spatial pattern. A suggested redesign of the distribution of obstetrics-gynaecology care is produced using the sectorgram technique.

1969

A. I. KISCH, J. W. KOVNER, L. J. HARRIS, G. KLINE, 'New proxy measure for health status'
HSR, Fall, 1969, 4(3), pp. 223–30.
See 862.

610   R. L. MORRILL, R. EARICKSON, 'Locational efficiency of Chicago hospitals: an experimental model'
HSR, Summer, 1969, 4(2), pp. 128–41.
A simulation model is constructed combining an interactance model and a transport model (distance minimising). Applied to Chicago, the model suggests that a relocation of beds would considerably reduce the costs of patient travel. However, the same improvements could be achieved by a relaxation of existing constraints on choice imposed by income and race.

611   E. SAVAS, 'Simulation and cost-effectiveness analysis of New York's ambulance service'
MS, August, 1969, 15(12), pp. 608–27.
A computer simulation was used to examine possible improvements in the ambulance service of New York City that would result from proposed changes in numbers and location patterns of ambulances. Cost-effectiveness evaluation of the various solutions suggested the superiority of dispersed configurations of ambulances – smaller numbers of ambulances were as effective in terms of response time in a dispersed system as in a satellite system, and at a much lower incremental cost per call.

612   G. W. SHANNON, R. L. BASHUR, C. A. METZNER, 'The concept of distance as a factor in accessibility and utilization of health care'
MCR, February, 1969, 26(2), pp. 143–61.
Traces the development of work on the distance between, and spatial distribution of, patients and health care providers. A bibliography of 58 items is provided.

1970

613   W. J. CARR, 'Economic efficiency in the allocation of hospital resources: central planning versus evolutionary development'
In H. E. Klarman (ed.) *Empirical Studies in Health Economics*, pp. 195–221 (18).
See 426.

614   J. E. MILLER, 'An indicator to aid management in assigning programme priorities'
PHR, August, 1970, 85(8), pp. 725–31.
See 868.

R. L. MORRILL, R. J. EARICKSON, P. REES, 'Factors influencing distances travelled to hospitals'
EG, April, 1970, 46(2), pp. 161–71.

Examines the influence of the physician and of racial, income and religious factors on distance travelled to hospital by patients. Reduced access to facilities, because of race and income, considerably increases distance travelled.

G. P. SCHULTZ, 'The logic of health care facility planning'
Soc.-Econ.Plan.Sciences, September, 1970, 4(3), pp. 383–93.

Drawing on the concepts of central place theory, a model is presented to enable the generation of an optimal facility pattern for a metropolitan region. The model has three levels of care: health centre, general hospital and medical centre (intensive care). The model takes into account service costs, travel costs, a social benefit function (benefits derived from utilisation) and the possibility of economies of scale in provision of care.

1971

R. GRUER, 'Economics of outpatient care'
Lancet, February 20th, 1971, 1(7695), pp. 390–4.

Estimates are made of the costs of consultant time and cost of patient time under a variety of different arrangements of locating outpatient clinics in the Scottish borders. Seven arrangements from complete centralisation to a system of peripheral clinics in cottage hospitals are costed.

1972

W. J. ABERNATHY, J. C. HERSHEY, 'A spatial-allocation model for regional health services planning'
OR, May–June, 1972, 20(3), pp. 629–42.

A model is presented that enables the determination of location and capacity of a specified number of health care centres within a region. The locations can be optimised according to a number of criteria: maximise utilisation, minimise distance per capita, minimise distance per encounter. The model operates on the presumption that the population can be stratified in such a way that each stratum has relatively homogeneous patterns of health-care utilisation.

619   J. R. LAVE, S. LEINHARDT, 'The delivery of ambulatory care to the poor: a literature review'
MS, December, 1972, 19(4), pp. 78–99.
See 122, 1243.

1973

620   A. B. CALVO, D. H. MARKS, 'Location of health care facilities: an analytical approach'
Soc.-Econ.Plan.Sciences, October, 1973, 7(5), pp. 407–22.
The problem of optimal location of medical facilities is considered. Optimisation according to three objective functions, minimisation of distance or travel time, minimisation of user costs and maximisation of demands upon a facility, is examined. A tentative utility maximisation approach is also outlined.

621   A. DONABEDIAN, *Aspects of Medical Care Administration: Specifying Requirements for Health Care*
Cambridge, Massachusetts: Harvard University Press, 1973, p. 649.
The last part of section 4 (pp. 419–85) is devoted to an extensive review of work on accessibility and locational efficiency of health facilities.
See 35.

622   C. HIMATSINGAN, 'Approaches to health and personal social services planning in the National Health Service and the place of health indices'
IJE, March, 1973, 2(1), pp. 15–21.
See 917.

623   R. S. KAPLAN, S. LEINHARDT, 'Determinants of physician office location'
MC, September–October, 1973, 11(5), pp. 406–15.
A study of Pittsburgh revealed that the proximity of short-term hospitals and the presence of extensive commercial zoning were the principal factors affecting physicians' office location. After controlling for these two factors, median income of the population was found to exert no influence on the number of physicians in an area, although physicians were scarce near large concentrations of Blacks.

D. S. LEVINE, D. E. YETT, 'A method for constructing proxy measures of health status'
In R. L. Berg (ed.) *Health Status Indexes*, pp. 12–22 (906).
See 923.

R. D. MUSTIAN, J. J. SEE, 'Indications of mental health needs: an empirical and pragmatic evaluation'
JHSB, March, 1973, 14, pp. 23–7.
See 926.

G. POVEY, D. UYENO, I. VERTINSKY, 'Social impact index for evaluation of regional resource allocation'
In R. L. Berg (ed.) *Health Status Indexes*, pp. 104–15 (906).
See 928.

1974

G. N. BERLIN, J. C. LIEBMAN, 'Mathematical analysis of emergency ambulance location'
Soc.-Econ.Plan.Sciences, December, 1974, 8(6), pp. 323–8.
Combines two models sequentially: first a static optimisation model to determine the location of depots; then a stochastic simulation model to evaluate the utilisation of ambulances to determine allocation of ambulances to depots.

U. CHRISTIANSEN, 'Demand for emergency health care and regional systems for provision of supply'
In M. Perlman (ed.) *The Economics of Health and Medical Care*, pp. 248–71 (44).
A study to design a new emergency care system for Greater Copenhagen. Information from a casualty survey on the value of patients' time and condition was used in a linear simulation model to determine the location and number of ambulances. The location of the emergency treatment units was constrained by existing location of hospitals.

J. MEADE, 'A mathematical model for deriving hospital service areas'
IJHS, Spring, 1974, 4(2), pp. 353–64.

630 A. D. WOLFSON, *A Health Index for Ontario*

Toronto: Ministry of Treasury, Economics and Intergovernmental Affairs, Ontario Statistical Centre, 1974, pp. 49.

See 948.

4 Evaluating the Contribution of Health Services

The use of the term 'contribution' carries the implication that the existence of health services 'makes something (or someone) better off'. But it is, properly, vague. The study of who is made better off, in what ways, and by how much, by the provision of health services in particular magnitudes and on particular terms is beset with difficulties. These are partly philosophical (what do we mean by 'better off', and hence by 'contribution'?), and partly practical: how do we identify and measure the 'contribution' of the health services, or of given changes therein. The two issues are clearly related; there is a different value-system for each distinct philosophical position.

Our four sub-divisions cover distinguishable types of valuation situations, but are intimately related by their common concern with the central question of the 'contribution' of health service provision to some kind of 'output'.

(a) Estimating the Cost of Disease, Cost-Effectiveness, Cost–Benefit Analyses of Particular Health-Care Programmes

At the beginning of the 1960s, anyone wishing to see how the cost–benefit type algorithms had been applied in health studies would have found little useful material. Since then the growth rate, whether measured by quantity or, to a lesser extent, by quality, has been very fast. Moreover, the obvious difficulties have not daunted researchers from tackling mental illness as well as apparently more tractable topics such as varicose veins.

Most of the work continues to identify the value of healthy (or working) time saved as the principal benefit together with, in the analysis of preventive programmes, treatment costs avoided. Almost all studies have commented (a) on the difficulties arising from the lack of satisfactory

155

epidemiological models to provide the underlying input–output relations and (b) on the difficulty of identifying an output unit on which to standardise cost-effectiveness studies. Although some progress has now been made with regard to the latter (see especially Torrance (704) and Bush *et al.* (728)), the former has in many cases proved intractable (even in the varicose veins case there is argument about whether the patients were really equally well off under either programme: Piachaud and Weddell, 745).

In this area economists and epidemiologists have a particular identity of interest and it is not altogether surprising that the best work, and the least qualified results, come from joint research projects.

1920

631   L. I. DUBLIN, J. WHITNEY, 'On the cost of tuberculosis'
JASA, December, 1920, 17, pp. 441–50.

A pioneering effort in measuring the economic costs of a disease. An estimate is made of total years of life lost due to tuberculosis by comparing life expectancy when all forms of death are included and life expectancy with tuberculosis deaths excluded. The value of a year of life lost was estimated to be $100, and the total loss in the population was estimated to be $26,500 million.

1946

632   L. I. DUBLIN, A. J. LOTKA, *The Money Value of a Man*
New York: Ronald Press, 1946, pp. xvii, 214.
See 823.

1950

633   B. MALZBURG, 'Mental illness and the economic value of a man'
Ment.Hyg., October, 1950, pp. 582–91.

An attempt to measure the indirect costs of various types of mental illness in New York State by estimating the number of years of productive activity lost due to incapacity caused by mental illness, and the earnings loss consequent upon the loss of working years.

1956

D. J. REYNOLDS, 'The cost of road accidents'
JRSS A, 1956, 119(4), pp. 393–408.

The costs calculated are those relating to damage of property, medical costs, administrative costs and the net reduction in output due to the loss of output from people killed and injured (minus the output that those would have themselves consumed). An appendix is included on the return to be gained from installation of pedestrian crossings and adequate rear lighting on vehicles.

1957

M. S. BLUMBERG, 'Evaluating health screening procedures'
OR, June, 1957, pp. 351–60.
See 843.

1958

R. FEIN, *Economics of Mental Illness*
New York: Basic Books, Joint Commission on Mental Illness and Health, Monograph Series No. 2, 1958, pp. xx, 164.

1959

S. J. MUSHKIN, F. d'A. COLLINGS, 'Economic costs of disease and injury'
PHR, September, 1959, 73(9), pp. 795–809.

The costs of disease and injury are viewed as being of three types: resource costs of providing health services; costs represented by the transfer of income and resources from the well to the sick; and production losses.

1961

638   C. E. RICE, 'Measuring social restoration performance of public psychiatric hospitals'
PHR, May, 1961, 76(5), pp. 437–46.
See 847.

639   B. A. WEISBROD, *Economics of Public Health*
Philadelphia: University of Pennsylvania Press, 1961, pp. xvi, 127.
The major part of the study is concerned with identifying and estimating the economic losses resulting from poor health. Three types of losses or costs are estimated: costs resulting from premature death, costs from sickness and treatment costs. These costs are calculated for the diseases cancer, tuberculosis and poliomyelitis in the United States for the year 1954. A major element in the costs is the output loss resulting from the diseases, which is measured by the discounted present value of future earnings.
See 987.

1962

640   S. J. MUSHKIN, 'Health as an investment'
JPE, October, 1962, 70(5 part 2), pp. 129–57. Also in M. H. Cooper, A. J. Culyer (eds.) *Health Economics*, pp. 93–134 (33).
See 46.

641   OFFICE OF HEALTH ECONOMICS, *Studies on Current Health Problems*
London: Office of Health Economics, 1962–
See 4.

642   E. E. PYATT, P. P. ROGERS, 'On estimating benefit–cost ratios for water supply investments'
AJPH, October, 1962, 52(10), pp. 1729–42.
The economic value of health gains from water supply improvements is viewed as the gain in contribution to productive activity resulting from reductions in mortality, morbidity and debility. An illustrative benefit–cost ratio calculation relating to the Puerto Rican water supply system is presented. Mortality benefits greatly exceeded other benefits.

1963

M. S. FELDSTEIN, 'Economic analysis, operational research, and the National Health Service'
OEP, March, 1963, 15(1), pp. 19–31.
The fear is expressed that operations research and systems analysis will be applied in the health field where economic analysis, and cost–benefit analysis in particular, is the appropriate framework within which to consider the problem.

S. KATZ, A. B. FORD, R. W. MOSKOWITZ, B. A. JACKSON, M. W. JAFFE, 'Studies of illness in the aged: the index of ADL – a standardized measure of biological and psychosocial function'
JAMA, 1963, 185(12), pp. 914–19.
See 849.

J. WISEMAN, 'Cost–benefit analysis and health service policy'
SJPE, February, 1963, 10(1), pp. 128–45. Also in B. F. Kiker (ed.)
Investment in Human Capital, Columbia South Carolina: University of South Carolina Press, 1971, pp. 433–51.
The role that cost–benefit studies (investment in health) of health programmes might play in the formulation of public policies is examined. The approach adopted in a number of studies is briefly outlined, and it is concluded that these studies present major problems of interpretation from the point of view of policy. Two possible approaches to making the studies policy-relevant are examined, the first based on the concepts and criteria of welfare economics, the second involving explicit recognition of the government as a decision-taking entity and endeavouring to develop analyses that are relevant to the value system of that entity.

1964

G. S. BECKER, *Human Capital*
New York: National Bureau of Economic Research, 1964, pp. xvi, 187.
See 48.

A. F. CONARD, J. MORGAN, R. PRATT, C. VOLTZ, R. BOMBAUGH,
Automobile Accident Costs and Payments – Studies in the Economics of Injury Reparation
Ann Arbor: University of Michigan Press, 1964, pp. xxviii, 506.
See 825, 1348.

648   R. FEIN, 'Health programmes and economic development'
In S. J. Mushkin (Chairman) *The Economics of Health and Medical Care*, pp. 271–82 (8).
See 826, 951.

649   A. G. HOLTMANN, 'Estimating the demand for public health services: the alcoholism case'
PF, 1964, 19(4), pp. 351–8.
The present value of losses due to decreased life expectancy, unemployment, absenteeism, imprisonment, hospitalisation for mental illness, and automobile accidents of male alcoholics in the U.S.A. in 1959 was estimated. The average loss per male alcoholic was considerably higher than the cost of treatment.

650   M. L. INGBAR, S. S. LEE, 'Economic analysis as a tool of programme evaluation: costs in a home care programme'
In S. J. Mushkin (Chairman) *The Economics of Health and Medical Care*, pp. 173–210 (8).
The costs of the home care programme of a Boston hospital are calculated separately for each of the services provided. The implications of such cost calculations for resource allocation are discussed.

651   U.S. DEPARTMENT OF HEALTH, EDUCATION AND WELFARE, *Economic Benefits from Public Health Services: Objectives, Methods, and Examples of Measurement*
Washington D.C.: USDHEW, Public Health Service Publication No. 1178, 1964, p. 31.
Five short papers on the use of cost–benefit analysis in the health field, the problems with the approach and possible ways forward.
1   C. C. Linnenberg, 'How shall we measure economic benefits from public health services?' pp. 1–12.
2   A. P. Ruderman, 'Lessons from Latin American experience', pp. 13–17.
3   G. E. Mitchell, 'The false economy of dental neglect', pp. 18–23.
4   D. D. Beckman, 'Vocational rehabilitation of the mentally disabled pays off in dollars and sense', pp. 24–8.
5   J. J. Hanlon, 'Can accounting sell health', pp. 29–31.

1965

652   R. W. CONLEY, *The Economics of Vocational Rehabilitation*
Baltimore: The Johns Hopkins Press, 1965, pp. xii, 177.

The Study examines the characteristics and costs of disability, approaches to the problem of rehabilitating the disabled, and the history of vocational rehabilitation in the United States. The major part of the study is an attempt to determine the material benefits and costs of the state–federal programme of vocational rehabilitation which restores over 100,000 people a year to gainful activity. The major benefit from rehabilitation is the increase in output of rehabilitants. Because of data limitations the study is forced to approximate the increase in output by the change in earnings of rehabilitants.
See 687, 769.

A. G. HOLTMANN, R. RIDKER, 'Burial costs and premature death'
JPE, June, 1965, 73(3), pp. 284–6.

An estimate is made of the costs of burial of those who die prematurely. Using estimates of the average cost of burial in the United States, it is shown that burial cost is a significant part of the total cost of disease.

H. E. KLARMAN, *The Economics of Health*
New York: Columbia University Press, 1965, pp. viii, 200.
See 11.

H. E. KLARMAN, 'Conference on the economics of medical research'
In *Report to the President, A National Programme to Conquer Heart Disease, Cancer and Stroke*, Vol. 2, February 1965, pp. 631–44.
Washington D.C.: U.S. Government Printing Office, 1965.

A summary of a discussion between seven distinguished U.S. economists and members of the De Bakey Commission. The discussion is centred around six questions, which relate to how much the United States can afford to spend on medical research, how the research funds should be allocated, and the role the various levels of government should play in funding research.

H. E. KLARMAN, 'Syphilis control programmes'
In R. Dorfman (ed.) *Measuring Benefits of Government Investments*, Washington D.C.: The Brookings Institution, 1965, pp. 367–414.

The first section of the paper critically reviews techniques used by economists to measure the cost of a disease. The second section of the paper measures the costs of cases infected in 1962. These costs are calculated for each group of cases classified by stage of discovery and treatment (four cost elements are included: medical care expenditures, output loss, reduction in earnings due to 'stigma' and loss of consumer benefit). The final section of the paper compares benefits of an eradication programme and programmes to reduce and control the disease.

657   D. P. RICE, 'Economic costs of cardiovascular diseases and cancer, 1962' In *Report to the President, A National Programme to Conquer Heart Disease, Cancer and Stroke*, Vol. 2, February 1965, pp. 439–630. Washington D.C.: U.S. Government Printing Office, 1965.

A massive study submitted by the health economics branch of the Department of Health, Education and Welfare to the De Bakey Commission. The study brings together a large amount of epidemiological and economic data. The costs are measured as the sum of direct medical costs and lost output resulting from morbidity and premature mortality, a technique used in a large number of more recent health cost–benefit studies.

1966

658   R. A. CRYSTAL, A. W. BREWSTER, 'Cost benefit and cost effectiveness analyses in the health field: an introduction' *Inquiry*, December, 1966, 3(4), pp. 3–13.

A simple introduction to cost–benefit and cost-effectiveness techniques.

659   S. ENKE, 'The economic aspects of slowing population growth' *EJ*, March, 1966, 76(1), pp. 44–56. Also in M. H. Cooper, A. J. Culyer (eds.) *Health Economics*, pp. 357–72 (33). *See* 954.

660   R. KOHN, 'Health objectives for the evaluation of health services and operational research' *CJPH*, January, 1966, 57(1), pp. 13–17.

Tables are constructed illustrating the contribution of seventeen major diagnostic classes of the ICD to deaths, premature mortality, disabling illness and non-disabling illness. These statistics are then compared to the share of those diagnostic categories in the present health budget to give some basic assistance for guiding the allocation of funds.

661   K. M. McCAFFREE, 'The cost of mental health care under changing treatment methods' *AJPH*, July, 1966, 56(7), pp. 1013–25.

A comparison of the costs of traditional custodial care and of intensive treatment therapies in Washington State. The undiscounted costs of intensive therapy were 30 per cent less than those of custodial care.

2   D. P. RICE, *Estimating the Cost of Illness*
    Washington D.C.: USDHEW, Public Health Service Publication No.
    947–6, May, 1966, pp. xii, 132.
    The case is developed for measuring the costs of illness as a sum of the costs of
    medical care (direct costs) and of the lost productivity due to morbidity and
    premature mortality (indirect costs). The problems of the approach, such as
    measuring the value of housewives' services, dealing with transfer payments,
    unemployment and a number of methodological difficulties, are discussed. A
    series of calculations of these costs for the United States in 1963 (for all disease,
    and for each broad diagnostic group separately) is presented.

3   G. TEELING-SMITH (ed.) *Surveillance and Early Diagnosis in General
    Practice*
    London: Office of Health Economics, May, 1966, p. 52.
    The report of a colloquium on health screening. Eight short papers were
    presented and discussed. The papers were intended to throw light on both
    economic and clinical issues, although most of those present had medical
    qualifications. Topics covered were multiphasic screening, chemical health
    screening, detection of cancer of the cervix, anaemia and diabetes, and
    detecting disease in clinical geriatrics. As a result of this colloquium, a series of
    short papers was commissioned, to be written by experts in the various clinical
    fields for general practitioners, outlining the current state of knowledge on
    selected common disorders. To date, eight of these 'early diagnosis papers'
    have been written and published by the Office of Health Economics. The
    papers deal with raised arterial blood pressure, visual defects, cancer of the
    cervix, depression, diseases of the lung, ischaemic heart disease, anaemia and
    urinary tract infection.

1967

R. BARLOW, 'The economic effects of malaria eradication'
AER, May, 1967, 57(2), pp. 130–48.
The study involves the specification of a fairly detailed model of the entire
economy because the eradication of malaria has far-reaching macro-economic
consequences that make conventional partial equilibrium cost–benefit analysis
inappropriate. The methodology developed is applied to the case of malaria
eradication in Ceylon. Preliminary results are presented indicating the course
that per capita income would have followed had the 1947 eradication programme not been implemented.
See 672.

665   R. W. CONLEY, M. CONWELL, M. B. ARRILL, 'An approach to measuring the cost of mental illness'
AJP, December, 1967, 124(6), pp. 755–62.

The object of the study is to estimate the total cost of mental illness in the United States. The costs are viewed as being a combination of tangible items (production loss, treatment costs, etc.) and intangible items (pain, grief, suffering). The distribution of the cost burden between the mentally ill and non-mentally ill is also examined. The tangible items are found to total over $20,000 million in 1966, 3 per cent of G.N.P.

666   H. CORREA, 'Health planning'
Kyklos, 1967, 20(4), pp. 909–23.
See 1379.

667   R. F. F. DAWSON, *Cost of Road Accidents in Great Britain*
London: Ministry of Transport, Road Research Laboratory Report LR 79, 1967. Excerpts are reprinted in M. H. Cooper, A. J. Culyer (eds.) *Health Economics*, pp. 336–56 (33).
See 802, 827, *833.*

668   H. E. KLARMAN, 'Present status of cost–benefit analysis in the health field'
AJPH, November, 1967, 57(11), pp. 1948–53.

An introduction to the nature and scope of cost–benefit analysis. Includes a brief survey of the achievements in the health field and a discussion of the major problems that remain to be solved.

669   D. P. RICE, 'Estimating the cost of illness'
AJPH, March, 1967, 57(3), pp. 424–40.

The total costs of illness, disability and death in the U.S.A. in a single year are calculated. Estimates are provided for eight major diagnostic groups and a further ten groups from the ICDA are lumped together. Direct costs are estimated by allocating national health expenditures to the diagnostic groups according to utilisation by diagnosis of specific services. Indirect costs were measured as losses in productive activity resulting from morbidity and mortality.

670   R. L. ROBERTSON, 'Issues in measuring the economic effects of personal health services'
MC, November–December, 1967, 5(6), pp. 362–8.
See 856.

S. ROTTENBERG, 'The allocation of biomedical research'
AER, May, 1967, 57(2), pp. 109–18.

A review of some of the problems involved in determining the correct
allocation of resources to research, and of some of the properties of research as
an activity that affects resource allocative decisions.

1968

R. BARLOW, *The Economic Effects of Malaria Eradication*
Ann Arbor, Michigan: Bureau of Public Health Economics, Research
Series No. 15., 1968, pp. viii, 167.
See 664.

M. B. BOND, J. E. BUCKWALTER, D. K. PERKIN, 'An occupational health
program – costs versus benefits'
AEH, September, 1968, 17, pp. 408–15.

An attempt to assess the benefits to a company of 27,000 employees of an
occupational health programme. Although the benefits of all medical activities
are not calculated, estimates are made of the savings from particular services.
Savings in sickness absence costs for the years of the programme appeared to
be substantial.

R. N. GROSSE, 'Planning, programming, and budgeting'
Bull.N.Y.Acad.Med., February, 1968, 44(2), pp. 125–30.

A brief presentation of work carried out by the United States Department of
Health, Education and Welfare. The problems of setting goals and determining
priorities are discussed using as illustrations work done on maternal and child
care and on disease control programmes.

J. B. HALLAN, B. S. H. HARRIS, 'The economic cost of end stage uremia'
Inquiry, December, 1968, 5(4), pp. 20–5.

Data are presented on the average and total cost per annum of centre dialysis,
on the cost of treating undialysed patients, and on the indirect costs of end
stage uremia in terms of the present value of lifetime earnings forgone of people
who die.

H. E. KLARMAN, J. O'S. FRANCIS, G. D. ROSENTHAL, 'Cost effectiveness
analysis applied to the treatment of chronic renal disease'
MC, January–February, 1968, 6(1), pp. 48–54. Also in M. H. Cooper,
A. J. Culyer (eds.) *Health Economics*, pp. 230–40 (33).

The paper examines the problem of choice of treatment for chronic kidney disease. It is concluded that kidney transplantation is the most effective way to increase life expectancy at given cost and is only slightly more expensive per case in present value terms than home dialysis, a treatment not practicable in all cases.

677   D. A. LE SOURD, M. E. FOGEL, D. R. JOHNSTON, *Benefit–Cost Analysis of Kidney Disease Programmes*
Washington D.C.: USDHEW, Public Health Service Publication No. 1941, 1968.

The study evaluates possible comprehensive kidney disease programmes (containing both curative and preventive elements). The costs and returns of two preventive and three treatment programmes are calculated. The study also examines the feasibility of regional nephrology programmes.

678   A. L. LEVIN, 'Cost-effectiveness in maternal and child health'
NEJM, May 9th, 1968, 278(19), pp. 1041–7.

The results of a cost-effectiveness analysis of maternal, infant and child health programmes are set out. The analysis proposed the 'general objective of making needed maternal and child health services available and accessible to all', and three subordinate objectives of reducing infant mortality, reducing unmet dental needs and reducing preventable handicapping conditions. Ten programmes are evaluated in terms of their success in meeting these objectives and their costs.

679   L. LIPWORTH, 'Estimating the need for facilities for renal dialysis'
PHR, August, 1968, 83(8), pp. 669–72.

An examination of the causes of death of persons aged 15–64 in San Francisco was used to estimate the number of persons who would benefit from long-term dialysis. It is estimated that there are 41 per million such persons aged 15–64, and 26 per million among all age groups (compared to Committee on Chronic Kidney Disease, 33 per million). Assuming an average survival of 5 years, this would eventually mean a total of 90 patients per million, or more than 10,000 persons in the U.S.A. who would benefit from long-term dialysis.

680   K. M. MCCAFFREE, 'The economic basis for the development of community mental health programmes'
MC, July–August, 1968, 6(4), pp. 286–99.

A comparison of the costs of mental health care in three institutions, two community oriented – day care treatment centre and psychiatric ward of a general hospital – the third a state mental hospital. The problems caused by dissimilarities in output in drawing firm conclusions from the analysis are discussed.

T. MᴄKᴇᴏᴡɴ (Chairman) *Screening in Medical Care*
London: Oxford University Press, for the Nuffield Provincial Hospitals Trust, 1968, pp. x, 173.

A collection of thirteen essays mainly concerned with assessing the medical effectiveness of screening procedures, although the paper by Pole deals specifically with the economic considerations in determining what screening programmes are put into effect.

1   T. McKeown, 'Validation of screening procedures', pp. 1–13.
2   J. M. G. Wilson, 'Bacteriuria in pregnancy', pp. 15–31.
3   C. R. Lowe, 'Breast cancer', pp. 33–41.
4   E. G. Knox, 'Cervical cancer', pp. 43–54.
5   E. G. Knox, 'Deafness in childhood', pp. 55–64.
6   W. J. H. Butterfield, 'Diabetes mellitus', pp. 65–80.
7   A. L. Cochrane, P. A. Graham, J. Wallace, 'Glaucoma', pp. 81–8.
8   A. L. Cochrane, P. C. Elwood, 'Iron deficiency anaemia', pp. 89–96.
9   J. M. G. Wilson, 'Evaluation of prescriptive screening for phenyl-ketonuria', pp. 97–115.
10   A. L. Cochrane, V. H. Springett, 'Pulmonary tuberculosis', pp. 117–22.
11   E. G. Knox, 'Rhesus haemolytic disease of the new born', pp. 123–40.
12   J. D. Pole, 'Economic aspects of screening for disease', pp. 141–58.
13   T. McKeown, E. G. Knox, 'The framework required for validation of prescriptive screening', pp. 159–73.
See 683.

A. H. Pᴀᴄᴋᴇʀ, 'Applying cost-effectiveness concepts to the community health system'
OR, March–April, 1968, 16(2), pp. 227–53.

The paper investigates the possibilities of planning the community health system using the techniques of systems analysis, model building and digital computer simulation, and approaches to measuring the output and the costs of treatment alternatives. See also A. H. Packer, G. D. Shellard, 'Measures of health-system effectiveness', *OR*, November–December, 1970, 18(6), pp. 1067–70.

J. D. Pᴏʟᴇ, 'Economic aspects of screening for disease'
In T. McKeown (Chairman) *Screening in Medical Care*, pp. 141–58 (681).

The first part of the paper considers the financial aspects of the screening programmes considered in the earlier chapters of this collection of essays. The second part of the paper considers the problems of carrying out cost–benefit analyses of screening programmes. Setting out the costs and benefits in a formal way is seen as a useful exercise even if all the items cannot be quantified.

684   W. F. SMITH, 'Cost-effectiveness and cost–benefit analyses for public health programmes'
PHR, November, 1968, 83(11), pp. 899–906.

An introduction to cost-effectiveness and cost–benefit analysis illustrated by reference to two studies carried out by the U.S. Department of Health, Education and Welfare; one study examined several ways of preventing motor accidents, the other study considered alternative treatments of kidney disease.

1969

685   R. AUSTER, I. LEVESON, D. SARACHEK, 'The production of health: an exploratory study'
JHR, Fall, 1969, 4(4), pp. 411–36. Also in V. R. Fuchs (ed.) *Essays in the Economics of Health and Medical Care*, pp. 135–58 (27).
See 49.

686   N. W. AXNICK, S. M. SHAVELL, J. J. WITTE, 'Benefits due to immunization against measles'
PHR, August, 1969, 84(8), pp. 673–80.

The total economic benefits of measles immunisation in the U.S.A., as measured by medical resources saved and working time saved, are calculated at $532 million for the years 1963–8; the total cost of the immunisation programme was $108 million.

687   R. W. CONLEY, 'A benefit–cost analysis of the vocational rehabilitation programme'
JHR, Spring, 1969, 4(1), pp. 226–52.

Extends earlier evaluation of the state–federal rehabilitation programme up to 1967 (R. W. Conley, *The Economics of Vocational Rehabilitation*, 1965). Estimates are made of the total increased lifetime earnings of more than 170,000 disabled workers assisted to obtain or retain productive employment in 1967. The benefits to the general taxpayer from the scheme are also calculated. From the point of view of increased lifetime earnings per dollar cost of the service, the most efficient allocation of resources appears to be towards the

most disabled and other least advantaged groups.
See 652, 1353.

G. E. HOGARTY, W. GUY, M. GROSS, G. GROSS, 'An evaluation of
community-based mental health programs: long-range effects'
MC, July–August, 1969, 7(4), pp. 271–80.

A comparison of the effects of a psychiatric day hospital and an outpatient
clinic. Patients were randomly assigned between the two facilities, evaluation
took place two and twelve months after treatment and a number of different
scales were used to assess patient improvement. For schizophrenic patients, day
hospital care appeared to be better, providing after-care facilities were utilised,
while for non-schizophrenics outpatient chemotherapy appeared to be as
effective and cheaper than day hospital treatment.

L. LIPWORTH, 'Cost effectiveness of a preventive program in renal disease'
MMFQ, July, 1969, 47, pp. 70–4.

Presents estimates of the costs of a national screening programme for kidney
disease among vulnerable groups in the U.S.A. (pregnant women, diabetics,
schoolgirls aged 6–9 years), the costs of treating detected cases and the number
of lives saved.

D. P. RICE, 'Measurement and application of illness costs'
PHR, February, 1969, 84(2), pp. 95–101.

Illness costs are measured as total direct expenditures plus indirect costs (the
discounted present value of future earnings lost with imputation of this value
for groups like housewives). Cost–benefit analysis of health care and the
difficulties and objections to the approach for measuring illness costs are then
discussed.

D. H. STIMSON, 'Utility measurement in public health decision-making'
MS, 1969, 16(2), pp. B-17–B-30.
See 865.

1970

D. B. AST, N. C. CONS, S. T. POLLARD, J. GARFINKEL, 'Time and cost
factors to provide regular, periodic dental care for children in a
fluoridated and non-fluoridated area: final report'
JADA, 1970, 80(4), pp. 770–6.

A report on a six-year study to compare dental care costs and chair time needed to provide dental care for children from age six years in fluoridated and non-fluoridated areas. The cost of dental care for children who drank fluoridated water from infancy was less than half that for those who did not.

693   M. BERKOWITZ, W. G. JOHNSON, 'Towards an economics of disability: the magnitude and structure of transfer and medical costs'
JHR, Summer, 1970, 5(3), pp. 271–97.
Transfer payments to the disabled, payments to survivors of the deceased, and medical costs, were used (with some adjustment to account for differences between size of transfers and the level of income the transfers were designed to replace) to provide a conservative estimate of the total costs of disability in the U.S.A. The estimated total loss was $43,000 million in 1967.
See 1355.

694   G. CALABRESI, *The Cost of Accidents: A Legal and Economic Analysis*
New Haven: Yale University Press, 1970, pp. 340.
Divided into five parts concerning: theoretical foundations of the law; techniques for reducing the costs of accidents; problems in reducing primary accident costs; the analysis of the 'fault system'; and justice and the 'fault system'. The objectives relate to reductions in both accidents and accident costs, the evaluation of costs and the assignment of liability.

695   A. J. CULYER, A. K. MAYNARD, 'The costs of dangerous drugs legislation in England and Wales'
MC, November–December, 1970, 8(6), pp. 501–9.
The study attempts to quantify the difference between the amounts of time needed to prescribe, obtain and use dangerous as opposed to non-dangerous drugs. The exercise indicated that if a non-dangerous drug with similar analgesic properties could replace dangerous drugs substantial resource savings could result.

696   J. A. DOWIE, 'Valuing the benefits of health improvement'
AEP, June, 1970, 9(14), pp. 21–41.
An examination of two particular issues in cost–benefit analysis: 'should the unconsumed production of the dead be deducted from the social loss of production incurred by their decease?' and 'do the so-called "intangible" costs of death, illness, and disability – pain, suffering, anxiety – constitute a separate element to be included in the cost–benefit analysis?' It is concluded that the first issue is resolved by careful specification of 'society', and in the second case it is suggested that only in the presence of market imperfections is it justifiable to include a separate element in addition to direct and indirect costs.

S. Fanshel, J. W. Bush, 'A health-status index and its application to health-service outcomes'
OR, November–December, 1970, 18(5), pp. 1021–66.
See 867.

G. R. Ford, 'Economic aspects of the treatment of varicose veins'
HT, 1970, 2(2), pp. 38–40.
Presents and discusses a variety of estimates of the treatment costs of varicose veins both by surgery and by injection compression therapy.

R. N. Grosse, 'Problems of resource allocation in health'
In R. H. Haveman, J. Margolis (eds.) *Public Expenditures and Policy Analysis*, Chicago: Markham Publishing Company, 1970, pp. 518–48.
The problems of achieving a better allocation of resources in health care are discussed. The development of programme budgeting, and the use of cost–benefit and cost–effectiveness analysis by the United States Department of Health, Education and Welfare are outlined, and studies carried out on screening for cancer, treatment of kidney disease and child health programmes are reviewed.

W. Malenbaum, 'Health and productivity in poor areas'
In H. E. Klarman (ed.) *Empirical Studies in Health Economics*, pp. 31–54 (18).
See 960.

P. R. A. May, 'Cost-efficiency of mental health delivery systems. 1. A review of the literature on hospital care'
AJPH, November, 1970, 60(11), pp. 2060–7.

P. R. A. May, 'Cost-effectiveness of mental health care. 2. Sex as a parameter of cost in the treatment of schizophrenia'
AJPH, December, 1970, 60(12), pp. 2269–72.

P. R. A. May, 'Cost-efficiency of mental health care. 3. Treatment method as a parameter of cost in the treatment of schizophrenia'
AJPH, January, 1971, 61(1), pp. 127–9.
The first paper reviewed and found wanting the literature on treatment costs; in particular there was no controlled research on the comparative costs of treating schizophrenic patients.

The second paper presents information, by sex, on the costs of different treatments, numbers of treatments given, length of stay and total cost per case, taken from a study of 288 first admission schizophrenic patients without significant prior treatment.

The third paper presents information on the costs and success of five treatment methods for schizophrenic patients.

702   P. NEWMAN, 'Malaria control and population growth'
JDS, January, 1970, 6(2), pp. 133–58.
See 962.

703   K. R. REINHARD, F. W. FELSMAN, L. F. MOODY, 'Time loss and in-direct economic costs caused by disease among Indians and Alaska natives. A comparison with the general U.S. population'
PHR, May, 1970, 85(5), pp. 397–411.

Estimates are made of the size of the disparity between the minority groups and the general population by comparing life expectancy and morbidity patterns. An estimate is also made of earnings loss as a result of morbidity and premature mortality.

704   G. W. TORRANCE, *A Generalized Cost-Effectiveness Model for the Evaluation of Health Programmes*
Hamilton, Ontario: Faculty of Business, McMaster University, Research Series No. 101, 1970.
See 871.

705   W. D. WOOD, H. F. CAMPBELL, *Cost–Benefit Analysis and the Economics of Investment in Human Resources – An Annotated Bibliography*
Kingston, Ontario: Industrial Relations Centre, Queen's University, 1970, pp. viii, 211.
See 1482.

1971

706   R. BROOKS, 'A cost–benefit analysis of the treatment of rheumatic diseases'
AE, 1971, 3(1), pp. 35–53.

The study is a cost–benefit analysis of treatment by surgery of patients with rheumatic disease. The costs in the calculation are medical costs; the benefits are measured as the discounted present value of future earnings of those who returned to work, with an imputed value for housewives. In the absence of a controlled clinical trial it was assumed that any observed return to work was a result of the treatment. No other treatment alternative is considered in the analysis. See also R. Brooks in *Annals of Rheumatic Disease*, November, 1969, pp. 655–61, and R. Brooks, W. W. Buchanan, *HB*, April, 1970, 28(2), pp. 42–3.

J. W. BUSH, M. M. CHEN, J. ZAREMBA, 'Estimating health programme outcomes using a Markov equilibrium analysis of disease development' *AJPH*, December, 1971, 61(12), pp. 2362–75.
See 875.

R. W. CHORBA, J. L. SANDERS, 'Planning models for tuberculosis control programmes'
HSR, Summer, 1971, 6(2), pp. 144–64.

A simulation model of tuberculosis is presented, with sub-models for different types of preventive intervention. Four simulations for different levels of disease prevalence are carried out to determine the cost-effective strategies for control in different situations. In low and moderate prevalence situations mass screening is difficult to justify; at high levels rescreening appeared to be justified.

A. L. COCHRANE, W. W. HOLLAND, 'Validation of screening procedures'
BMB, January, 1971, 27(1), pp. 3–8.

Existing screening methods are divided into three categories: conditions for which tests are acceptable, conditions for which there is insufficient evidence to justify routine tests, and conditions for which there may be some benefit from the use of tests. The value of a screening test, it is suggested, may be assessed according to seven criteria: simplicity, acceptability, accuracy, cost, precision, sensitivity and specificity. The last three criteria are discussed at some length.

A. J. CULYER, R. J. LAVERS, A. WILLIAMS, 'Social indicators: health'
ST, 1971, 2, pp. 31–42.
See 877.

R. FEIN, 'On measuring economic benefits of health programmes'
In G. McLachlan, T. McKeown (eds.) *Medical History and Medical Care*, London: Oxford University Press, 1971, pp. 181–220.

The first part of the paper reviews the development of human capital theory from the work of Sir William Petty to the rate of return studies carried out in the 1960s. The second part of the paper considers some of the particularly troublesome problems in the area of benefit measurement.

712   J. T. GENTRY, 'The planning of community health services: facilitating rational decision making'
Inquiry, September, 1971, 8(3), pp. 4–21.
See 1396.

713   B. GRAB, B. CVJETANOVIC, 'Simple method for rough determination of the cost–benefit balance point of immunization programmes'
WHO Bulletin, 1971, 45(4), pp. 536–41.
An illustration of the construction of nomograms for determining the cost–benefit balance point for immunisation programmes. The costs are taken to be the costs of vaccination programmes; the benefits are the costs of treating people who without vaccination would have become sick that are saved.

714   A. W. GROGONO, D. J. WOODGATE, 'Index for measuring health'
Lancet, November 6th, 1971, pp. 1024–6.
See 878.

715   P. R. A. MAY, 'Cost efficiency of treatments for the schizophrenic patient'
AJP, April, 1971, 127(10), pp. 1382–5.
The service costs of five alternative treatment regimes are calculated. For most schizophrenic patients, milieu care, in the absence of additional treatment, was found to be both expensive and relatively ineffective.

716   F. C. MENZ, 'Economics of disease prevention: infectious kidney disease'
Inquiry, December, 1971, 8(4), pp. 3–18.
The problems of carrying out a cost–benefit analysis of infectious kidney disease prevention programmes are examined, and an illustrative hypothetical calculation of costs and benefits is carried out.

717   D. R. MEYER, 'Disability equivalences: a logic system for comparison of alternate health programmes'
AJPH, August, 1971, 61(8), pp. 1514–17.
See 880.

718   W. B. NEENAN, 'Distribution and efficiency in benefit–cost analysis'
CJE, May, 1971, 4(2), pp. 216–24.
An evaluation of an X-ray tuberculosis screening programme in Michigan. The major part of the article is devoted to discovering the implicit distributional objectives of the programme by geographical area and by race; these distributional

weights being calculated on the assumption that any deviation from the efficiency maximisation criteria is redistributional.

J. ORTIZ, R. PARKER, 'A birth–life–death model for planning and evaluation of health service programmes'
HSR, Summer, 1971, 6(2), pp. 120–43.
A Markovian model of the birth–life–death process is constructed in which probabilities of death from various causes in each age group and specific fertility rates for each age interval are set out. By simulation it is possible to examine the effect of various programmes that have an impact on mortality and fertility.

J. D. POLE, 'Mass radiography: a cost–benefit approach'
In G. McLachlan (ed.) *Problems and Progress in Medical Care, Fifth Series*, pp. 45–56 (24).
An application of cost–benefit analysis to a screening technique for which good data exist on the detection of cases of tuberculosis, success of treatment and prevention of secondary cases. The results of the analysis support the decision to abandon mass screening for pulmonary tuberculosis in the United Kingdom. *See 748.*

D. ROBINSON, 'Cost and effectiveness of a program to prevent rheumatic fever'
HSMHA Health Rep., April, 1971, 86(4), pp. 385–9.
A study of the Massachusetts throat culture programme to prevent rheumatic fever. Information is presented on the extent of the medical problem, the cost per prevented case of acute rheumatic fever and the utilisation of the service by different income groups and different types of community.

C. T. STEWART, 'Allocation of resources to health'
JHR, Winter, 1971, 6(1), pp. 104–22.
See 965.

V. VIKRAMAN, O. SETH, 'Programme for control of pulmonary T.B. in India 1971–80. A cost–benefit analysis'
Indian J. Tuberc., 1971, 18(3), pp. 73–83.
An estimate is presented of the total monetary loss resulting from premature mortality and morbidity caused by pulmonary tuberculosis. The costs and benefits of a more limited control programme are then calculated. The benefits are measured as the gains in years of productivity activity resulting from reduced mortality and morbidity, valued at average earnings.

724   B. A. WEISBROD, 'Costs and benefits of medical research: a case study of poliomyelitis'
JPE, May–June, 1971, 79(3), pp. 527–44.

The study involves a calculation of the rate of return to the research effort that led to the development of vaccines against poliomyelitis. Calculated in the study are the time streams of research expenditures, the time streams of benefits resulting from application of the knowledge (the reduction in productive effort lost and medical costs of victims of polio), and the costs of the vaccination programme. In the case of polio the rate of return was high and was found to be heavily influenced by the costs of application of the findings. The paper closes with a discussion of the likely allocative efficiency of the private market when a collective-consumption good requires the use of an individual-consumption good (vaccination) for its application.

725   J. M. G. WILSON, 'Screening in the early detection of disease'
In G. McLachlan (ed.) *Portfolio for Health, Problems and Progress in Medical Care, Essays on Current Research, Sixth Series*, pp. 47–59 (25).

The paper considers the problems of screening for cancer of the cervix, diabetes, chronic glaucoma, asymptomatic bacteriuria, and phenylketonuria. The questions of whom to screen and how to do the screening, and the need to carry out cost-effectiveness studies and the problems facing such studies are also discussed.

1972

726   B. ABEL-SMITH, 'Health priorities in developing countries: the economist's contribution'
IJHS, February, 1972, 2(1), pp. 5–12.

With no acceptable measure of health output, complex health planning models and systems such as programme budgeting cannot be used in developing countries. The greatest contribution the economist can make to health planning is in cost-effectiveness studies.

727   D. M. BELLANTE, 'A multivariate analysis of a vocational rehabilitation programme'
JHR, Spring, 1972, 7(2), pp. 226–41.

Estimates are made of cost–benefit ratios of rehabilitation of various sub-groups of the disabled population. The conclusion of Conley (*JHR*, Spring, 1969) that it may be desirable in terms of economic efficiency to rehabilitate uneducated, middle aged, non-white and other less productive groups is tested

and is substantially contradicted; only the conclusion about non-whites is verified. With the exception of race, the variables studied bear about the same type of relationship to rehabilitation outcome as they do to earnings in the general labour market. The benefit–cost ratios do indicate, however, the desirability of expanding investment in rehabilitation for all groups.
See 687.

J. W. BUSH, S. FANSHEL, M. M. CHEN, 'Analysis of a tuberculin testing programme using a health status index'
Soc.-Econ.Plan.Sciences, 1972, 6(1), pp. 49–68.
See 884.

A. L. COCHRANE, 'The history of the measurement of ill-health'
IJE, June, 1972, 1(2), pp. 89–93.
See 876.

A. L. COCHRANE, *Effectiveness and Efficiency: Random Reflections on Health Services*
London: The Nuffield Provincial Hospitals Trust, 1972, pp. xii, 92.

It is argued that cost–benefit analysis of health services is not yet feasible and that two preliminary steps are necessary before it can become a practical possibility. The two preliminary steps are the main subject of the monograph. The first step is to measure medical effectiveness (the effect of a medical action), and the appropriate approach to this problem is the randomised controlled trial. The second step is to achieve optimal use of personnel and materials to achieve levels of effectiveness comparable to those achieved in controlled trials (efficiency). In addition to the main theme the monograph contains a chapter examining the relationship between changing inputs to the British National Health Service and changing mortality and morbidity patterns, and a chapter on inequality in the health services, both regional inequality and inequality between social classes in access to services.

E. J. COHN, 'Assessment of malaria eradication: costs and benefits'
AJTMH, September, 1972, 21(5), pp. 663–7.

The need for discounting the costs and benefits of disease control programme is discussed with reference to the Indian choice of an eradication rather than a control programme. Assessment of the costs and benefits of malaria eradication suggests that the output increases from a population free from disease may be offset in terms of its effect on development by increased population growth.
See 967.

732   A. J. Culyer, R. J. Lavers, A. Williams, 'Health indicators'
In A. Shonfield, S. Shaw (eds.) *Social Indicators and Social Policy*,
London: Heinemann Educational Books, for the Social Science
Research Council, 1972, pp. 94–118.
See 877.

733   L. Dickinson, 'Evaluation of the effectiveness of cytologic screening for
cervical cancer. III Cost–benefit analysis'
Mayo Clin.Proc., August, 1972, 47(8), pp. 550–5.
The costs and benefits of a screening programme are estimated. Benefits are
measured as the increased years of life expectancy; costs are measured as the
costs of screening and treatment, minus the income tax on additional earnings
resulting from extended life, minus the additional costs of treating those who
are unscreened.

734   S. Enke, R. A. Brown, 'Economic worth of preventing death at different
ages in developing countries'
J.Biosoc.Sci., July, 1972, 4(3), pp. 299–306.
See 969.

735   S. Fanshel, 'A meaningful measure of health for epidemiology'
IJE, 1972, 1(4), pp. 319–37.
See 888.

736   D. A. T. Griffiths, 'Economic evaluation in the health services'
ASBMT, 1972, 52(3), pp. 215–34.
Shows that economic evaluation cannot rely on market rules in the health
sphere and proceeds, with illustrations, to show the kinds of question concerning costs and outcomes that economists can usefully ask and, sometimes,
answer.

737   R. N. Grosse, 'Cost–benefit analysis of health service'
AAAPSS, January, 1972, 399, pp. 89–99.
Two studies carried out by the U.S. Department of Health, Education and
Welfare are reviewed, the first concerned with disease control programmes,
particularly control of various types of cancer, the second concerned with
maternal and child health programmes.

J. HALPERN, P. R. BINNER, 'A model for an output value analysis of mental health programmes'
AMH, Winter, 1972, pp. 40–51.

J. A. KING, C. G. SMITH, 'The treatment milieu and prediction of mental hospital effectiveness'
JHSB, June, 1972, 13(2), pp. 180–94.
See 894.

D. KODLIN, 'A note on the cost–benefit problem in screening for breast cancer'
Meth.Inform.Med., 1972, 11(4), pp. 242–7.

W. A. LAING, *The Costs and Benefits of Family Planning*
London: Political and Economic Planning, Broadsheet 534, February, 1972, pp. ii, 23.
The study examines the extra demand for health and welfare services likely to be made by various groups of 'unwanted' children over the 16–18 years of their dependency (services like education are not included). The total costs of excess usage are compared with the estimated cost of family planning per prevented birth in order to derive cost–benefit ratios.

R. J. LAVERS, 'The implicit valuation of forms of hospital treatment'
In M. M. Hauser (ed.) *The Economics of Medical Care*, pp. 190–205.
See 481.

M. S. LEVITT, 'Problems of efficiency'
In M. M. Hauser (ed.) *The Economics of Medical Care*, pp. 33–41.
See 1032.

G. L. MADDOX, 'Interventions and outcomes: notes on designing and implementing an experiment in health care'
IJE, 1972, 1(4), pp. 339–45.
See 896.

S. MAIDLOW, H. BERMAN, 'The economics of heroin treatment'
AJPH, October, 1972, 62(10), pp. 1397–406.
An analysis is provided of heroin treatment alternatives. A cost–benefit

analysis is carried out comparing residential therapeutic communities and drug substitution (methadone maintenance). On economic grounds methadone maintenance appeared the better treatment choice.

746   D. PIACHAUD, J. M. WEDDELL, 'The economics of treating varicose veins' *IJE*, 1972, 1(3), pp. 287–94.

A comparison of treatment of varicose veins by surgery with treatment by injection–compression sclerotherapy. The output of treatment was assumed to be the same for both methods (on the basis of a clinical trial). The costs of surgical treatment were, however, significantly higher both in health service costs and in loss of earnings resulting from surgical patients being away from work for a longer period.
See 747.

747   D. PIACHAUD, J. M. WEDDELL, 'Cost of treating varicose veins' *Lancet*, December 2nd, 1972, pp. 1191–2.
See 746.

748   J. D. POLE, 'The economics of mass radiography' In M. M. Hauser (ed.) *The Economics of Medical Care*, pp. 105–14 (28).

A discussion of the economic techniques required for evaluating a screening programme. The costs and benefits that should be considered are enumerated. The case of screening for pulmonary tuberculosis is examined but quantitative results are not presented. See also the comment by J. R. Shannon pp. 115–18.
See 720.

749   B. M. POPKIN, 'Economic benefits from the elimination of hunger in America' *PP*, Winter, 1972, 20(1), pp. 133–53.

The total benefits that would result from the elimination of malnutrition in the U.S.A., measured as the additions to the present value of the lifetime earnings of the poor population resulting from improved educational achievement, worker productivity, greater resistance to disease, reduced premature mortality and intergenerational effects, are calculated to be worth $14–50,000 million.

750   P. C. REYNELL, M. C. REYNELL, 'The cost–benefit analysis of a coronary care unit' *BHJ*, 1972, 34, pp. 897–900.

The study calculates the costs per life saved (survival to leave hospital) in a five-bedded coronary care unit. The costs calculated are of two types: the costs of the unit (direct cost), and cost resulting from a changing pattern of care, in particular the admission of patients who would otherwise have been treated at home.

R. M. ROSSER, V. C. WATTS, 'The measurement of hospital output'
IJE, December, 1972, 1(4), pp. 361–7.
See 897.

J. SCHNEIDER, L. B. TWIGGS, 'The costs of carcinoma of the cervix'
OG, December, 1972, 40(6), pp. 851–9.
Literature relevant to estimating the medical cost of carcinoma of the cervix is surveyed, and tentative cost estimates are put forward for screening programmes and the costs of treatment of the cases detected by them.

G. TEELING-SMITH, 'Health, wealth, and happiness'
SEA, May, 1972, 6(2), pp. 135–48.
An outline is provided of the way medical decision-taking and patient expectations, and the interaction between them, may act to frustrate rational allocation of resources. The evaluation of existing services using randomised control trials is regarded as a necessary step in obtaining an efficient allocation of resources.

G. TEELING-SMITH, 'A cost–benefit approach to medical care'
In M. M. Hauser (ed.) *The Economics of Medical Care*, pp. 146–58 (28).
A survey of cost–benefit studies undertaken by the Office of Health Economics. It is concluded that there are few cases where therapeutic progress has yielded great economic savings and it is even more difficult to find cases in clinical preventive medicine (diphtheria is one exception). It is also concluded that most screening for presymptomatic diagnosis appears to be of limited value, largely because the benefits of early diagnosis have not yet been established. See also the comment by J. Wiseman, pp. 159–61.

G. W. TORRANCE, W. H. THOMAS, D. L. SACKETT, 'A utility maximisation model for evaluation of health care programmes'
HSR, Summer, 1972, 7(2), pp. 118–33.
See 899.

C. UPTON, W. SILVERMAN, 'The demand for dental services'
JHR, Spring, 1972, 7(2), pp. 250–61.
Estimates are presented of the direct costs of fluoridating the public water supply and of the reduction in dental bills expected from fluoridation. The

estimates are made for a hypothetical town of one million population with the same age distribution as that projected for the whole population of U.S.A. in 1975.

757   R. WAGER, *Care of the Elderly – an Exercise in Cost–Benefit Analysis*
London: Institute of Municipal Treasurers and Accountants, 1972, p. 74.

A study comparing institutional care with domiciliary care of the elderly in which every attempt is made to estimate real resource costs to the community rather than just financial costs. A major element in the study is the construction of an 'index of incapacity' – clients score points for fourteen components relating to sensory perception, intellectual processes, personal care, physical mobility and domestic duties, and on the basis of these points are classified according to five grades of incapacity.

758   J. E. WEINRICH, 'Direct economic costs of deafness in the United States'
American Annals of the Deaf, August, 1972, pp. 446–54.

An estimate is made of the expected loss in lifetime earnings for a person born deaf or who becomes deaf before acquiring the power of speech. The method used involves comparison of the educational attainments of the deaf population with those of the non-deaf population.

1973

759   B. ABEL-SMITH, B. BENJAMIN, W. W. HOLLAND, J. W. PEARSON, D. F. PIACHAUD, O. GOLDSMITH, J. D. POLE, *Accounting for Health*
London: King Edward's Hospital Fund, 1973, p. 63.
See 32.

760   J. R. ASHFORD, G. FERSTER, D. M. MAKUC, 'An approach to resource allocation in the reorganised National Health service'
In G. McLachlan (ed.) *The Future – and Present Indicatives, Problems and Progress in Medical Care, Essays on Current Research, Ninth Series*, pp. 57–90.
See 1412.

761   A. B. ATKINSON, J. L. SKEGG, 'Anti-smoking publicity and the demand for tobacco in the U.K.'
Man. School, September, 1973, 41(3), pp. 265–82.

Econometric analysis suggested that publicity had a small effect on the number of cigarettes consumed – a sudden fall in consumption was followed by a gradual return towards the previous level of consumption, the eventual fall being small and accounted for entirely by male smokers. There has, however, been a downward trend in the weight of tobacco consumed. The price elasticity of demand was found to be low.

J. H. BABSON, *Disease Costing*
Manchester: University Press, 1973, pp. viii, 151.

Data generated by hospital costing systems are used to estimate the cost of individual cases; these costs are then aggregated by diagnostic category. A preliminary study attempts to cost two diagnoses, appendicitis and inguinal hernia. The results lend support to the view that costs of specific illnesses provide an indication of the overall costliness of a hospital. The technique is then used to examine the cost of treating cases of inguinal hernia and varicose veins, in a day care unit and as inpatients in the same hospital, and to estimate the cost of four types of maternity confinement.

An earlier outline of some parts of this study is provided in J. H. Babson, 'Hospital costing in Great Britain', *The Hospital*, April, 1971, 67(4), pp. 106–11.

R. L. BERG, 'Establishing the values of various conditions of life for a health status index'
In R. L. Berg (ed.) *Health Status Indexes*, pp. 120–7.
See 905.

A. BLUMSTEIN, R. G. CASSIDY, 'Benefit–cost analysis of family planning'
Soc.–Econ.Plan.Sciences, April, 1973, 7(2), pp. 151–60.

An introduction to cost–benefit analysis of family planning. A model is presented for the evaluation of alternative family planning programmes by weighing the programme costs against the benefits of unwanted births. Long range effects are considered using a sequential application of a dynamic model.

D. B. BROWN, 'Cost/benefit of safety investments using fault tree analysis'
J.Saf.Res., June, 1973, 5(2), pp. 73–81.

The use of fault tree analysis in achieving an efficient allocation of resources available for safety measures is outlined. The technique allows quantification of the effect of a particular safety measure in reducing the probability of an undesirable event.

J. W. BUSH, M. M. CHEN, D. L. PATRICK, 'Health status index in cost effectiveness: analysis of a PKU programme'
In R. L. Berg (ed.) *Health Status Indexes*, pp. 172–94.
See 908.

767 C. L. CHIANG, R. D. COHEN, 'How to measure health: a stochastic model for an index of health'
IJE, March, 1973, 2(1), pp. 7–13.
See 910.

768 E. J. COHN, 'Assessing the costs and benefits of anti-malaria programmes: the Indian experience'
AJPH, December, 1973, 63(12), pp. 1086–96.
Detailed estimates are provided of the costs of the Indian eradication programme. The benefits from the programme are difficult if not impossible to quantify, and as the programme benefits have already been almost completely exhausted a retrospective effort to value them is not worthwhile. The conceptual issues underlying benefit measurement are however discussed. At any reasonable discount rate it is concluded that there is very little difference between eradication and control programmes from the point of view of cost.

769 R. W. CONLEY, *The Economics of Mental Retardation*
Baltimore: The Johns Hopkins Press, 1973, pp. xiii, 377.
An extensive review of the problems of mental retardation. The study examines the epidemiology and etiology of retardation, programmes for the mentally retarded in the United States and the effects of retardation, particularly the effect on earnings. The sixth chapter of the book is a benefit–cost analysis of mental retardation programmes and contains a long discussion of the problems and limitations of the analysis. The final chapter deals with improving services for the mentally retarded, determining the size and scope of programmes and deciding on the balance of types of employment (sheltered or market) and types of accommodation (sheltered or institutional) for the retarded.
See 652.

770 G. N. DAVIES, 'Fluoride in the prevention of dental caries: a tentative cost–benefit analysis'
BDJ, July 17th, August 7th, August 21st, September 4th, September 18th, October 2nd, 1973.
This series of papers begins by reviewing several fluoridation trials and goes on to carry out cost-effectiveness and cost–benefit studies of fluoridation. A comparison of the costs of implementing a scheme for the fluoridation of school water supplies with the savings in dental treatment costs yielded cost–benefit ratios of 1:15.4 for the United States, and 1:6.0 for the United Kingdom.

771 M. S. FELDSTEIN, M. A. PIOT, T. K. SUNDARESAN, *Resource Allocation Model for Public Health Planning: A Case Study of Tuberculosis Control*

Geneva: World Health Organisation, 1973, p. 110.

A pioneering cost–benefit analysis of tuberculosis control integrating epidemiological and economic analysis and data. The analysis is applied in a case study of the Republic of Korea. Output concepts used include years of temporary disability avoided, permanent impairment avoided and deaths averted.

B. E. FORST, 'Quantifying the patient's preferences'
In R. L. Berg (ed.) *Health Status Indexes*, pp. 209–21.
See 913.

N. J. GLASS, 'Cost–benefit analysis and health services'
HT, August, 1973, 5, pp. 51–6.

A survey of the application of cost–benefit and cost-effectiveness analysis in the health field. Studies of a wide variety of health problems are examined.

P. F. GRINER, 'Medical intensive care in the teaching hospital: costs versus benefits: the need for an assessment'
Ann.Intern.Med., 1973, 78(4), pp. 581–5.

Sketches the problems of carrying out a cost–benefit analysis of medical care, the information available and that needed. The problems are particularly acute in a teaching hospital where the impact is not only on the health of patients treated but also on teaching and research.

J. E. GROGAN, M. C. SMITH, 'The economic cost of ulcerative colitis: a notional estimate for 1968'
Inquiry, June, 1973, 10(2), pp. 61–8.

The total costs of the disease for the United States in 1968 were calculated to be $216.1 million, of which the direct medical costs constituted $67.4 million.

C. HIMATSINGANI, 'Approaches to health and personal social services planning in the National Health Service and the place of health indices'
IJE, March, 1973, 2(1), pp. 15–21.
See 917.

A. G. HOLTMANN, 'On the optimal timing of research expenditures'
Inquiry, March, 1973, 10(1), pp. 47–9.

Examines the level and time pattern of research expenditures on polio and suggests that acceleration would probably have been worthwhile. The exercise suggests simulation to determine whether it is justifiable to increase expenditure to speed up research in any particular area.

778   A. G. HOLTMANN, 'The size and distribution of benefits from U.S. medical research: the case of eliminating cancer and heart disease'
PF, 1973, 28(3–4), pp. 354–61.
Estimates of the benefits from reducing the probability of death from cancer and heart disease are made from data on the present value of future earnings of white and black males.

779   N. P. KNEPPRETH, D. H. GUSTAFSON, J. H. ROSE, R. P. LEIFER, 'Techniques for the assessment of worth'
In R. L. Berg (ed.) *Health Status Indexes*, pp. 228–38.
See 920.

780   E. G. KNOX, 'A simulation system for screening procedures'
In G. McLachlan (ed.) *The Future – and Present Indicatives, Problems and Progress in Medical Care, Essays on Current Research, Ninth Series*, pp. 17–55 (38).

781   G. L. MARTIN, I. M. NEWMAN, 'Costs and effects of a student health-aide programme'
JACHA, February, 1973, 21, pp. 237–40.
Information is provided on the University of Nebraska's programme using students trained as health aides to reduce pressure on the University health centre. The costs of the programme, the number and type of cases treated, the number of cases referred to the medical centre and the amount of medical resources at the health centre saved by the programme, are outlined.

782   D. L. PATRICK, J. W. BUSH, M. M. CHEN, 'Methods for measuring levels of well-being for a health status index'
HSR, Fall, 1973, 8(3), pp. 228–45.
See 927.

783   J. D. POLE, 'The use of outcome measures in health service planning'
IJE, 1973, 2(1), pp. 23–30.
See 928.

784   H. S. RUCHLIN, D. C. ROGERS, *Economics and Health Care*
Springfield, Illinois: Charles C. Thomas Publisher, 1973, pp. xvii, 317.
See 39.

K. C. STEINER, H. A. SMITH, 'Application of cost–benefit analysis to a
PKU screening programme'
Inquiry, December, 1973, 10(4), pp. 34–40.
Making fairly standard assumptions (average instead of marginal costs, using
forgone earnings as a measure of potential benefit) it is calculated that the
benefit–cost ratio for a phenylketonuria screening programme for Mississippi is
in excess of 1.37.

J. H. STEWART, N. D. TOPP, S. MARTIN, E. SCHAWROWAS, Y. FLAUS,
G. R. SHIEL, J. F. MAHONY, 'The costs of domiciliary maintenance haemo-
dialysis. A comparison with alternative renal replacement regimes'
MJA, January 27th, 1973, pp. 156–9.
A comparison of the medical care costs of home and hospital fibre and Kiil
dialysis, and cadaveric renal transplantation. In Australia, home dialysis was
not markedly more expensive than alternative treatment regimens.

G. W. TORRANCE, D. L. SACKETT, W. H. THOMAS, 'Utility maximization
model for programme evaluation: a demonstration application'
In R. L. Berg (ed.) *Health Status Indexes*, pp. 156–65.
See 933.

J. F. WEBB, R. S. KHAZEN, *et al.*, 'PKU screening – is it worth it?'
CMAJ, February 3rd, 1973, 108, pp. 328–9.
A consideration of Ontario's programme for PKU screening of newborn
infants. A comparison is made of the costs of detecting PKU and treating it and
the costs of institutionalising a severely retarded child for life.

B. A. WEISBROD, R. L. ANDREANO, R. E. BALDWIN, A. C. KELLEY,
E. H. EPSTEIN, *Disease and Economic Development: the Impact of Parasitic
Diseases in St. Lucia*
Madison, Wisconsin: University of Wisconsin Press, 1973.
See 978.

1974

R. L. AKEHURST, 'Regulating the use of asbestos'
In D. S. Lees, S. Shaw (eds.) *Impairment, Disability, and Handicap*, pp.
81–93 (809).
The paper discusses the information on costs and benefits needed to evaluate

the regulations introduced in the United Kingdom in 1970 to control the use of asbestos.
See 791, 1365.

791   R. L. AKEHURST, 'Optimal control of disease-inducing work conditions'
In A. J. Culyer (ed.) *Economic Policies and Social Goals*, pp. 199–215 (41).

Discusses the problems in measuring the costs of controlling industrial diseases and the benefits from so doing.
See 790, 1365.

792   A. B. ATKINSON, 'Smoking and the economics of government intervention'
In M. Perlman (ed.) *The Economics of Health and Medical Care*, pp. 428–41 (44).

The welfare economic implications of government intervention to reduce smoking are explored in the light of a model of individual smoking behaviour. The choice between taxation and health education as a means of reducing smoking is considered, and it is shown that there is a point beyond which further information on the effects of smoking is undesirable, even if it can be provided at zero costs to the smoking population.
See 1359.

793   A. B. ATKINSON, T. W. MEADE, 'Methods and preliminary findings in assessing the economic and health services consequences of smoking, with particular reference to lung cancer'
JRSS A, 1974, 137(3), pp. 297–312, 333–46.

A framework for considering the economic and health services consequences of smoking is outlined. Detailed consideration is given to the medical care costs, and the information available and that needed for their quantification is discussed.

794   R. E. BALDWIN, B. A. WEISBROD, 'Disease and labor productivity'
EDCC, April, 1974, 22(3), pp. 414–35.
See 978.

795   D. F. BERGWALL, P. N. REEVES, N. B. WOODSIDE, *Introduction to Health Planning*
Washington D.C.: Information Resources Press, 1974, pp. vii, 231.

A chapter providing an introduction to cost–benefit and cost-effectiveness analysis is included.
See 1418.

M. Berkowitz, W. G. Johnson, 'Health and labor force participation'
JHR, Winter, 1974, 9(1), pp. 117–128.
See 979.

N. H. Bryant, L. Candland, R. Loewenstein, 'Comparison of care and cost outcomes for stroke patients with and without home care'
Stroke, January–February, 1974, 5, pp. 54–9.

E. D. Charles, J. G. Van Matre, J. M. Miller, 'Spinal cord injury— a cost–benefit analysis of alternative treatment modals'
Paraplegia, 1974, 12(3), pp. 222–31.
A brief report of a project evaluating a special treatment centre for patients with spinal cord injury. A preliminary cost–benefit analysis using only reduced medical costs as a measure of benefit is presented in the paper.

A. J. Cheadle, R. Morgan, 'The economics of rehabilitation'
BJP, 1974, 125, pp. 193–201.
The study measures the direct cost of a psychiatric rehabilitation service for long-stay patients by studying a rehabilitation unit's first 200 consecutively admitted patients and their careers over the years 1961–70. The study also details the tax and insurance contributions of those patients successfully resettled in the community. The study concentrates on measurement of financial flows including transfers, rather than real resource costs.

J. E. Cohen, 'Potential economic benefits of eliminating mortality attributed to schistosomiasis in Zanzibar'
SSM, July, 1974, 8(7), pp. 383–98.
An estimate is made of the potential economic benefits to males in Zanzibar in 1960 of eliminating mortality due to urinary schistosomiasis. The measurement of benefit is the increase in output due to the extension of working lives. Separate estimates are made of the benefits from curative and preventive programmes.

A. J. Culyer, 'Economics, social policy and disability'
In D. S. Lees, S. Shaw (eds.) *Impairment, Disability and Handicap*, pp. 17–29 (809).

A paper intended to introduce the non-economist to the economist's approach to health and welfare problems. The paper discusses the underlying rationale of cost–benefit analysis and approaches to compensating the disabled.

802   R. F. F. DAWSON, 'The cost of human impairment from road accidents'
In D. S. Lees, S. Shaw (eds.) *Impairment, Disability and Handicap*, pp. 94–105 (809).

The paper discusses earlier work by the Road Research Laboratory on measurement of the cost of road accidents, other possible approaches to the valuation of life, and some possible ways of reducing impairment in road accidents.
See 827, 833.

803   K. DUNNELL, L. IDE, 'An attempt to assess the cost of home care'
In D. S. Lees, S. Shaw (eds.) *Impairment, Disability and Handicap*, pp. 106–22 (809).

A study to compare the costs of caring for responauts (individuals requiring regular mechanical respiratory support) at home as opposed to care in a hospital or care in a Cheshire Home (charitably supported homes for the disabled). The study dealt with a sample of only eighteen patients; those in the Cheshire Home were in the least disabled group of the patients considered.

804   P. J. FITZPATRICK, 'Cost-effectiveness in cancer'
CMAJ, October 5th, 1974, 111(2), pp. 652–8.

805   E. T. FUJII, 'Public investment in the rehabilitation of heroin addicts'
SSQ, June, 1974, 55(1), pp. 39–51.

The four major programmes in the United States dealing with the heroin problem – detoxification, civil commitment, imprisonment and parole, and methadone maintenance – are evaluated. By any set of assumptions about crime, discount rate, or age group, methadone maintenance is the preferred treatment. Methadone maintenance is then compared to heroin maintenance and heroin legalisation. If it were possible to change the laws, heroin maintenance is the preferred alternative. It is also concluded that with the current market structure activities further to reduce the supply of heroin would be socially very costly.

806   N. J. GLASS, I. T. RUSSELL, 'Cost–benefit analysis in the health service: a case study of elective herniorrhaphy'
BJPSM, February, 1974, 28(1), p. 68.

An outline of a paper presented at the Society for Social Medicine, Annual

Meeting, 1973. The paper evaluates a proposal for a national policy to develop specialist units for elective herniorrhaphy.

F. L. GOLLADAY, 'Patient participation and productivity in the medical care sector'
In J. Rafferty (ed.) *Health Manpower and Productivity*, pp. 85–105 (329).
Reviews literature on the contribution of the patient to the delivery of health care. This includes work on preventive medicine, compliance with prescribed medical treatments, utilisation of health services and health educational activities.

H. E. KLARMAN, 'Application of cost–benefit analysis to the health services and the special case of technologic innovation'
IJHS, Spring, 1974, 4(2), pp. 325–52.
A review of the state of the art in health cost–benefit and cost-effectiveness analysis. The paper examines completed studies in which 'both the benefits and costs of specified programmes are measured and valued simultaneously, with their respective present values juxtaposed and compared', which leaves only a fairly short list of studies. The paper then goes on to examine the way in which changes in technology affect costs and benefits of health services and in particular to consider capital investment in hospitals and automated multiphasic screening. The paper closes with a discussion of the barriers to systematic analysis of expenditures for health systems technology and the prospects of overcoming these barriers. An excellent bibliography is provided.

D. S. LEES, S. SHAW (eds.) *Impairment, Disability and Handicap*
London: Heinemann Educational Books Ltd., 1974.
The nine papers in the volume were written as contributions to a working conference on 'The Cost of Human Impairment'. The first three papers deal with the general issues underlying the economic and legal approaches to the problems of costing impairment and disability and to compensating those who suffer physical damage. The final six papers are detailed studies that attempt to measure the costs of impairment in a variety of different settings.
See 790, 801, 802, 803, 813, 837, 937, 942, 1368.

A. MAYNARD, R. TINGLE, 'The mental health services: a review of the statistical sources, and a critical assessment of their usefulness'
BJP, April, 1974, 124, pp. 317–26.
A review of the available data sources on the British mental health services. The rationale of data collection and publication is examined, and it is concluded

that the available statistics are inadequate for evaluation of the limited objectives for mental health provision fixed so far, let alone to meet the needs of the radical reforms of the services that are planned.

811   M. PAGLIN, 'Public health and development: a new analytical framework' *EC*, November, 1974, 41(4), pp. 432–41.

Presents a model for evaluating public health programmes that integrates consumer gains in the form of increased life expectancy with the investment gains in the form of increases in output (which have usually formed the sole basis for the evaluation).

812   D. I. PLESSAS, 'Environmental pollution, social costs, and health policy in the U.S.'
IJHS, Spring, 1974, 4(2), pp. 273–84.

The problems of establishing health damage functions relating disease to pollution are discussed. Recent studies of the costs of pollution, the resulting mortality and morbidity, and the health care resource costs, are outlined, and how these estimates might be incorporated into environmental policy discussed.

813   P. SAINSBURY, J. GRAD DE ALARCON, 'The cost of community care and the burden on the family of treating the mentally ill at home'
In D. S. Lees, S. Shaw (eds.) *Impairment, Disability and Handicap*, pp. 123–40 (809).

A study comparing a service area whose policy was to treat patients at home as far as possible with an area with a more conservative hospital centred approach. A large amount of evidence was collected on the patients and their families, although most of it is qualitative rather than quantitative.

814   R. M. SCHEFFLER, J. LIPSCOMB, 'The consumption and investment benefits of disease programs'
GC, July, 1974, 5(3), pp. 8–16.
See 815.

815   R. M. SCHEFFLER, J. LIPSCOMB, 'Alternative estimations of population health status: an empirical example'
Inquiry, September, 1974, 11(3), pp. 220–8.

Sample survey data are used in the calculation of two indices, one reflecting the physiological emotional cost, and the other the monetary costs of disability. Two sets of weights are used in the indices: monetary value weights of

occupying defined disability function levels derived by multiple regression analyses, examining the effects of variables such as age, sex and health status on income; and subjective utility weights for various disability states derived by subjecting 15 experts to a von Neumann–Morgenstern standard gamble experiment.
See 814.

S. O. SCHWEITZER, 'Cost effectiveness of early detection of disease'
HSR, Spring, 1974, 9(1), pp. 22–32.

A framework for evaluation of diagnostic tests for mass screening is outlined. The framework is applied to the 'Pap' test for cervical cancer. The results of the study, taking the expected lifetime earnings approach to the value of life, suggest that as a one-time screening device the test is cost-effective.

B. STARFIELD, 'Measurement of outcome: a proposed scheme'
MMFQ, 1974, 52(1), pp. 39–50.
See 945.

D. TAYLOR, (ed.) *Benefits and Risks in Medical Care*
London: Office of Health Economics, 1974, pp. xii, 104.

The seven short papers in this collection are concerned with assessing the value of different aspects of modern medical care. They bring together a good deal of information and discuss the limitations of that information for evaluating care. The papers do suggest, however, that a good deal of morbidity and premature mortality in Britain could be avoided.
1 H. Campbell, 'Changes in mortality in England and Wales at adult ages between 1940 and 1971', pp. 1–15.
2 D. L. Crombie, 'Changes in patterns of recorded mortality', pp. 17–41.
3 M. Shepherd, 'Progress and problems in mental health', pp. 43–52.
4 W. L. Laing, 'The benefits and risks for children', pp. 53–69.
5 G. Teeling-Smith, 'Adverse reactions and the harmful misuse of medicines', pp. 71–83.
6 J. P. Bunker, 'Risks and benefits of surgery', pp. 85–91.
7 W. M. Wardell, 'Assessment of the benefits, risks and costs of medical progress', pp. 93–104.

T. J. TRUSSELL, 'Cost versus effectiveness of different birth control methods'
Population Studs., March, 1974, 28(1), pp. 85–106.

A study of current British family planning delivery systems. The methods of birth control costed in the study are the condom, spermicides, oral contraceptives, the IUD, the diaphragm, vasectomy and abortion. The effectiveness of the methods is measured in terms of pregnancies and births prevented, but use effectiveness rather than theoretical effectiveness of different methods is used, i.e. the reliability of the method when used in everyday situations by a given population.

820   A. WILLIAMS, 'The cost–benefit approach'
BMB, 1974, 30(3), pp. 252–6.

Discusses what commitment to cost–benefit analysis as a planning tool implies. The type of problem for which cost–benefit analysis might prove useful is outlined, and some applications in the health field are discussed. The paper includes a check list of questions that should be asked whenever a study recommending a particular use of resources is carried out.

821   A. WILLIAMS, 'Measuring the effectiveness of health care systems'
In M. Perlman (ed.) *The Economics of Health and Medical Care*, pp. 361–76. Also in *BJPSM*, 1974, 28(3), pp. 196–202.
See 947.

(b)   The Valuation of Life

The valuation (statistical, marginal or other) of human life is one of the more provoking (especially to non-economists) of the issues that health economists have tackled with some sophistication. The literature ranges between approaches that treat human lives as though they could be equated with the lives of machines (in which case the problem ought to be seen as one of determining their optimal rate of obsolescence!) and studies of the behaviour of sophisticated – but at least human – 'rational calculators', well-trained in such matters as the von Neumann–Morgenstern standard gamble. The most thoughtful treatments of the general issues are probably Schelling (829) and Mishan (834): these may help convince the sceptics that economists are not always the ghouls they sometimes seem to wish to appear, and that they may even have a serious contribution to make to the understanding of a far from trivial aspect of human behaviour.

1927

E. A. WOODS, C. B. METZGER, *America's Human Wealth. The Money Value of Human Life*
New York: Crofts, 1927.

1946

L. I. DUBLIN, A. J. LOTKA, *The Money Value of a Man*
New York: Ronald Press, 1946, pp. xvii, 214.
A revision of the work that originally appeared in 1930. The valuation process is centred around the calculation of the present value of future lifetime earnings at different ages. The revision was necessitated because of a substantial lowering of the interest rate and an increase in the average length of life of the American population. The second chapter of the book provides a survey of early work on human capital. Other chapters deal with the American family, the cost of bringing up a child, the burden of the handicapped, valuation of indemnity for personal injury or death, disease and the depreciation of the money value of a man, applications to public health and life insurance, and the implications for social insurance.
See 45.

1956

D. J. REYNOLDS, 'The cost of road accidents'
JRSS A, 1956, 119(4), pp. 393–408.
See 634.

1964

A. F. CONARD, J. MORGAN, R. PRATT, C. VOLTZ, R. BOMBAUGH, *Automobile Accident Costs and Payments – Studies in the Economics of Injury Reparation*
Ann Arbor: University of Michigan Press, 1964, pp. xxviii, 506.
Estimates are presented of the economic loss suffered by victims of automobile

accidents in Michigan, including medical expenses, property damage, costs of collecting compensation and income loss.
See 1348.

826 R. FEIN, 'Health programmes and economic development'
In S. J. Mushkin (Chairman) *The Economics of Health and Medical Care*, pp. 271–82 (8).
A review of early attempts by Petty, Chadwick, Farr and others to estimate the value of a man.
See 951.

1967

827 R. F. F. DAWSON, *Cost of Road Accidents in Great Britain*
London: Ministry of Transport, Road Research Laboratory Report LR 79, 1967. Excerpts are reprinted in M. H. Cooper, A. J. Culyer (eds.) *Health Economics*, pp. 336–56 (33).
The objective of the study is to calculate the economic consequences of road accidents that occurred in 1963. The method used involves an estimate of the loss of future production by the individual involved in the accident, minus future consumption in the case of a fatality, plus an arbitrary value for the 'subjective' costs of a death or serious accident.
See 802, 833.

828 D. P. RICE, B. S. COOPER, 'The economic value of human life'
AJPH, November, 1967, 57(11), pp. 1954–66.
Tables of the present value of lifetime earnings (discounted at 4 per cent) of individuals by age, sex, colour and three levels of schooling are presented. The figures are calculated from cross-section data for 1964 on the United States population.
See 657, 662, 669, 690.

1968

829 T. C. SCHELLING, 'The life you save may be your own'
In S. B. Chase (ed.) *Problems in Public Expenditure Analysis*, Washington D.C.: The Brookings Institution, 1968, pp. 127–62. Also in M. H. Cooper, A. J. Culyer (eds.) *Health Economics*, pp. 295–321 (33).

The approaches that have been used in attempting to value life and the problems associated with them are discussed. It is pointed out that the most difficult problems lie in attempting to estimate the worth of the individual's life to himself. It is suggested that some of the problems a consumer faces in evaluating avoidance of a single awesome event may be overcome by the use of risk scaling procedures.

1969

M. JONES-LEE, 'Valuation of reduction in the probability of death by road accident'
JTEP, 1969, 3(1), pp. 37–47. Also in M. H. Cooper, A. J. Culyer (eds) *Health Economics*, pp. 322–35 (33).

It is suggested that the problems encountered in trying to obtain an estimate of the value to an individual of a change in the probability of losing his life may be overcome by getting the individual to reveal his preferences in the abstracted context of a von Neumann–Morgenstern experiment. The assumptions underlying such an approach are spelled out, and as an illustration of the approach the analysis is carried out for a university lecturer aged 30 (not the author).

1970

G. CALABRESI, *The Cost of Accidents: A Legal and Economic Analysis*
New Haven: Yale University Press, 1970, pp. x, 340.
See 694.

J. A. DOWIE, 'Valuing the benefits of health improvement'
AEP, June, 1970, 9(14), pp. 21–41.
See 696.

1971

R. F. F. DAWSON, *Current Cost of Road Accidents in Great Britain*
London: Ministry of Transport, Road Research Laboratory Report LR 396, 1971.
See 827.

834   E. J. MISHAN, 'Evaluation of life and limb: a theoretical approach'
JPE, 1971, 79(4), pp. 687–705. Also in R. Layard, *Cost–Benefit Analysis*, Harmondsworth, Middlesex: Penguin Books, 1972, pp. 219–42.

It is argued that most of the methods used to evaluate the loss of saving of life have serious conceptual difficulties, and none are consistent with the approach normally used in cost–benefit analysis. The correct approach, by reference to the Pareto principle, should be in terms of what each member of the community is willing to pay or receive for estimated changes in risk. The paper goes on to specify the types of risk that must be evaluated, pointing out that some personal (voluntary) risks must be disregarded by the cost–benefit analyst, the individual having decided that the utility derived from an action outweighs the risks involved (e.g. smoking).

1973

835   R. L. BERG, 'Establishing the values of various conditions of life for a health status index'
In R. L. Berg (ed.) *Health Status Indexes*, pp. 120–7.
See 905.

1974

836   R. L. AKEHURST, A. J. CULYER, 'On the economic surplus and the value of life'
YB, November, 1974, 26(2), pp. 63–78.

An approach for estimating a minimum value of human life is developed. It is argued that the conceptually correct measure of the benefit from working is not the present value of earnings but that of the economic surplus from working. The approach suggests that an appropriate measure of the value of human life in cost–benefit studies concerning projects expected to change longevity is, in general, one half of earned income plus some additional amounts to allow for transfer payments, overtime payments, and other features of everyday life.

837   D. R. HARRIS, 'The legal system of compensation for death and personal injury suffered in personal accidents'
In D. S. Lees, S. Shaw (eds.) *Impairment, Disability and Handicap*, pp. 30–55 (809).

The paper gives an account of how the legal system arrives at the size of damages awarded for personal injury or death.

M. JONES-LEE, 'The value of changes in the probability of death or injury' *JPE*, July–August, 1974, 82(4), pp. 835–49.

The paper develops results concerning the value to an individual, in the form of Hicksian compensating variations in wealth, of current period changes in the risk of his death. A section is included on how the analysis might be modified to cover outcomes of death or injury to others, to non-fatal accidents, and to cover changes in risk over more than a single period.

(c) Measuring the Output of Health Services

The literature on output measurement reflects two characteristics of the state of research in this field: the need for a disciplinary convergence among researchers on the one hand and decision-makers on the other, and the relative paucity of contributions from 'mainstream' economists. The literature is a spreading one, and marginal decisions as to what to include have not been easy. The criterion has been that the contribution should concern output in an economist's context (that is, should be related to resource allocation in conditions of scarcity). We have interpreted this, perhaps liberally, to *include* indices of health status of a purely descriptive kind, but have *excluded* studies of intermediate outputs (such as patient flows through a system), even though we are aware that the latter have commonly been treated as 'output', for example in hospital cost studies.

It is of interest, given that this is a field that might be expected to be of central concern to economists, lying as it does at the heart of questions concerning the objectives (and hence the efficiency) of health services, to observe that perhaps the best work has been done by specialists in operational research, particularly in Canada and the U.S.A. The literature reveals a growing concern with, and sophistication in the handling of, the problems of social choice inherent in combining various dimensions of health (or more usually, ill-health) to form an index. Examples are provided by the work of Bush (U.S.A.), Torrance (Canada), and their associates.

1914

839   E. A. CODMAN, 'The product of a hospital'
SGO, January–June, 1914, 18, pp. 491–6.
See 339.

1939

840   K. STOUMAN, I. S. FALK, 'Health indices: a study of objective indices of health in relation to environment and sanitation'
Bulletin of Health: League of Nations, 1939, 8, pp. 901–96.
An early attempt to derive descriptive indices of a community's health in terms of mortality, morbidity, environment and public health provisions.

1950

841   E. R. WEINERMAN, 'Appraisal of medical care programmes'
AJPH, September, 1950, 40(9), pp. 1129–34.
Eight criteria are suggested for appraising medical care programmes, including assessment of the relationship between objectives and accomplishments of a programme and the needs of the area, assessment of administrative and financial structures, professional assessment of the competence of the providers, and assessment of the quality of care by reference to the number of times particular clinical procedures are carried out.

1955

842   M. C. SHEPS, 'Approaches to the quality of hospital care'
PHR, September, 1955, 70(9), pp. 877–86.
A review of the problems of measurement of hospital quality and the types of indices that have been used. Four main techniques of quality appraisal are identified, based on set standards of care, elements of performance, effects of care and clinical evaluations.

1957

M. S. BLUMBERG, 'Evaluating health screening procedures'
OR, June, 1957, pp. 351–60.
A survey of the issues to consider in evaluating screening procedures. The difficulties are illustrated by reference to a study of diabetes screening by blood sugar level. A model is postulated for selecting the optimal screening level. Eight other formulae that have been used for evaluating screening procedures are also included.

L. S. ROSENFELD, 'Quality of medical care in hospitals'
AJPH, July, 1957, 47(7), pp. 856–65.
Evaluation of quality of care is carried out on the basis of the judgement by specialists of the way the hospitals manage a particular set of illnesses and operations.

S. SWAROOP, K. UEMURA, 'Proportional mortality of 50 years and above: a suggested indicator of the component "health, including demographic conditions" in the measurement of levels of living'
WHO Bulletin, 1957, 17, pp. 439–81.
Discriminant function analysis is applied to mortality data to derive an international index of health status.

1958

WORLD HEALTH ORGANISATION, *The First Ten Years of the World Health Organisation*
Geneva: WHO, 1958.
Chiefly famous for its quite impossible, but invariably quoted, definition of 'health'.

1961

C. E. RICE, 'Measuring social restoration performance of public psychiatric hospitals'
PHR, May, 1961, 76(5), pp. 437–46.
Two cohorts of patients are used in the study for measurement of the social

restoration performance of psychiatric hospitals: an admission cohort and a resident cohort, patients already in the hospital when the study began. Social restoration is measured at three levels: by the number of patients who return to the community, by their length of stay in the community, and by the post-hospital adjustment of those returned to the community.

1962

848 H. R. KELMAN, A. WILLNER, 'Problems in measurement and evaluation of rehabilitation'
APMR, April, 1962, 43, pp. 172–81.
A modification of the Katz activities of daily living (ADL) scale, which does not use a dichotomous scaling of performance in the dimensions in which the index is measured.

1963

849 S. KATZ, A. B. FORD, R. W. MOSKOWITZ, B. A. JACKSON, M. W. JAFFE, 'Studies of illness in the aged: the index of ADL – a standardized measure of biological and psychosocial function'
JAMA, 1963, 185(12), pp. 914–19.
A much-referred-to index based upon a Guttman-scaling of function and independence of elderly persons in the first instance, but subsequently broadened to a sample of chronically ill and relatively healthy persons of all ages. It has been used in prognostic studies and as an outcome measure.

1964

850 R. F. L. LOGAN, 'Assessment of sickness and health in the community: needs and methods'
MC, July–September, 1964, 2(3), pp. 173–90, and *MC*, October–December, 1964, 2(4), pp. 218–25.
See 64.

851 C. M. WYLIE, B. K. WHITE, 'A measure of disabilities'
AEH, June, 1964, 8, pp. 834–9.
A description of the Maryland Disability Index (also called the Barthel Index)

of daily living, and its use in three chronic disease hospitals in Maryland. Notably, the paper finds that the weights used in constructing the index are not always those used by doctors in, for example, deciding to discharge patients.

1965

C. L. CHIANG, *An Index of Health: Mathematical Models*
Washington D.C.: USDHEW, Public Health Service, National Center for Health Statistics, Series 2, No. 5, 1965, p. 19.

Mathematical models are developed of the distribution and duration of illness episodes, and of mortality. A macro index of the mean duration of sickness is calculated.

F. I. MAHONEY, D. W. BARTHEL, 'Functional evaluation: the Barthel Index'
MSMJ, February, 1965, 14, pp. 61–5.

Points are assigned to patients according to whether they can perform each of ten basic functions independently or whether they require help. The points awarded are summed, so that a patient who can perform all of the functions independently scores 100 on the Barthel Index.

1966

R. A. BAUER (ed.) *Social Indicators*
Cambridge, Massachusetts: The M.I.T. Press, 1966, pp. xxii, 357.

The volume resulted from an attempt to appraise the social impact of outer space exploration. The subject matter of the volume is the entire set of social indicators and statistical series that have been used, or might be used, to assess the degree of achievement of societal goals or evaluate specific programmes. There is very little discussion specifically on the topic of health indicators.

D. F. SULLIVAN, *Conceptual Problems in Developing an Index of Health*
Washington D.C.: Vital and Health Statistics, Public Health Service Publication No. 1000; Series 2, No. 17, 1966.

An early survey of some issues presaging much subsequent development in the health index field. A useful starting point for those interested in a pragmatic approach to the problem.

1967

856 R. L. ROBERTSON, 'Issues in measuring the economic effects of personal health services'
MC, November–December, 1967, 5(6), pp. 362–8.

Describes a proposal to measure the effects of different health insurance plans in the United States on utilisation of health services and time off work. Conceptual difficulties in identifying specific inputs and outputs are noted but not resolved.

857 S. SHAPIRO, 'End result measurements of quality of medical care'
MMFQ, 1967, 45(2), pp. 7–30.

A description of follow-up studies of morbidity, mortality, utilisation and disability among participants in the New York Health Insurance Plan.

1968

858 I. M. MORIYAMA, 'Problems in the measurement of health status'
In E. Sheldon, W. Moore (eds.) *Indicators of Social Change*, New York: Russell Sage Foundation, 1968.

A useful review of macro indicators in the United States (with some international comparisons) before the 'take-off' of the health indicators movement.

859 A. H. PACKER, 'Applying cost-effectiveness concepts to the community health system'
OR, March–April, 1968, 16(2), pp. 227–53.
See 682.

860 P. J. SANAZARO, J. W. WILLIAMSON, 'End results of patient care: a provisional classification based on reports by internists'
MC, 1968, 6(2), pp. 123–30.

Applies a version of the 'critical incident' technique used in psychology to derive 'beneficial' and 'detrimental' outcomes of physician care, as assessed by physicians from their recent case experience.

1969

H. C. CHASE, 'Ranking countries by infant mortality rates'
PHR, January, 1969, 84(1), pp. 19–27.

Description of a technique for ranking countries by their infant mortality rates developed by three U.S. health agencies.

A. I. KISCH, J. W. KOVNER, L. J. HARRIS, G. KLINE, 'New proxy measure for health status'
HSR, Fall, 1969, 4(3), pp. 223–30.

A proxy measure of ill-health is proposed based on days of hospitalisation, drug consumption and acute and chronic conditions.

V. NAVARRO, 'Systems analysis in the health field'
Soc.-Econ.Plan.Sciences, 1969, 3, pp. 179–89.
See 1385.

M. W. REDER, 'Some problems in the measurement of productivity in the medical care industry'
In V. R. Fuchs (ed.) *Production and Productivity in the Service Industries*, New York: National Bureau of Economic Research, 1969, pp. 95–131.

The need to define output of medical services independently of inputs is recognised. It is suggested that output be measured as a weighted number of individuals enrolled in a comprehensive health plan, the plan being care of a specified quality, changes or differences in quality between plans being accounted for by adjustment using a measurement of quality based on a ranking according to degree of attainment of a number of objectives such as lower age-specific mortality and lower rates of undetected illness.
See 165.

D. H. STIMSON, 'Utility measurement in public health decision-making'
MS, 1969, 16(2), pp. B-17–B-30.

The Churchman–Ackoff method is used to assign priorities, as seen by public administrators, to the objectives of a health care agency and to some alternative means of achieving them.

1970

866   D. M. DuBois, 'Evaluation of health service systems, with special emphasis on college health services'
JACHA, February, 1970, 18(3), pp. 182–91.
Discusses the general problems of evaluating health systems. A system for assessing effectiveness based upon chargeable health impairment units saved (percentage impairment multiplied by number of days of impairment) is suggested.

867   S. FANSHEL, J. W. BUSH, 'A health-status index and its application to health-service outcomes'
OR, November–December, 1970, 18(5), pp. 1021–66.
A short review of the extant approaches in 1970 is followed by the development of an index that has since become a classic. Equivalence in time and equivalence in population are the two methods of paired comparison used to generate weights for the disability dimensions of ill-health. The technique is applied tentatively to a tuberculosis screening and treatment programme.

868   J. E. MILLER, 'An indicator to aid management in assigning programme priorities'
PHR, August, 1970, 85(8), pp. 725–31.
The paper in which Miller's 'Q' index for use in the U.S. Indian Health Service is described. The index combines mortality and morbidity data and assigns priority to disease control according to the divergence between Indian experience and that of the rest of the United States population.

869   J. P. NEWHOUSE, 'Determinants of days lost from work due to sickness'
In H. E. Klarman (ed.) *Empirical Studies in Health Economics*, pp. 59–70 (18).
An attempt to estimate a production function for the reduction of days lost from work because of sickness. The limitations of straightforward multiple regression analysis and of principal components analysis, which is used as a supplement, are set out. Policy conclusions are limited. Desirable reallocations cannot be recommended because the study is concerned with only one output of a number of medical care and other inputs. Some of the variables affect only particular age groups, but the data are not sufficiently disaggregated in this respect, and of all the variables considered the only one to which cost can easily be assigned is food.

M. SILVER, 'An economic analysis of variations in medical expenses and work loss rates'

In H. E. Klarman (ed.) *Empirical Studies in Health Economics*, pp. 121–40 (18).

See 98.

G. W. TORRANCE, *A Generalized Cost-Effectiveness Model for the Evaluation of Health Programmes*

Hamilton, Ontario: Faculty of Business, McMaster University, Research Series No. 101, 1970.

A pioneering review of the outcome side of cost-effectiveness studies in the health territory including exposition of the 'standard gamble' and 'time trade-off' approaches to weighting the components of an index. The approach is applied to programmes in prevention (haemolytic disease and T.B.) and treatment (coronary emergency and kidney dialysis). A major source.

D. J. TRANTOW, 'An introduction to evaluation. Programme effectiveness and community needs'

RL, January, 1970, 31(1), pp. 2–9.

An introductory article discussing the nature and process of evaluation and the need to shift from input and throughput to output measurement as a basis for allocating resources.

1971

C. J. AUSTIN, 'Selected social indicators in the health field'

AJPH, August, 1971, 61(8), pp. 1507–13.

It is argued that social indicators should be examined with reference to a conceptual model of how change occurs. The article looks at some models of this type: systems approaches, cybernetic self-regulating models.

N. B. BELLOC, L. BRESLOW, J. R. HOCHSTIM, 'Measurement of physical health in a general population survey'

AJE, 1971, 93(5), pp. 328–36.

See 99.

J. W. BUSH, M. M. CHEN, J. ZAREMBA, 'Estimating health programme outcomes using a Markov equilibrium analysis of disease development'

AJPH, December, 1971, 61(12), pp. 2362–75.

The stochastic movement of patients through function levels and disease states is represented by a stationary Markov chain. The idea is (data permitting) to build a macro-model of the disease process in a population in order to estimate the impact of health care programmes.

876   A. L. COCHRANE, 'The history of the measurement of ill-health'
IJE, June, 1972, 1(2), pp. 89–93.

Makes the simple, but revolutionary, point that indicators for medical intervention should be based not on the arbitrary selection of some moment of a distribution of symptoms but on evidence about the effectiveness of treatment at various points on the distribution.

877   A. J. CULYER, R. J. LAVERS, A. WILLIAMS, 'Social indicators: health'
ST, 1971, 2, pp. 31–42.

An analytical examination of the logic and application of indicators of health status, need and effectiveness.
See 886.

878   A. W. GROGONO, D. J. WOODGATE, 'Index for measuring Health'
Lancet, November 6th, 1971, pp. 1024–6.

A simple index based on ten dimensions of function is proposed.

879   E. A. HEFFERIN, A. H. KATZ, 'Issues and orientations in the evaluation of rehabilitation programmes. A review article'
RL, March, 1971, 32(3), pp. 66–74, 95; April, 1971, 32(4), pp. 98–107, 113.

The article consists of three main parts: an examination of the problems of evaluation, a survey of approaches to measurement, and a review of some evaluative studies. Although the economic implications of rehabilitation programmes are not directly considered, the approaches to evaluation considered are concerned with the measurement of outcomes, clinical, social, psychological or vocational.

880   D. R. MEYER, 'Disability equivalences: a logic system for comparison of alternate health programmes'
AJPH, August, 1971, 61(8), pp. 1514–17.

Suggests a system based on disability units (professional assessment of disability multiplied by a time dimension) for evaluation of health programmes.

D. F. SULLIVAN, *Disability Components for an Index of Health*
Data Evaluation and Methods Research Series 2, No. 42, USDHEW,
Rockville, 1971, p. 35.

A development of Sullivan's earlier advocacy of comprehensive macro-health
indicators. This study measures the total volume of disability by categories
based on, e.g., client groups, institutional groups and period of disablement.
See 855.

D. F. SULLIVAN, 'A single index of mortality and morbidity'
HSMHA Health Rep., April, 1971, 86, pp. 347–54.

An adaptation of life tables to produce health indicators in terms of expectation of life free from disability and expectation of disability. 'Disability' was
defined in various ways, all relating to restriction of activity. The indices are
applied to age, sex and race comparisons, but not longitudinally, for which
comparisons they were conceived.

1972

L. BRESLOW, 'A quantitative approach to the WHO definition of health:
physical, mental and social well-being'
IJE, 1972, 1(4), pp. 347–55.

A social survey method of constructing scales of physical, mental and social
health is presented.

J. W. BUSH, S. FANSHEL, M. M. CHEN, 'Analysis of a tuberculin testing
programme using a health status index'
Soc.-Econ.Plan.Sciences, 1972, 6(1), pp. 49–68.

A health status index is constructed based upon several levels of function from
well-being (1.0) to death (0.0). The utility numbers between 0 and 1 are called
function weights (cardinal scale of function weights). Using a set of function
weights the function status of a person or population can be computed over
time. The output of a health programme can be measured as the difference
between two functions: the function status with the programme, and the
function status without the programme. The index is illustrated by reference to
a tuberculin testing programme on children.

A. J. CULYER, 'Appraising government expenditure on health services: the
problems of "need" and "output"'
PF, 1972, 27(2), pp. 205–11.

The problems of developing an operational concept of need are discussed. A concept similar to the concept of demand is suggested, based on the preferences of publicly accountable officials. To make the concept operational requires measurement of the output of health agencies. One possible approach to measuring output is outlined. *See 877.*

886 A. J. CULYER, R. J. LAVERS, A. WILLIAMS, 'Health indicators'
In A. Shonfield, S. Shaw (eds.) *Social Indicators and Social Policy*, London: Heinemann Educational Books, for the Social Science Research Council, 1972, pp. 94–118.
See 877.

887 D. W. DUNLOP, 'The development of an output concept for analysis of curative health services'
SSM, June, 1972, 6(3), pp. 373–85.
The suggested output measure focuses on the individual or set of individuals who have consumed the curative health services being considered. The measure of output is the number of persons initially demanding service, adjusted according to the relative success with which they are treated. The application of the measure in an analysis of health services in Uganda is briefly discussed.

888 S. FANSHEL, 'A meaningful measure of health for epidemiology'
IJE, 1972, 1(4), pp. 319–37.
The theory of a health index, capable of charting health status through time and having weights determined by the 'population-equivalence' method, is expounded. It is applied to the question of maximising the health benefits of a VD control programme with a given budget.

889 S. B. GOLDSMITH, 'The status of health status indicators'
Health Services Reports, March, 1972, 87(3), pp. 212–20.
A succinct critical review of the concept of health, health indices (up to 1972) and their application.
See 914.

890 J. HALPERN, P. R. BINNER, 'A model for an output value analysis of mental health programmes'
AMH, Winter, 1972, pp. 40–51.

1 A. I. HARRIS, J. R. BUCKLE, C. R. W. SMITH, E. HEAD, E. COX, *Handicapped and Impaired in Great Britain*
London: HMSO, Office of Population Censuses and Surveys, Parts I and II, 1971, Part III, 1972, p. 600.

A milestone in the measurement of disability on a large scale. Disability was identified in several dimensions, which were combined into an overall classification of handicap and need. The second volume of the survey went on to examine the work and housing of impaired persons in Great Britain. The final volume is a survey of income and entitlement to supplementary benefit of impaired people in Great Britain.

2 J. D. HENNES, 'The measurement of health'
MCR, December, 1972, 29(11), pp. 1268–88.

A review of work on health indices. Most of the major contributions up to late 1972 are included. A useful bibliography of 87 items is provided.

3 B. S. HETZEL, 'The implications of health indicators: a comment'
IJE, December, 1972, 1(4), pp. 315–18.

Argues, contrary to the prevailing view, that mortality data can usefully chart the health status of both underdeveloped and developed countries.

4 J. A. KING, C. G. SMITH, 'The treatment milieu and prediction of mental hospital effectiveness'
JHSB, June, 1972, 13(2), pp. 180–94.

The paper first considers a set of scales that attempt to measure the therapeutic orientation of the treatment milieu. The second part of the paper demonstrates that a significant relationship exists between the therapeutic orientation of the treatment milieu and both in-hospital and in-community measures of effectiveness. The findings suggest that the 'humanistic' tradition of therapy is not necessarily the most appropriate from the point of view of in-community patient rehabilitation.

5 W. A. LAING (ed.) *Evaluation in the Health Services*
London: Office of Health Economics, May, 1972, p. 38.

The report of a symposium bringing together clinicians, social scientists and planners. Short papers were presented by W. A. Laing outlining the field, M. Jefferys on 'The contribution of the health services to social welfare', J. Algie on 'Evaluation and social service departments', A. L. Cochrane on 'Effectiveness and efficiency in medical treatment', A. J. Culyer on 'Indicators of health', and B. H. Dawson on 'The responsibilities of clinical freedom'. The discussions between the participants are also recorded.

896   G. L. MADDOX, 'Interventions and outcomes: notes on designing and implementing an experiment in health care'
IJE, 1972, 1(4), pp. 339–45.

An outline of an experiment in measuring the outcome of non-institutional care of elderly persons.

897   R. M. ROSSER, V. C. WATTS, 'The measurement of hospital output'
IJE, December, 1972, 1(4), pp. 361–7.

A numerical index of health status in two (not combined) dimensions, disability and distress, was applied to patients at admission and on the first subsequent outpatient visit to a London hospital. Most patients seemed to improve.
See 942.

898   S. SHAPIRO, R. FINK, C. ROSENBERG, 'A programme to measure the impact of multiphasic health testing on health differentials between poverty and non-poverty groups'
MC, May–June, 1972, 10(3), pp. 207–14.

A description of a project to test the extent of reductions in certain ill-health characteristics of poverty and non-poverty groups in the Health Insurance Plan of New York. The populations would be tested by the Automated Multiphasic Health Test (AMHT) and asked to answer questionnaires relating, amongst other things, to disability and restriction of activity.

899   G. W. TORRANCE, W. H. THOMAS, D. L. SACKETT, 'A utility maximisation model for evaluation of health care programmes'
HSR, Summer, 1972, 7(2), pp. 118–33.

A linear health utility scale is described that allows the assignment of utility values to health states for any disease or treatment programme. Measurement of utility is achieved by either von Neumann–Morgenstern 'standard gamble' approach or a 'time trade-off' technique. The use of the index cost-effectiveness analysis is discussed, and an example illustrating its use in the evaluation of three hypothetical programmes is provided.

900   R. WAGER, *Care of the Elderly – an Exercise in Cost–Benefit Analysis*
London: Institute of Municipal Treasurers and Accountants, 1972, p. 74.

1 L. D. WILCOX, R. M. BROOKS, G. M. BEAL, G. E. KLONGLAN, *Social Indicators and Societal Monitoring*
Amsterdam: Elsevier Scientific Publishing Company, 1972, p. 464.

An annotated bibliography that references most of the important contributions to the social indicators field up to 1972. A paper by Brooks at the beginning of the book discusses the development of the social indicators movement, the major contributions to the field and current activities in different countries and international agencies.

2 A. D. WOLFSON, *A Health Index for Ontario*
Toronto: Ministry of Treasury, Economics and Intergovernmental Affairs, Economic Planning Branch, 1972.

A preliminary run for the fuller report by Wolfson.
See 948.

1973

3 J. R. ASHFORD, K. L. O. READ, V. C. RILEY, 'An analysis of variations in perinatal mortality amongst local authorities in England and Wales.
IJE, Spring, 1973, 2(1), pp. 31–46.

Five measures of performance or output were used in this study of the maternity services in England and Wales: Perinatal mortality in the less than 2,501 grams birthweight, perinatal mortality in the above 2,500 grams birthweight group, overall perinatal mortality, the proportion of live births and late foetal deaths of less than 2,500 grams birthweight, and a perinatal mortality standardised for national variations in birthweight distribution.
See 498.

4 M. BERDIT, J. W. WILLIAMSON, 'Function limitation scale for measuring health outcomes'
In R. L. Berg (ed.) *Health Status Indices*, pp. 59–65 (906).

A six-point ordinal scale of physical function is developed for use as a measure of outcome in community health care.

5 R. L. BERG, 'Establishing the values of various conditions of life for a health status index'
In R. L. Berg (ed.) *Health Status Indices*, pp. 120–7 (906).

An experiment using both the 'standard gamble' and 'equivalent' approaches to deriving the value of life. The results obtained from the sample display a large variance.

906   R. L. BERG (ed.) *Health Status Indices*
Chicago: Hospital Research and Educational Trust, 1973, p. 262.
The proceedings of a conference conducted by Health Services Research, which took place in Tucson, Arizona, October 1–4, 1972. The papers in the collection are described elsewhere in the bibliography. The discussions at the conference are reported in the volume.
See 904, 905, 908, 909, 913, 918, 919, 920, 922, 923, 924, 929, 931, 933, 934.

907   R. H. BROOK, F. A. APPEL, 'Quality-of-care assessment: choosing a method for peer review'
NEJM, 1973, 288(25), pp. 1323–9.
A good example of outcome, rather than process, orientation in the clinical context. Amongst other things, the empirical results reveal interestingly that a higher proportion of care seems successful when judged by outcome than by process, and that the outcome indicators used were not significantly correlated with process indicators.

908   J. W. BUSH, M. M. CHEN, D. L. PATRICK, 'Health status index in cost-effectiveness: analysis of a PKU programme'
In R. L. Berg (ed.) *Health Status Indices*, pp. 172–94 (906).
A model using a function index in a prognostic setting for evaluating the cost-effectiveness of a phenylketonuria programme.

909   M. K. CHEN, 'The G index for programme priority'
In R. L. Berg (ed.) *Health Status Indices*, pp. 28–34.
A modification of Miller's 'Q index' for use in planning the United States Indian health service or other sub-groups of the population having special morbidity and/or mortality characteristics.

910   C. L. CHIANG, R. D. COHEN, 'How to measure health: a stochastic model for an index of health'
IJE, March, 1973, 2(1), pp. 7–13.
A continuous time Markov model with stationary transition probabilities is applied to a notion of ill-health based on the fraction of a year an individual spends in a particular state of health.

911   A. DONABEDIAN, *Aspects of Medical Care Administration: Specifying Requirements for Health Care*
Cambridge, Massachusetts: Harvard University Press, 1973, p. 649.
The book contains extensive reviews of work on indicators of need and measurement of health service outcomes.
See 35.

M. S. FELDSTEIN, M. A. PIOT, T. K. SUNDARESAN, *Resource Allocation Model for Public Health Planning: A Case Study of Tuberculosis Control*
Geneva: World Health Organisation, 1973, p. 110.
See 771.

B. E. FORST, 'Quantifying the patient's preferences'
In R. L. Berg (ed.) *Health Status Indices*, pp. 209–21 (906).
The 'standard gamble' technique is employed to suggest the plausibility of constructing preference functions based on consumers' values.

S. B. GOLDSMITH, 'A re-evaluation of health status indicators'
Health Services Reports, December, 1973, 88(10), pp. 937–41.
An updating of his previous review.
See 889.

A. W. GROGONO, 'Measurement of ill-health: a comment'
IJE, 1973, 2(1), pp. 5–6.
A brief review of the state of the art.

L. D. HABER, 'Some parameters for social policy in disability: a cross national comparison'
MMFQ, Summer, 1973, 51(3), pp. 319–40.
The policy problems presented by disability are examined in the light of two major and several minor U.S. surveys, and of studies from Australia, Denmark, Great Britain and Israel. Wide differences in the estimates highlight the problems of definition and measurement. A switch in measurement to emphasis on behavioural processes of adaptation and normalisation, rather than on medical aspects of disability, is recommended.
See 1362.

C. HIMATSINGANI, 'Approaches to health and personal social services planning in the National Health Service and the place of health indices'
IJE, March, 1973, 2(1), pp. 15–21.
A planner's (sympathetic) assessment of the health index research programme.

D. C. HOLLOWAY, 'Evaluating health status for utilization review'
In R. L. Berg (ed.) *Health Status Indices*, pp. 89–98 (906).
An index of 'clinical status' is developed as a measure of physician 'concern',

and applied to hyperthyroidism. Its role was seen mainly in determining the extent to which a patient needed physician care and hence needed to be in one kind of health facility rather than another.

919 S. KATZ, C. A. AKPOM, J. A. PAPSIDERO, S. J. WEISS, 'Measuring the health status of populations'
In R. L. Berg (ed.) *Health Status Indexes*, pp. 39–52 (906).

A short review of the development of epidemiological and demographic statistics and the role of social surveys of health status, leading up to the activities of daily living index (ADL) developed by Katz and his colleagues. *See 849.*

920 N. P. KNEPPRETH, D. H. GUSTAFSON, J. H. ROSE, R. P. LEIFER, 'Techniques for the assessment of worth'
In R. L. Berg (ed.) *Health Status Indices*, pp. 228–38 (906).

A survey of some alternative ways of incorporating values into indices: ranking, equivalance grouping, magnitude estimation, graphical, preference ratio, gambling methods and indifference curves.

921 M. M. LAW, R. STEELE, A. S. KRAUS, 'Measuring the impact of a district health unit – a baseline study'
CJPH, January–February, 1973, 64(1), pp. 13–24.

A study to assess the current health status and utilisation of health services of a population prior to the setting up of a new public health service. The study employed both household interview and clinical examinations to assess health status.

922 M. LERNER, 'Conceptualization of health and social well-being'
In R. L. Berg (ed.) *Health Status Indices*, pp. 1–6 (906).

A general review of the objectives and difficulties of constructing health indices, of the broadest kind.

923 D. S. LEVINE, D. E. YETT, 'A method for constructing proxy measures of health status'
In R. L. Berg (ed.) *Health Status Indices*, pp. 12–22 (906).

Uses factor analysis to identify indicators of medical under-service for regional health planning.

924 J. E. MILLER, 'Guidelines for selecting a health status index'
In R. L. Berg (ed.) *Health Status Indices*, pp. 243–7 (906).

Offers some adminstrative criteria for evaluating health indices.

25 C. MOSER, 'Social indicators—systems, methods and problems'
RIW, June, 1973, 19(2), pp. 133–42.

A review of the nature and development of social indicators, and their relationship to the whole body of social statistics.

26 R. D. MUSTIAN, J. J. SEE, 'Indicators of mental health needs: an empirical and pragmatic evaluation'
JHSB, March, 1973, 14, pp. 23–7.

A brief analysis of criteria of need currently utilised by six states in the United States Public Health Service.

27 D. L. PATRICK, J. W. BUSH, M. M. CHEN, 'Methods for measuring levels of well-being for a health status index'
HSR, Fall, 1973, 8(3), pp. 228–45.

This study explores the valuation problem in health index construction by experiments with category rating, magnitude estimation and equivalence rating. Experiments were performed on students and public health administrators. The results using different methods tended to converge.

28 J. D. POLE, 'The use of outcome measures in health service planning'
IJE, 1973, 2(1), pp. 23–30.

A general review of the role of economic logic and techniques such as health status measurement.

29 G. POVEY, D. UYENO, I. VERTINSKY, 'Social impact index for evaluation of regional resource allocation'
In R. L. Berg (ed.) *Health Status Indices*, pp. 104–15 (906).

An index is developed using a simulation model to identify regional shortages and surpluses of resources in terms of 'ecological' indicators of need. The equations of the model are not presented.

30 S. SAINSBURY, *Measuring Disability*
London: Occasional Papers on Social Administration No. 54, G. Bell and Sons Ltd., 1973, p. 125.

The book opens with an examination of current methods of defining and assessing disability for the purposes of providing services or financial benefits. The second part of the book reviews techniques that have been developed by social scientists for identifying and assessing disabled persons. The final part of the book describes a pilot study (by interview) undertaken to explore the social concept of disability. An index is devised based on capacity to perform a number of tasks or activities. A small subsidiary study was also carried out to explore the relationship between assessment of capacity made in the interview with observed performance.

931   D. E. SKINNER, D. E. YETT, 'Debility index for long-term-care patients'
In R. L. Berg (ed.) *Health Status Indices,* pp. 69–82 (906).
A Guttman scale of restriction in activities of daily living is developed to provide a measure of case-mix in cost studies of long-term inpatient care.

932   B. STARFIELD, 'Health services research: a working model'
NEJM, July 19th, 1973, 289(3), pp. 132–6.
A formulation of health services research is proposed that takes into account the relations between the structure of medical care (the setting and instruments), the process of medical care (the overlap between medical practice and patient behaviour) and the outcome of medical care (the impact on the health of the patients). The proposed framework is then used to classify current research in health services.

933   G. W. TORRANCE, D. L. SACKETT, W. H. THOMAS, 'Utility maximization model for programme evaluation: a demonstration application'
In R. L. Berg (ed.) *Health Status Indices,* pp. 156–65 (906).
The 'standard gamble' and 'time trade-off' techniques are used on a small sample of G.P.s to derive measures of health outcomes of a T.B. screening programme, a haemolytic disease programme and a kidney disease programme.

934   G. A. WHITMORE, 'Health state preferences and the social choice'
In R. L. Berg (ed.) *Health Status Indices,* pp. 135–45 (906).
A decision theoretic analysis of some of the issues involved in health index construction. Particular emphasis is put on the problems of interpersonal comparisons in a social welfare function.

1974

935   R. DOLL, 'Surveillance and monitoring'
IJE, December, 1974, 3(4), pp. 305–14.
Discusses measures that can be used to monitor health services. These are principally related to the outcome rather than the process of care. Medical efficiency measures such as mortality and morbidity, social acceptability

measures such as public opinion surveys, and the use of cost–benefit analyses to measure economic efficiency, are all approved.

36 J. P. DUPUY, 'On the social rationality of health policies'
In M. Perlman (ed.) *The Economics of Health and Medical Care*, pp. 481–509 (44).

The paper falls into two parts. The first part seeks to demonstrate the rationality of decision-takers in the health-care sector. Examples of irrationality are held to be the product of crudely drawn indicators of the outputs of the health system. The second part of the paper considers the results of a study of the consumption of medicines in France. The growth in drug consumption has been explained on purely technical grounds (innovations in the drugs produced), but it is suggested here that the growth can be explained by the 'significative' function of medicines in the doctor–patient relationship.

37 J. GARRAD, 'Impairment and disability: their measurement, prevalence and psychological cost'
In D. S. Lees, S. Shaw (eds.) *Impairment, Disability and Handicap*, pp. 141–56 (809).

The paper describes the use of interview techniques to identify and assess the severity of disability and to identify impairment in a population.

38 D. L. KLEMMACK, J. R. CARLSON, J. N. EDWARDS, 'Measures of well-being – an empirical and critical assessment'
JHSB, September, 1974, pp. 267–70.

An enquiry to determine the empirical relations between three measures of well-being: a 'life satisfaction' scale, a 'social isolation' scale and a 'willingness to live' scale. The first two measures were not statistically separable.

9 J. LAVE, L. B. LAVE, S. LEINHARDT, 'Modelling the delivery of medical services'
In M. Perlman (ed.) *The Economics of Health and Medical Care*, pp. 326–51 (44).
See 1422.

0 E. LEVY, 'Health indicators and health systems analysis'
In M. Perlman (ed.) *The Economics of Health and Medical Care*, pp. 377–401 (44).

The paper discusses the reasons for constructing health indicators and reviews previous work on health indicators. It is concluded that present work on health indicators falls into two camps: indicators that are operational but analytically unsatisfactory; and indicators that are the product of a conceptual and analytical approach but to which, at least for the present, there is no prospect of attaching numbers. An approach falling between the two camps is proposed. An analysis of the health care system and its sub-systems suggests that the appropriate approach in the absence of a unique indicator is a battery of indicators, the battery characterised by three dimensions: indicators of vulnerability, indicators of morbidity and indicators of mortality.

941   C. E. LEWIS, 'The state of the art of quality assessment – 1973'
MC, October, 1974, 12(10), pp. 799–806.

Traces development of quality assessment in the United States since 1900. He argues that until the method of payment becomes goal-oriented (viz. towards outcomes) assessment of quality will continue to focus on process rather than outcome.

942   R. M. ROSSER, V. C. WATTS, 'The development of a classification of the symptoms of sickness and its use to measure the output of a hospital'
In D. S. Lees, S. Shaw (eds.) *Impairment, Disability and Handicap*, pp. 157–70.
See 897.

943   R. M. SCHEFFLER, J. LIPSCOMB, 'Alternative estimations of population health status: an empirical example'
Inquiry, September, 1974, 11(3), pp. 220–8.
See 815.

944   S. B. SLATER, C. VUKMANOVIC, P. MACUKANOVIC, T. PRVULOVIC, J. L. CUTLER, 'The definition and measurement of disability'
SSM, 1974, 8, pp. 305–8.

A brief description of a WHO and Federal Institute of Public Health (Belgrade) project to measure the prevalence of disability in a population. Six different measures of disability were devised. The study will hopefully have implications for cross-national comparisons.

945   B. STARFIELD, 'Measurement of outcome: a proposed scheme'
MMFQ, 1974, 52(1), pp. 39–50.

Suggests an approach to health status measurements based on a health profile with seven categories of outcome arrayed in parallel rather than reduced to a single index.

16 D. Taylor, (ed.) *Benefits and Risks in Medical Care*
London: Office of Health Economics, 1974, pp. xii, 104.
See 818

17 A. Williams, 'Measuring the effectiveness of health care systems'
In M. Perlman (ed.) *The Economics of Health and Medical Care*, pp.
361–76 (44). Also in *BJPSM*, 1974, 28(3), pp. 196–202.
Sketches out a measure, based on the general social functioning of the patient,
that will allow movement from measures of effectiveness based on throughput
or workload to measures based on the health status of the individual. A
proposed field trial relating to the care of the elderly is outlined.

18 A. D. Wolfson, *A Health Index for Ontario*
Toronto: Ministry of Treasury, Economics and Intergovernmental
Affairs, Ontario Statistical Centre, 1974, p. 49.
Uses the 'standard gamble' method to construct a disease specific index of ill-
health (using doctors' preferences) for regions within the province of Ontario.
Demonstrates the possibility of constructing indices, which have sometimes
been described as mere theoretical toys, and is therefore important for this as
well as its substantive results.

19 K. G. Wright, 'Alternative measures of the output of social programmes:
the elderly'
In A. J. Culyer (ed.) *Economic Policies and Social Goals*, pp. 239–72
(41).
A comprehensive review of outcome measurement in programmes for the
elderly with a description of a Markov-type research project into changes in
health status among the elderly receiving different regimes of treatment.

(d) The Role of Health Care in Economic Growth and Development

The inclusion of a separate section on the role of health care in economic
growth and development is a recognition that health service provision
may have an impact and an importance for the rate of growth of
community output that is significantly different in developing countries. A
large proportion of the literature in this section is concerned with three
problems. One problem examined is the impact of health services on

population growth: Enke (954), Leibenstein (957) and Fucaraccio (974) discuss the impact of birth control programmes on population growth; Newman (962) discusses the effect of malaria control on population growth. The second major question examined is the impact of debilitating disease on the productive effort of the population; the contributions of Malenbaum (960), Conly (967), Weisbrod *et al.* (977) and Baldwin and Weisbrod (978), fall into this category. The final concern of economists in this area has been to question the relevance of Western medicine, with its emphasis on curative rather than preventive services, in developing countries; papers dealing with this sort of question are: Gish (958), Stewart (965) and Rifkin and Kaplinsky (976).

1957

950   S. SWAROOP, K. UEMURA, 'Proportional mortality of 50 years and above: a suggested indicator of the component "health, including demographic conditions" in the measurement of levels of living'
WHO Bulletin, 1957, 17, pp. 439–81.

1964

951   R. FEIN, 'Health programmes and economic development'
In S. J. Mushkin (Chairman) *The Economics of Health and Medical Care*, pp. 271–82 (8).

After reviewing early attempts to measure the money value of a man, the question of whether health measures may be undesirable in underdeveloped countries is examined, and answered in the negative. Comment by R. Goode pp. 282–5.
See 826.

952   M. PERLMAN, 'Some economic aspects of public health programmes in underdeveloped areas'
In S. J. Mushkin (Chairman) *The Economics of Health and Medical Care*, pp. 286–98 (8).

The major part of the paper is a description of public health programmes in Latin America believed by the author to have been successful or unsuccessful. Comment by A. P. Ruderman.

1965

53 CENTRE FOR DEVELOPMENT STUDIES OF THE CENTRAL UNIVERSITY OF VENEZUELA, CARACAS IN CO-OPERATION WITH THE PAN AMERICAN SANITARY BUREAU, *Health Planning: Problems of Concept and Method*
Washington D.C.: Pan American Health Organisation and World Health Organisation, 1965, pp. v, 77.

A review, first, of the need to relate objectives to the means of achieving them to produce feasible, consistent and economically efficient planning. This is followed by a survey of the available real resources in the Venezuelan health sector, and various disease programmes are then costed. Problems of predicting future health status of the population are discussed and data needs identified. Finally, the preceding analysis and data form the basis for making regional and national health care targets and plans.

1966

54 S. ENKE, 'The economic aspects of slowing population growth'
EJ, March, 1966, 76(1), pp. 44–56. Also in M. H. Cooper, A. J. Culyer (eds.) *Health Economics*, pp. 357–72 (33).

It is argued that the increase in per capita income resulting from birth control programmes is very much higher than that resulting from equivalent investment in industrial capital. A cost-effectiveness analysis of various methods of birth control is carried out, and the use of bonuses to encourage family planning is discussed.
See 957.

1967

5 R. BARLOW, 'The economic effects of malaria eradication'
AER, May, 1967, 57(2), pp. 130–48.
See 664, 672.

6 WORLD HEALTH ORGANISATION, *National Health Planning in Developing Countries*
Geneva: World Health Organisation, Technical Report Series No. 350, 1967, p. 40.
See 1382.

1969

957 H. LEIBENSTEIN, 'Pitfalls in benefit–cost analysis of birth prevention'
Population Studs., 1969, 23(2), pp. 161–70.
A criticism of Enke's approach.
See also S. Enke, 'Leibenstein on the benefits and costs of birth control programmes', *Population Studs.*, 1970, 24(1), pp. 115–16, and the reply by Leibenstein, pp. 117–19.
See 954.

1970

958 O. GISH, 'Health planning in developing countries'
JDS, July, 1970, 6(4), pp. 67–76.
It is argued that in developing countries much greater reductions in mortality and morbidity can be achieved by an improved system of distribution of health care than by any advances in medical science. Health centres are argued to be the best institutions on which to spend the low health-care budget, and the medical assistant the appropriate type of manpower to train.
See 1138.

959 M. A. KATOUZIAN, 'The development of the service sector: a new approach'
OEP, November, 1970, 22(3), pp. 362–82.
A reappraisal of Fisher–Clark Theory of stages of development, the weakest link of which is the extension of the basic argument for the development pattern of the 'primary' and 'secondary' sectors to services. To aid in the appraisal the service sector is sub-divided into three sectors and the production and consumption characteristics of the components of these sub-divisions examined.

960 W. MALENBAUM, 'Health and productivity in poor areas'
In H. E. Klarman (ed.) *Empirical Studies in Health Economics*, pp. 31–54 (18).
A fairly strong relationship was found between health and productivity in a group of twenty-two less developed countries for which there are United Nations data, and for Mexico for which more detailed census material is available; the results for Thailand and India were less satisfactory. Several health variables were used in the analysis. The results most favourable to the case for health improvement were obtained when infant mortality was used as

the summary measure of health conditions. See also the comment by R. Goode, pp. 55–7.

1 J. E. MILLER, 'An indicator to aid management in assigning programme priorities'
PHR, August, 1970, 85(8), pp. 725–31.
See 867.

2 P. NEWMAN, 'Malaria control and population growth'
JDS, January, 1970, 6(2), pp. 133–58.

A study investigating the effects of malaria control on mortality and fertility rates in Ceylon. The results indicated that malaria control accounted for 60 per cent of the population explosion in Ceylon.

3 H. L. STETTLER, 'The New England throat distemper and family size'
In H. E. Klarman (ed.) *Empirical Studies in Health Economics*, pp. 17–27 (18).

Evidence is presented that suggests that changes in the child death rate in the 1734–40 diphtheria epidemic resulted in adjustments in the birth rate. The evidence is not adequate to demonstrate that family size was adjusted in anticipation of higher infant mortality. See also the comment by M. Perlman, pp. 28–30.

1971

---

4 V. NAVARRO, A. P. RUDERMAN (EDS.) *Health and Socio-economic Development*
IJHS, August, 1971, 1(3), pp. 187–292.

A brief review of the role of health in economic development by Wolf, five articles, and a research report constitute this special issue of the *IJHS*. The articles are as follows:

R. Cibotti, 'Introduction to the analysis of development and planning', pp. 201–24.

W. Scott, 'Cross-national studies of the impact of levels of living on economic growth: an example', pp. 225–32.

A. Waterson, 'An operational approach to development planning', pp. 233–52.

D. H. S. Griffith, D. V. Romana, H. Mashaal, 'Contribution of health to development', pp. 253–70.

T. Dahl, 'Operations research on health care in Chile: an experiment', pp. 271–84.
Research Report:
A. Kühner, 'The impact of public health programmes on economic development. Report of a study of malaria in Thailand', pp. 285–92.

965   C. T. STEWART, 'Allocation of resources to health'
JHR, Winter, 1971, 6(1), pp. 104–22.

A four part classification of resources devoted to health is developed (treatment, prevention, information and research) and the relationships between resources devoted to the different sub-systems is discussed. Using life expectancy as the dependent variable the effects of treatment variables, literacy (information) and potable water (prevention) are measured for nations in the Western hemisphere. The last two variables were significant; the treatment variables were insignificant suggesting that a re-allocation of resources away from treatment is desirable, especially for underdeveloped countries. Comment by E. Meeker (*JHR*, Spring, 1973, 8(2), pp. 257–9).

966   V. VIKRAMAN, O. SETH, 'Programme for control of pulmonary T.B. in India 1971–80. A cost–benefit analysis'
Indian J. Tuberc., 1971, 18(3), pp. 73–83.
See 723.

1972

967   G. N. CONLY, 'The impact of malaria on economic development'
AJTMH, September, 1972, 21(5), pp. 668–74.

A description of a study of Eastern Paraguay where a serious epidemic prompted an eradication programme. A basic problem is the separation of the effects of a change in the endemicity of malaria from the effects of other changes. There was a serious shortage of economic information; the sorts of economic indicators on which information was collected are discussed, although the actual information is not tabulated in the article.
See 731.

968   D. W. DUNLOP, 'The development of an output concept for analysis of curative health services'
SSM, June, 1972, 6(3), pp. 373–85.
See 887.

9 S. Enke, R. A. Brown, 'Economic worth of preventing death at different ages in developing countries'
J.Biosoc.Sci., July, 1972, 4(3), pp. 299–306.
Sample calculations are presented to show the economic worth of preventing the death of individuals of different ages, worth of the individual being measured as the discounted value of the stream of differences between individual consumption and production at different ages. The implications of the calculations for health programmes in developing countries are discussed.

0 H. E. Hilleboe, A. Barkhuus, W. C. Thomas, *Approaches to National Health Planning*
Geneva: World Health Organisation, Public Health Papers No. 46, 1972, p. 108.
See 1407.

1973

A. Blumstein, R. G. Cassidy, 'Benefit–cost analysis of family planning'
Soc.-Econ.Plan.Sciences, April, 1973, 7(2), pp. 151–60.
See 764.

E. J. Cohn, 'Assessing the costs and benefits of anti-malaria programmes: the Indian experience'
AJPH, December, 1973, 63(12), pp. 1086–96.
See 768.

M. S. Feldstein, M. A. Piot, T. K. Sundaresan, *Resource Allocation Model for Public Health Planning: A Case Study of Tuberculosis Control*
Geneva: World Health Organisation, 1973, p. 110.
See 771.

A. Fucaraccio, 'Birth control and the argument of saving and investment'
IJHS, Spring, 1973, 3(2), pp. 133–44.
The argument that birth control will increase saving and investment is rejected in a Latin American context. The argument that capital is scarce is rejected, and in any case, those at whom the birth control programme is aimed are those

unable to save. The savings on public health and educational expenditures are likely to be minimal.

975   W. Malenbaum, 'Health and economic expansion in poor lands'
IJHS, Spring, 1973, 3(2), pp. 161–73.

The author argues that existing theory and experience do not provide a basis for policy on economic development, population growth or investment in health. Motivational elements are seen as important in development, and health schemes may have a greater influence in this way than in their impact on mortality and morbidity statistics.

976   S. B. Rifkin, R. Kaplinsky, 'Health strategy and development planning: lessons from the People's Republic of China'
JDS, January, 1973, 9(2), pp. 213–32.

The relationship of health care services to the socio-political-economic system, and the pattern of provision in less-developed countries are examined. A study of the history of provision of health services in China after 1949 reveals, in contrast to other less-developed countries, an emphasis on preventive programmes, and the delivery system has been designed to aid this end: the use of medical auxiliaries, traditional medical practitioners and public health programmes integrated with development programmes.

977   B. A. Weisbrod, R. L. Andreano, R. E. Baldwin, A. C. Kelley, E. H. Epstein, *Disease and Economic Development: the Impact of Parasitic Diseases in St. Lucia*
Madison, Wisconsin: University of Wisconsin Press, 1973.
See 978.

1974

978   R. E. Baldwin, B. A. Weisbrod, 'Disease and labor productivity'
EDCC, April, 1974, 22(3), pp. 414–35.

A study of plantation workers in St. Lucia to examine the effect of schistosomiasis and other parasitic diseases on productivity. Regression analysis was used to examine the effect of disease on earnings per week, choice of more or less demanding work, productivity per day and number of days worked per week. The findings suggested that the diseases had few significant effects on total productivity, reduced productivity per day of sick workers being offset by more days of work.
See 977.

⟩ M. BERKOWITZ, W. G. JOHNSON, 'Health and labor force participation'
JHR, Winter, 1974, 9(1), pp. 117–28.

A variety of factors affecting labour force participation were examined to assess the significance of health variables being included independently in a model to explain participation. Participation of blacks was more likely to be reduced by health factors than that of whites. Education and marital status were not suitable as proxies for health in explaining participation.

0 J. E. COHEN, 'Potential economic benefits of eliminating mortality attributed to schistosomiasis in Zanzibar'
SSM, July, 1974, 8(7), pp. 383–98.
See 800.

1 R. M. HARTWELL, 'The economic history of medical care'
In M. Perlman (ed.) *The Economics of Health and Medical Care*, pp. 3–20 (44).

The history of medical care is seen to be divided into two periods separated by the industrial revolution. For most of history medical care has had a negligible impact on aggregate social indicators such as mortality and morbidity.

2 M. PAGLIN, 'Public health and development: a new analytical framework'
EC, November, 1974, 41(4), pp. 432–41.
See 810.

3 M. PERLMAN, 'Economic history and health care in industrialized nations'
In M. Perlman (ed.) *The Economics of Health and Medical Care*, pp. 21–33 (44).

Provides a historical perspective to demonstrate the varying perceptions of the problems of health care. The point is made that the present emphasis of health care is on delivery of care, whereas historically nutritional aspects and sanitary control have been more important. The need to collect more sophisticated morbidity data if health care is to be properly assessed is discussed. Two methods used by economists to assess health care, human capital theory and production function analysis, are examined and found to have logical deficiencies.

5 Finance and Organisation of Health Services

Previous sections have looked at the literature of health economics from the viewpoint of the standard characteristics of the economic problem: demand, supply, value, output, cost. The present section, in contrast, is concerned with institutional arrangements and their implications. Systems of financing and organising health-care delivery can and do vary greatly between countries: from private initiative supported by varying degrees of state finance and/or intervention, to a preponderance of provision by state agencies largely without charge to the consumer. The comparison and evaluation of systems is complicated by the fact that individuals attach values to the delivery system itself: they are concerned about the way health care is delivered in a manner, and for reasons, that they would think inappropriate to a discussion of the delivery of their morning milk. The fact that people attach values to activities that elsewhere would be thought of as means rather than ends combines with the very real practical difficulties of identifying causal relationships between inputs and outputs within any given delivery system to make this one of the most difficult fields imaginable for fruitful comparative study. At the same time, the attraction of financing and organisational studies is considerable, since although individuals exhibit strong preferences for one system of delivery rather than another, these co-exist with a widespread belief that actual systems exhibit significant weaknesses, whether in level of provision, breadth of access or costs to users.

The general topic divides naturally into those studies that are concerned with the role of the public sector and those concerned with the characteristics and problems of particular systems. The two are closely related, the conceptual distinction being between what might be called *externally oriented* studies, where the focus of attention is the identification of the market failure etc., reasons for state intervention, and the specification of the type of action needed to deal with the identified problem, and *internally oriented* studies, concerned with the operation of particular
230

systems. At the practical level, the distinction leads to some arbitrariness of classification.

The final sub-section is somewhat diffuse. It is concerned with the consequences of different delivery systems for labour force participation, health preservation and compensation.

(a) The Role of the Public Sector

We include here those studies whose concern is with the general issues affecting the suitability and deficiencies of the market for the delivery of health care, and/or with the methods (provision, legislation, insurance, etc.) that the state might use to remedy the postulated deficiencies.

This sub-section also includes the various contributions to the discussion of the supply of blood. This literature could have been classified elsewhere. Our reason for placing it here is that the major contribution of this literature, in our view, is less the contribution made to our understanding of the characteristics of the market for blood than the consequential elucidation and debate about principles, objectives, logic and evidence in the delivery of health care generally.

1951

J. ROTHENBERG, 'Welfare implications of alternative methods of financing medical care'
AER, May, 1951, 41(2), pp. 676–87.

An early discussion of four different systems of financing medical care: private medicine – no insurance; private medicine – voluntary sickness insurance; private medicine – compulsory sickness insurance; and socialised medicine.

1960

D. S. LEES, 'The economics of health services'
LBR, 1960, 56, pp. 26–40.

The first part of the paper examines the growth and distribution between services of expenditure on the National Health Service from the time of its inception to 1958/59. The second part of the paper considers the case for public provision and concludes that a return to a properly functioning market system would offer a number of advantages.

1961

986   D. S. Lees, *Health Through Choice*
London: Institute of Economic Affairs, Hobart Paper No. 14, 1961.
The National Health Service is examined in relation to the principles of a free society. It is concluded that the N.H.S. is incompatible with these principles. It is also argued that the N.H.S. is incapable of producing a rising standard of care for patients and unable to maintain the continuing freedom of the medical profession. Building a free market in medical care to replace the N.H.S. is canvassed.

987   B. A. Weisbrod, *Economics of Public Health*
Philadelphia: University of Pennsylvania Press, 1961, pp. xvi, 127.
The third and fourth chapters examine the nature of the commodity 'better health', and the problems of determining the public's demand for health-producing activities.
See 639.

1962

988   D. S. Lees, 'The logic of the British National Health Service'
JLE, October, 1962, 5, pp. 111–18.
The arguments against the use of prices and personal payment in medical care are examined and found to be 'based on strong feelings and weak logic'. It is argued that the proponents of the National Health Service are attempting to enforce equality of consumption of medical care, and that equality may be being pressed at the expense of 'good' medical care.

1963

989   K. J. Arrow, 'Uncertainty and the welfare economics of medical care'
AER, December, 1963, 53(5), pp. 941–73. Also in M. H. Cooper, A. J. Culyer (eds.) *Health Economics*, pp. 13–48.
See 1161.

J. Jewkes, S. Jewkes, D. S. Lees, A. Kemp, 'Ethics and the economics of medical care – discussion'
MC, October–December, 1963, 1(4), pp. 234–44.

Three short critical discussions of R. M. Titmuss' original article (*MC*, 1963, 1(1), pp. 16–22). Jewkes and Jewkes criticise Titmuss' view of the British N.H.S. Kemp disputes Titmuss' interpretation and choice of facts about the deficiencies of the U.S. health-care system. Lees also disputes the choice of facts about the U.S. health-care system, but more fundamentally criticises Titmuss for misunderstanding the nature and functioning of markets.
See 992, 1003.

H. E. Klarman, 'The distinctive economic characteristics of health services'
JHHB, Spring, 1963, 4, pp. 44–9.

A list is provided of the characteristics that together distinguish medical services from other goods in the market: a person's need for medical care is asserted as the basis of the right to receive such care regardless of ability to pay; there is an uneven and unpredictable incidence of illness and hence demand for services; the consumer lacks knowledge of medical care; a large section of the medical care industry is non-profit; and finally some types of care generate large external benefits.

R. M. Titmuss, 'Ethics and economics of medical care'
MC, 1963, 1(1), pp. 16–22.

Principally a criticism of D. S. Lees (*Health Through Choice*, 1961). It is argued that for a number of reasons, and because of consumer ignorance in particular, the market is not able to produce a desirable solution to the problem of resource allocation in the health field. The case is supported by evidence on the deficiencies of the market in the U.S. health-care system.
See 986, 990.

J. Wiseman, 'Cost–benefit analysis and health service policy'
SJPE, February, 1963, 10(1), pp. 128–45. Also in B. F. Kiker (ed.) *Investment in Human Capital*, Columbia South Carolina: University of South Carolina Press, 1971, pp. 433–51.
See 645.

1964

994 J. JEWKES, S. JEWKES, A. KEMP, D. S. LEES, *Monopoly or Choice in Health Services?*
London: Institute of Economic Affairs, Occasional Paper No. 3, 1964.
A collection of papers criticising the case put forward by sociologists and social administrators for universal medical services financed from general taxation. *See 990, 992.*

1965

995 J. M. BUCHANAN, *The Inconsistencies of the National Health Service*
London: Institute of Economic Affairs, Occasional Paper No. 7, 1965, p. 24.
See 1100.

996 H. E. KLARMAN, 'The case for public intervention in financing health and medical services'
MC, 1965, 3(1), pp. 59–62.
A brief summary of the arguments adduced to support public intervention in financing public and personal health and medical services.

997 H. E. KLARMAN, 'Conference on the economics of medical research'
In *Report to the President, A National Programme to Conquer Heart Disease, Cancer and Stroke*, Vol. 2, February 1965, pp. 631–44. Washington D.C.: U.S. Government Printing Office, 1965.
See 655.

1967

998 BRITISH MEDICAL ASSOCIATION, *Is There an Alternative?*
London: British Medical Association, 1967, p. 74.
A collection of short articles and discussions relating to alternative methods of financing of the health service in the U.K., or reorganising the structure of the National Health Service. Four articles are by economists:

G. A. Duncan, 'Hospital sweepstakes in the Irish Republic'
C. Clark, 'Decentralizing administration'
A. Seldon, 'Prospects for private health insurance'
J. Wiseman, 'A health corporation?'
See 1000.

D. S. LEES, 'Efficiency in government spending social services: health'
PF, 1967, 22(1/2), pp. 176–89.

The paper examines the case for collective provision of personal health services. The arguments in favour of collective provision rest on the ability to reduce contract costs or the existence of significant externalities. Both, it is argued, are of minor quantitative significance. The paper then goes on to consider arguments for large-scale government provision of health services, the logic of zero prices, and arguments based on equality of consumption. See also the comment by D. Dolman pp. 190–4.

J. WISEMAN, 'A health corporation?'
BMJ, 8th April, 1967, 2, pp. 102–3.

The idea of converting the British National Health Service to a public corporation, of a type similar to the nationalised industries or to the British Broadcasting Corporation, is examined and found wanting.

1968

M. H. COOPER, A. J. CULYER, *The Price of Blood*
London: Institute of Economic Affairs, Hobart Paper No. 41, 1968, p. 47.

The paper is principally a theoretical analysis of the feasibility and desirability of pricing of blood, as empirical study is prevented by the dearth of statistics. It is concluded that blood is an economic good and is amenable to economic analysis, that pricing is feasible, and that the introduction of a dual pricing system would increase supply. Apart from offering prices (either direct payment or exemption from payment in the future on the basis of blood donated) there is also the possibility of increasing supply by removing obstacles in the way of potential donors. Which method of increasing supply would be the least costly is not clear.
See 1013.

R. M. TITMUSS, *Choice and 'the Welfare State'*
London: Fabian Society, Fabian Tract No. 370, 1968, p. 15.
See 1003, 1013.

1003   R. M. TITMUSS, *Commitment to Welfare*
London: George Allen and Unwin Ltd., 1968, p. 272.

A collection of twenty-one essays. Five essays are centred around the topic 'The Health and Welfare Complex' and four on the topic 'Dilemmas in Medical Care'. In the second group is the essay 'Ethics and the economics of medical care', which appeared in *Medical Care* in 1963, generating a debate on the role of government in health care provision. A postscript is added to the essay in this volume, and two more essays 'Welfare state and welfare society', and 'Choice and "the welfare state"', have a bearing on this issue. *See* 1107.

1969

1004   R. M. BAILEY, 'An economist's view of the health services industry'
Inquiry, March, 1969, 6(1), pp. 3–18.

A discussion of some of the characteristics of medical care that may make a free market for care undesirable and may necessitate government intervention.

1005   C. W. BAIRD, 'On the publicness of health care'
RSE, September, 1969, 27(2), pp. 109–20.

Government intervention in the health field can be justified either because of the existence of externalities or because it is an efficient way to deal with poverty (contributing to human capital formation). The real question to be considered is which form of intervention will produce a given level of health at least resource cost. A programme of subsidies and bounties to promote consumption of preventive services and a system of tax credits against medical expenditures are recommended. The need to maintain some control over supply in the face of expanded demand is stressed; a major aspect of such control in the U.S.A. would be to weaken the control of the American Medical Association.

1006   C. M. LINDSAY, 'Medical care and the economics of sharing'
EC, November, 1969, 36(144), pp. 351–62. Also in M. H. Cooper, A. J. Culyer (eds.) *Health Economics*, 75–89 (33).

A possible theoretical foundation for the institutional characteristics of the British National Health Service is devised. The basis for the approach is the presumption that a large segment of society believes that everyone should have 'equal access' to the medical resources available, that medical need and not economic status should determine eligibility for care. The paper explores the externalities generated by the desire for greater equality and the possible

approaches that might be employed to promote the desired extension of equality.
See 1018.

A. SELDON, A. J. CULYER, C. M. LINDSAY, *The Price of Health, an Economic Analysis of the Theory and Practice of Financing Health Services*
Melbourne: Office of Health Care Finance, 1969, p. 85.
Contains three articles concerning the debate over compulsory health insurance in Australia. A. Seldon, 'The economics of health service financing', argues that compulsory insurance is both costly and illiberal, its aims being better served by control of medical monopolies and by income redistribution. A. J. Culyer, 'Economics of health systems', uses externality theory to argue that the Scotton–Deeble proposals would be less preferred than a universal subsidy/tax system with free care for high risk clients. C. M. Lindsay, 'Compulsion and the provision of medical services', argues against government provision because of its 'stultifying effect' and against risk pooling on account of its inequities. He argues for a tax/subsidy scheme such that the taxes vary with the income of contributors, subsidies inversely with income and with the sickness of the individual.
See 1180, 1187, 1188, 1198, 1199.

J. WISEMAN, 'Some economic problems of medical care'
JRCGP, February, 1969, Supplement No. 1, 17(79), pp. 2–7.
A contribution to a symposium on 'Society and its general practitioners'. The nature of the commodity 'health' is taken as a starting point for discussion. Differences in the type of government intervention in the health market are then explored, and finally the position of doctors, their professional outlook, and the public interest are examined.

1970

C. W. BAIRD, 'A technique for analysing inaccurately estimated trade-offs'
RSE, September, 1970, 28(2), pp. 173–8.
Examines the situation that will arise in the health-care market if consumers underestimate the marginal product of preventive services relative to curative services. A subsidy to preventive services will save scarce resources. A simple diagrammatic analysis is provided to show the size of subsidy necessary.

1010   BRITISH MEDICAL ASSOCIATION, *Health Services Financing*
London, BMA, 1970, pp. xvi, 605.
See 1065, 1111.

1011   C. C. HAVIGHURST, 'Health maintenance organisations and the market for
health services'
Law Contemp.Probl., Autumn, 1970, 35(4), pp. 716–95.
See 1297.

1012   C. M. LINDSAY, J. M. BUCHANAN, 'The organisation and financing of
medical care in the United States'
Appendix Q of British Medical Association, *Health Services Financing*,
pp. 535–85 (1065).
The second section of the paper is entitled 'why not use free markets to organise
and finance medical services?' and discusses externalities, uncertainty in
demand, option demand and transactions costs.
See 1207.

1013   R. M. TITMUSS, *The Gift Relationship: from Human Blood to Social Policy*
London: George Allen and Unwin Ltd., p. 339.
The book concerns itself with the provision of blood for transfusion, docu-
menting the form of organisation in various countries but with particular
emphasis on the United States and England and Wales. The material on blood
policy is, however, viewed as being of wider significance, a point of departure
for considering the whole of social policy. The voluntary donation of blood
provokes fundamental issues: the provision of blood is an area of conflict
between altruistic and commercial values. Titmuss implies that the differences
in the form of organisation of blood supplies reflect differences between the
social values of the two societies. A particularly disputed proposition made
by Titmuss is that the effect of paying for blood will eventually lead to a
decrease in the supply and a lower quality of blood for transfusion.
See 528, 1001, 1002, 1021, 1026, 1028, 1033, 1036, 1039, 1040, 1041, 1046.

1971

1014   C. W. BAIRD, 'On profits and hospitals'
JEI, March, 1971, 5(1), pp. 57–66.
The two main arguments cited against profit-maximising hospitals are the
possibility of monopoly power being misused, and consumer ignorance about

the product. It is argued that in most urban areas there are adequate numbers of hospitals to maintain a competitive situation, and to dispel consumer ignorance it is argued that consumer journals could be developed and hospitals provide informative advertising. See also H. M. Goldstein, 'More on profits and hospitals', *JEI*, December, 1971, 5(4), pp. 113–23, C. W. Baird, 'Still more on profits and hospitals', *JEI*, 5(4), pp. 123–6.

R. R. CAMPBELL, *Economics of Health and Public Policy*
Washington D.C.: American Enterprise Institute for Public Policy Research, 1971, p. 108.
See 23.

M. H. COOPER, 'How to pay for the health service'
JRSH, 1971, 91(5), pp. 217–21.

Suggestions to break up the British National Health Service are, it is argued, unreasonable. The alternatives suggested offer at least as many possibilities of inefficiency. Limited adjustments to increase the efficiency of the N.H.S., and efforts to make tax-payers aware of the link between tax payments and health care, are canvassed.

A. J. CULYER, 'The nature of the commodity "health care" and its efficient allocation'
OEP, July, 1971, 23(2), pp. 189–211. Also in M. H. Cooper, A. J. Culyer (eds.) *Health Economics*, pp. 49–74 (33).

The paper examines the characteristics of health care that have been cited, in the 'market versus state' debate, as a justification for a particular form of organisation of health services. It is concluded that no *a priori* economic case can be made for one form of organisation rather than another. The major reason for this is that the institutions through which resource allocation and distribution are accommodated to individuals' preferences are all costly to operate. Choice of institutional form is therefore an empirical matter. It is suggested, however, that the efficiency of existing institutions could undoubtedly be improved by application of cost–benefit and cost-effectiveness techniques.

A. J. CULYER, 'Medical care and the economics of giving'
EC, August, 1971, 38(151), pp. 295–303.

Demonstrates that an approach in which the externality relationship relates to the quantity of suffering felt by people, rather than to the distribution of suffering as in the Lindsay sharing approach, is superior in that it does not require the introduction of special traits into the utility functions of individuals

and fits easily into, and is consistent with, the externality literature. The approach also suggests a number of implications that are broadly consistent with observable events.
See 1006.

1019 A. DONABEDIAN, 'Social responsibility for personal health services: an examination of basic values'
Inquiry, June, 1971, 8(2), pp. 3–19.

The issue of greater government involvement in medical care is considered from two archetypal and opposing viewpoints, characterised as 'libertarian' and 'egalitarian'. The article then goes on to consider whether medical care has any distinguishing characteristics that make removal from the market desirable. It is concluded that while medical care is not peculiar in any one property, it is peculiar in the combination of properties that characterise it.
See 35.

1020 R. FEIN, G. I. WEBER, *Financing Medical Education: An Analysis of Alternative Policies and Mechanisms*
New York: McGraw-Hill Book Company, 1971, p. 279.

A case is presented for greater federal government involvement in the financing of medical education in the U.S.A.
See 254.

1021 N. GLAZER, 'Blood'
PI, Summer, 1971, 24, pp. 86–94.

An article length review of Titmuss' *The Gift Relationship*.
See 1013.

1022 H. G. GRUBEL, 'Risk, uncertainty, and moral hazard'
JRI, March, 1971, 38(1), pp. 99–106.
See 1220.

1023 R. HARRIS, A. SELDON, *Choice in Welfare 1970*
London: The Institute of Economic Affairs, 1971, p. 84.
See 1119.

1024 L. MCCOY, 'The nursing home as a public utility'
JEI, March, 1971, 5(1), pp. 67–76.

A case is presented for giving nursing homes in the U.S.A. public utility status, with regulation under an appropriate state commission of entry to the market, classification of homes, standards and services and rate structures. The case is developed on the ground of similarities between nursing homes and other organisations that are already treated as public utilities.

M. V. PAULY, *Medical Care at Public Expense, A Study in Applied Welfare Economics*
New York: Praeger Publishers, 1971, pp. xvi, 160.

Having established a rationale for public involvement in the provision of medical care, the conditions for optimality in the public provision of medical care are derived. This ideal system is used as a basis from which to evaluate current and proposed public involvement in the provision of medical care in the United States. The techniques used are those of Paretian welfare economics. The chapter headings are as follows:

1 The meaning of efficiency in the public provision of medical care.
2 An approach to optimality in the public provision of medical care.
3 Optimal insurance against the cost of medical care.
4 Efficient national health insurance.
5 Medicare – public provision regardless of wealth.
6 Medicaid – public provision without controls.

R. M. SOLOW, 'Blood and thunder'
YLJ, July, 1971, 80(8), pp. 1696–711.

A review of Titmuss' *The Gift Relationship*, which is particularly critical of Titmuss' attack on the market as a mechanism for mobilising and allocating resources.
See 1013.

B. A. WEISBROD, 'Costs and benefits of medical research: a case study of poliomyelitis'
JPE, May–June, 1971, 79(3), pp. 527–44.
See 724.

1972

K. J. ARROW, 'Gifts and exchanges'
PPA, Summer, 1972, 1(4), pp. 343–62.

A series of penetrating comments on the issues raised by Titmuss in *The Gift Relationship*. Arrow concludes, as have other economist commentators, that many of Titmuss' points are not empirically established, with the exception of

the relation between the commercial blood supply and post-transfusion hepatitis.
See 1013.

1029 A. J. CULYER, 'On the relative efficiency of the National Health Service'
Kyklos, 1972, 25(2), pp. 266–87.

Certain of the issues thrown up in the theoretical arguments of the 1960s about the organisation and finance of medical care are examined. Most of the strong policy conclusions previously reached are shown to be not strictly tenable given conventional value judgements and given a purely qualitative approach. Among the questions tackled are: Is the N.H.S.-type of organisation likely to produce a Pareto-optimum allocation of resources compared with the market? Can one infer that the objective of the N.H.S. is equality of consumption? Does the existence of a private sector alongside the N.H.S. enable the attainment of a Pareto-optimum?

1030 A. J. CULYER, 'The "market" versus the "state" in medical care – a minority report on an empty academic box'
In G. McLachlan (ed.) *Problems and Progress in Medical Care, Essays on Current Research, Seventh Series*, pp. 1–31 (30).

The paper examines two related sets of issues. The first set of issues is concerned with the relative abilities of the N.H.S. form of organisation and a market system to approach a social welfare maximum, and whether the existence of observable deficiencies in one system or the other is evidence to support a choice between systems. The second set of issues deals with the question of whether the special characteristics of medical care make one form of organisation inherently superior (in terms of social welfare) to another.

1031 A. J. CULYER, P. JACOBS, 'The war and public expenditure on mental health care in England and Wales – the postponement effect'
SSM, February, 1972, 6(1), pp. 35–56.
See 1130.

1032 M. S. LEVITT, 'Problems of efficiency'
In M. M. Hauser (ed.) *The Economics of Medical Care*, pp. 33–41 (28).

The paper sets out to provide the non-economist with an outline of the requirements of an economically efficient system of medical care. The bulk of the paper is devoted to efficiency under present N.H.S. arrangements. See also the comment by A. J. Culyer, pp. 42–6.

S. ROTTENBERG, 'The production and exchange of used body parts'
In *Toward Liberty: Essays in Honour of Ludwig Von Mises* Vol. 2,
Merlo Park California: Institute for Humane Studies, 1972.

An uncompromising discussion of the advantages of organising markets for
exchanging human spare parts, including blood.
See 1013.

L. G. SGONTZ, 'The economics of financing medical care: a review of the
literature'
Inquiry, December, 1972, 9(4), pp. 3–19.

A survey of the debates on private versus public finance of medical care is
provided, and then alternative existing and proposed institutional arrangements for financing medical care in the United States are evaluated in terms of
their ability to satisfy various distributional externalities. A substantial
bibliography is provided. See also the comment by D. Whipple, 'Health care as
a right: its economic implications', *Inquiry*, March, 1974, 11(1), pp. 65–8.

1973

J. F. BLUMSTEIN, M. ZUBKOFF, 'Perspectives on government policy in the
health sector'
MMFQ, Summer, 1973, 51(3), pp. 395–426.

A review of many of the arguments in the market versus state provision of
medical services debate. It is argued that policies designed to increase the
effectiveness of the market mechanism should be considered. Forms of
intervention of this type are examined.

M. H. COOPER, A. J. CULYER, 'The economics of giving and selling blood'
In Institute of Economic Affairs, *The Economics of Charity*, pp. 109–43
(1039).

The first part of the paper critically examines the Titmuss view (as expressed in
The Gift Relationship). The second part of the paper extends Cooper and
Culyer's earlier analysis and suggests how some of the worst consequences
feared for the payment method might be mitigated.
See 1001, 1013.

A. J. CULYER, 'Should social policy concern itself with drug "abuse"?'
PFQ, October, 1973, 4(1), pp. 449–56.

The paper examines the Paretian significance of six arguments used to justify
the prohibition of drugs for non-therapeutic use. The only arguments of

Paretian significance are related to physical harm done to others and to corruption of minors.

1038   P. J. FELDSTEIN, *Financing Dental Care: An Economic Analysis*
Lexington: D. C. Heath and Company, 1973, pp. xvii, 260.
See 36.

1039   INSTITUTE OF ECONOMIC AFFAIRS, *The Economics of Charity*
London: The Institute of Economic Affairs, Readings No. 12, 1973, pp. xviii, 197.

Sub-titled 'Essays on the comparative economics and ethics of giving and selling, with applications to blood,' this is a collection of eight essays and some appendices of technical evidence. The first five essays deal with the theoretical principles and analysis of 'giving'; the last three essays consider the application to blood.
1   A. A. Alchian, W. R. Allen, 'The pure economics of giving', pp. 1–13.
2   G. Tullock, 'The charity of the uncharitable', pp. 15–32.
3   A. J. Culyer, 'Quids without quos – a praxeological approach', pp. 33–61.
4   T. R. Ireland, 'The calculus of philanthropy', pp. 63–78.
5   D. B. Johnson, 'The charity market: theory and practice', pp. 79–106.
6   M. H. Cooper, A. J. Culyer, 'The economics of giving and selling blood', pp. 109–43.
7   T. Ireland, J. Koch, 'Blood and American social attitudes', pp. 145–55.
8   D. B. Johnson, 'The U.S. market in blood', pp. 157–67.
Appendix A: M. J. Ireland, 'The legal framework of the market for blood', pp. 171–8.
Appendix B: A. J. Salsbury, 'Medical evidence: blood donation and the Australian antigen', pp. 179–82.
See 1013, 1036, 1040.

1040   T. R. IRELAND, J. V. KOCH, 'Blood and American social attitudes'
In Institute of Economic Affairs, *The Economics of Charity*, pp. 145–55 (1039).

A brief review of some of the features of the U.S. blood market and some possibilities for improving it.

1041   P. SINGER, 'Altruism and commerce: a defense of Titmuss against Arrow'
PPA, Spring, 1973, 2(3), pp. 312–20.

Particularly defends Titmuss' treatment of data against Arrow's criticisms and argues that he successfully shifted the burden of proof to defenders of the market.

1974

B. ABEL-SMITH, 'Value for money in health services'
SSB, July, 1974, 37(7), pp. 17–28.
Principally a review of three paths to intervention in the provision of health
services that a society might pursue. The first is the regulation of services that
are delivered; the second is the planning of the delivery system; the third is
action to change the behaviour of those who control the system.

P. D. CUMMING, E. L. WALLACE, D. M. SURGENOR, B. D. MIERZWA, F. A.
SMITH, 'Public interest pricing of blood services'
MC, September, 1974, 12(9), pp. 743–53.
See 528, 1013.

E. GINZBERG, 'The health services industry: realism in social control'
JEI, June, 1974, 8(2), pp. 381–94.
The deficiencies of markets in producing desirable results in the field of health
care are outlined. The development is traced of government intervention in the
U.S.A. in the financing of health care, in expanding the supply of health care
resources and in developing devices to control cost inflation. Gradual modifications are seen to be more desirable than wholesale restructuring of the health-
care system.

C. C. HAVIGHURST (ed.) *Regulating Health Facilities Construction*
Washington D.C.: American Enterprise Institute for Public Policy
Research, 1974, p. 314.
Of particular interest are the papers by C. C. Havighurst, 'Speculations on the
market's future in health care', pp. 249–69, who argues that the market is a
viable candidate for the job of straightening out the health-care industry; W. J.
Curran, 'A national survey and analysis of state certificate-of-need laws for
health facilities', pp. 85–111; and R. A. Posner, 'Certificates of need for health
care facilities: a dissenting view', pp. 113–21, who discusses the differences
between the health-care setting and the other areas in which public utility
regulation has been used.
See 1268.

R. A. KESSEL, 'Transfused blood, serum hepatitis, and the Coase theorem'
JLE, October, 1974, 17(2), pp. 265–89.
Titmuss' view that too low a quality of blood has been provided to patients in
the United States is supported. It is argued, however, that this is the result of

financial incentives being too small rather than too large. Doctors do not bear product liability for blood and this had hampered the development of low risk blood sources.
See 1013

1047   E. LIEFMANN-KEIL, 'Consumer protection, incentives and externalities in the drug market'
In M. Perlman (ed.) *The Economics of Health and Medical Care*, pp. 117–29 (44).

The paper follows the new approach to the theory of demand (Becker and Lancaster) in analysing the costs of the efforts to protect the consumer, and the externalities generated by the regulations introduced to reduce other externalities.

1048   D. NEUHAUSER, 'The future of proprietaries in American health services'
In C. C. Havighurst (ed.) *Regulating Health Facilities Construction*, pp. 233–47.
See 546.

1049   A. WILLIAMS, '"Need" as a demand concept (with special reference to health)'
In A. J. Culyer (ed.) *Economic Policies and Social Goals*, pp. 60–76 (41).
See 155.

(b)   Characteristics and Problems of Different Systems of Provision

---

The studies in this sub-section are grouped under four heads. (i) *Comparative Studies* includes works that compare different delivery systems. The entries form a somewhat heterogeneous set, differing in conceptual framework, in breadth of coverage and in depth (nature and extent of the characteristics examined). The other three sets, (ii)–(iv), relate to the important major systems of delivery. (ii) lists works concerned with state provision: it is heavily weighted by studies of the U.K. system and closely related to the works listed in 5(a). (iii) encompasses studies of insurance systems other than Medicare and Medicaid, which have a large enough literature to merit separate classification under (iv).

(i) *Comparative Studies*

1963

B. ABEL-SMITH, *Paying for Health Services: A Study of the Costs and Sources of Finance in Six Countries*
Geneva: World Health Organisation, Public Health Papers No. 17, 1963, p. 86.
The study was carried out principally to establish a methodology for the study of health-care costs. The six countries studied are Ceylon, Chile, Czechoslovakia, Israel, Sweden and the United States. No attempt was made to standardise among the six countries the particular year to which the figures of cost relate (the year of account selected varies from 1956 to 1959).

P. COWAN, 'The size of hospitals'
MC, January–March, 1963, 1(1), pp. 1–9.
See 357.

J. HOGARTH, *The Payment of the General Practitioner*
Oxford: Pergamon Press, 1963, pp. xii, 684.
See 177.

J. JEWKES, S. JEWKES, *Value for Money in Medicine*
Oxford: Basil Blackwell, 1963.
See 1095.

OFFICE OF HEALTH ECONOMICS, *Health Services in Western Europe*
London: Office of Health Economics, May, 1963, p. 16.
An early brief comparison of health service systems in Europe, looking at methods of payment, form of organisation and, where possible, numbers of doctors and hospital beds. The countries covered are Austria, Belgium, Denmark, Eire, Finland, France, Germany, Italy, Luxembourg, Netherlands, Norway, Portugal, Spain, Sweden, Switzerland and the United Kingdom.
See 4.

1965

B. ABEL-SMITH, 'The major patterns of financing and organisation of medical services that have emerged in other countries'
MC, January–March, 1965, 3(1), pp. 33–40.

Traces the development of medical care organisation in eastern and western Europe and the U.S.A. It is argued that the differences in the organisation and financing of medical care that have emerged have been influenced by long-established differences in attitudes to medical care, rather than by political ideologies of relatively recent origin.

1056   R. R. L. LOGAN, T. S. EIMERL, 'Case loads in hospital and general practice in several countries'
MMFQ, April, 1965, 43(2 part 2), pp. 302–10.

The problems of making international comparisons of health services are discussed. Information on hospital bed provision and admissions is provided for thirteen countries. More detailed information on types of admissions and average length of stay is provided for the U.S.A., Sweden, Israel, and England and Wales. Some information is provided on place and rates of general practitioner contact in ten countries.

1967

1057   B. ABEL-SMITH, *An International Study of Health Expenditure, and its Relevance for Health Planning*
Geneva: World Health Organisation, Public Health Papers No. 32, 1967, p. 127.

Thirty-three countries were included in the study. Most of the information in the study was drawn from replies to a questionnaire. The geographical distribution of the countries included was as follows: five from Africa, seven from the Americas, one from South-East Asia, eleven from Europe, four from the Eastern Mediterranean, and five from the Western Pacific. The final chapter attempts to show how the information collected can be used for health planning.

1058   O. W. ANDERSON, 'Toward a framework for analysing health services systems with examples from selected countries'
SEA, January, 1967, 1(1), pp. 16–31.

Two elements are seen to form the core of a health services system: the first is 'the elasticity of the perception of illness and what people do about it', and the second is 'the necessary discretionary judgement and authority that is required by physicians'. These elements are seen to force a high degree of necessary flexibility in the range of methods of delivering health services. The health systems of Sweden, United States and the United Kingdom are examined in this light.

J. S. DEEBLE, 'The costs and sources of finance of Australian health services'
ER, 1967, 43(4), pp. 518–43.
See 1179.

O. L. PETERSON, A. M. BURGESS, R. BERFENSTAM, B. SMEDBY, R. F. L. LOGAN, R. J. C. PEARSON, 'What is value for money in medical care? Experiences in England and Wales, Sweden, and the U.S.A.'
Lancet, April 8th, 1967, 1(7493), pp. 771–6.
Published data are examined to illustrate some of the important differences between these countries. Comparisons are made of health status (using mortality data), health expenditures, manpower, hospitals and the use of services.

1968

L. S. REED, W. CARR, 'Utilization and cost of general hospital care: Canada and the United States, 1948–1966'
SSB, November, 1968, 31(11), pp. 12–20.
Canada was found to have a higher admission rate, a longer average length of stay and more days of hospital care per 1000 population than the United States.

1969

T. W. BICE, K. L. WHITE, 'Factors related to the use of health services: an international comparative study'
MC, March–April, 1969, 7(2), pp. 124–33.
See 1449, *1461*.

M. I. ROEMER, *The Organisation of Medical Care Under Social Security*
Geneva: International Labour Office, Studies and Reports, New Series, No. 73, 1969, pp. viii, 241.
The study examines the organisation of medical care within the framework of the social security system in eight countries: Belgium, Canada, Ecuador, the

Federal Republic of Germany, India, Poland, Tunisia and the United Kingdom. The study reviews the experiences of these countries in organising the supply of medical resources, dealing with special problems such as disease prevention, safeguarding patient and provider of care and disability certification, in developing resources and in particular in meeting rural health needs, and finally in influencing quality and costs.

1970

1064   R. ANDERSEN, B. SMEDBY, O. W. ANDERSON, *Medical Care Use in Sweden and the United States: A Comparative Analysis of Systems and Behaviour*
Chicago: University of Chicago, Center for Health Administration Studies, Research Series, No. 27, 1970, pp. xiii, 174.

The monograph sets out to investigate differences between the United States and Sweden in the amounts and types of health services utilised. The analysis is based on comparable social surveys carried out in the two countries in 1964.

1065   BRITISH MEDICAL ASSOCIATION, *Health Services Financing*
London: BMA, 1970, pp. xvi, 605.

The second section contains fourteen papers examining the finance and organisation of health services in the developed world (Appendices D–Q).

D   A. Seldon, 'Organisation and financing of medical care in Australia', pp. 309–24.
E   H. Kohlmaier, 'The organisation and financing of health insurance in Australia', pp. 325–42.
F   A. P. Ruderman, 'The organisation and financing of medical care in Canada', pp. 343–58.
G   L. Sirc, 'Organisation and financing of medical care in East European Communist countries', pp. 359–72.
H   G. Rosch, 'The economics of medical care in France', pp. 373–402.
I   W. Schreiber, 'Health insurance in the German Federal Republic', pp. 403–20.
J   G. Duncan, 'The organisation and financing of medical care in Ireland', pp. 421–30.
K   H. Ahlbaun, 'Sickness insurance in the Grand Duchy of Luxembourg', pp. 431–8.
L   J. von Langendonc, 'Organisation and financing of medical care in the Netherlands and Belgium', pp. 439–70.
M   J. T. Ward, 'Organisation and financing of medical care in New Zealand', pp. 471–84.

N   K. Evang, 'The organisation and financing of health services in Norway', pp. 485–506.

O   T. Thorburn, 'Organisation and financing of medical services in Sweden', pp. 507–20.

P   M. Hauser, 'Organisation and financing of medical services in Switzerland', pp. 520–34.

Q   C. M. Lindsay, J. M. Buchanan, 'The organisation and financing of medical care in the United States', pp. 535–85.

See 1012, 1111, 1207.

W. A. GLASER, *Paying the Doctor: Systems of Remuneration and Their Effects*
Baltimore: The Johns Hopkins Press, 1970, pp. xii, 323.

A study of methods of payment of medical practitioners in Cyprus, Egypt, England, France, Germany, Greece, Israel, Italy, Lebanon, the Netherlands, Poland, Spain, Sweden, Switzerland, Turkey and the U.S.S.R.
See 237.

R. M. TITMUSS, *The Gift Relationship: from Human Blood to Social Policy*
London: George Allen and Unwin Ltd., 1970, p. 339.
See 1013.

1971

O. W. ANDERSON, 'Styles of planning health services. The United States, Sweden and England'
IJHS, May, 1971, 1(2), pp. 106–20.

Case studies of the styles of planning of health services in the three countries are presented. It is concluded that the nature of health services and the fact that they reflect the differing social and political contexts in which they operate makes standardising health services systems from country to country impossible.

O. GISH, *Doctor Migration and World Health*
London: G. Bell and Sons Ltd., Occasional Papers on Social Administration No. 43, 1971, p. 151.

The second part of the monograph examines the causes and the impact of large-scale doctor migration from developing countries. The countries examined in the study are India, Pakistan, Ceylon, Malaysia, Singapore, Hong Kong, the

Philippines, Thailand, Indonesia, Iran, Ethiopia, Sudan, Kenya, Ghana and Trinidad.
See 256.

1070 M. I. ROEMER (ed.) 'Social insurance as an influence on medical care patterns'
IJHS, November, 1971, 1(4), pp. 309–414.

Eight papers dealing with the impact of social insurance on the prevailing patterns of medical care in countries of western Europe, Latin America, North America and Australasia.

M. Pflanz, 'German health insurance: the evolution and current problems of the pioneer system', pp. 315–30.

R. F. Bridgman, 'Medical care under social security in France', pp. 331–41.

D. G. Gill, 'The British National Health Service: professional determinants of administrative structure', pp. 342–53.

M. I. Roemer, 'Social security for medical care: is it justified in developing countries?' pp. 354–61.

T. L. Hall, S. Diaz, 'Social security and health care patterns in Chile', pp. 362–77.

M. V. Bastos, 'Brazil's multiple social insurance schemes and their influence on medical care', pp. 378–89.

C. W. Dixon, 'Changes in hospitals and general practice under social security in New Zealand', pp. 390–7.

J. E. F. Hastings, 'Federal-provincial insurance for hospital and physician's care in Canada', pp. 398–414.

1071 E. R. WEINERMAN, 'Research on comparative health service systems'
MC, May–June, 1971, 9(3), pp. 272–90.

The objectives and the problems of cross-national studies of health-care systems are discussed. Sixty-five published studies are classified according to methodological approach, and several major pieces of unpublished work are mentioned. A typology for data-gathering and comparative analysis of total health service systems is presented.

1972

1072 O. W. ANDERSON, *Health Care: Can There Be Equity?*
New York: John Wiley and Sons, 1972, pp. xxii, 273.

Extensive comparisons are made between the health services of the United States, Sweden and England, the liberal–democratic context in which the services operate, their performance from 1950 to 1970, and the chronic problems and issues that to a different extent have beset all three systems. A substantial bibliography is provided. This book draws on earlier work by the author and others on the health services of these countries.

J. H. BABSON, *Health Care Delivery Systems: A Multinational Survey* London: Pitman and Sons Ltd., 1972, pp. vii, 128.

The study concentrates on three regulatory devices and their potential within various administrative environments to produce adequate health services, hospital financing mechanisms, patterns of hospital ownership and procedures for accreditation and licensing of hospitals. The countries studied are Denmark, Finland, Sweden, Switzerland and Belgium, which are considered representative of the basic organisational patterns found in Europe, and Great Britain and Yugoslavia, which are exceptions. The adequacy of the various health-care systems is judged by indicators of effectiveness (accessibility, quality, integration) and of efficiency. A large bibliography is provided.

R. D. FRASER, 'Health and general systems of financing health care' *MC*, July–August, 1972, 10(4), pp. 345–56.

Linear regression analysis is used to examine the relationship between infant mortality, used as a proxy for the level of health, and the number of physicians per 10,000 population, number of hospital beds per 1000, and GDP per capita in 18 countries. The estimated equation is then used to make predictions of infant mortality in 1950, 1955 and 1960. The differences between observed mortality and predicted mortality are then examined. An attempt to explain the differences by differences in degree of government involvement in the health sector was not successful, but a significant relationship was found between unexplained variations in infant mortality and the percentage of health-care resources devoted to the provision of non-personal public health. *See 1077.*

F. ILLUMINATI, 'The cost of health. (General medicine, hospitalization, medicaments, relations of the medical profession with social security)' *ISSR*, 1972, 25(4), pp. 376–94.

A set of international comparisons between twelve countries in Europe. Data are presented on the costs of hospital services and prescriptions, and on the number of hospital cases and the number of prescriptions. The nature of health service benefits and the beneficiaries' share in health-care costs is outlined, and the policies adopted to tackle rising costs discussed.

1973

1076 C. ALTENSTETTER, 'Planning for health facilities in the United States and in West Germany'
MMFQ, Winter, 1973, 51(1), pp. 41–71.
A study of the origins and nature of planning for health facilities in the two countries. In West Germany state and local government have long accepted public responsibility in the health field. In the United States comprehensive health planning appears to have been the outcome of several isolated decisions.

1077 R. D. FRASER, 'An international study of health, and general systems of financing health care'
IJHS, Summer, 1973, 3(3), pp. 369–97.
A follow-up to Fraser, *MC*, July–August, 1972. Data from twenty-five countries for 1955, 1960 and 1965 are used. Support is provided for the results of the original study. Size of government role and size of the personal health sector are not important determinants of levels of health, whereas non-personal public health does appear to be a significant determinant.
See 1074.

1078 L. D. HABER, 'Some parameters for social policy in disability: a cross national comparison'
MMFQ, Summer, 1973, 51(3), pp. 319–40.
See 916, 1362.

1079 R. KOHN, S. RADIUS, 'International comparison of health service systems, an annotated bibliography'
IJHS, Spring, 1973, 3(2), pp. 295–309.
See 1490.

1080 G. LAZARCIK, 'Defence, education, and health expenditures, and their relation to GNP in Eastern Europe, 1960–1970'
Amer.Econ., Spring, 1973, 17(1), pp. 29–34.
GNP and expenditure estimates were obtained for Bulgaria, Czechoslovakia, East Germany, Hungary, Poland and Rumania. Although the annual rate of growth in expenditure in the six countries was higher for defence (11.1 per cent) than the other categories, the average annual increase in health expenditure was 7.6 per cent.

1974

E. KLEIMAN, 'The determinants of national outlay on health'
In M. Perlman (ed.) *The Economics of Health and Medical Care*, pp. 66–81 (44).

Investigates international differences in per capital levels of health outlay, and their division between private and public components. The findings suggest that households, having decided on the amount of services they wish to consume, adjust their actual purchases to allow for free provision of similar services by government (the public sector behaves in a parallel manner with regard to private purchases).

V. NAVARRO, 'The underdevelopment of health or the health of underdevelopment: an analysis of the distribution of human health resources in Latin America'
IJHS, Winter, 1974, 4(1), pp. 5–27.

It is argued that the highly skewed distribution of health resources in Latin American countries is a symptom of the highly inequitable distribution of all resources and economic power, and not just a result of capital scarcity, the existence of dual economies or the lack of technological diffusion from rich to poor countries.

C. P. WEN, 'Health in the midst of economic development in Taiwan'
MC, January, 1974, 12(1), pp. 85–94.

Catalogues the failure of development planners in Taiwan to devote resources to health services, and compares a variety of statistics relating to provision of health services and indices of health status with similar data from Japan and some Western countries.

(ii)   *State Provision*

1951

S. E. HARRIS, 'The British health experiment: the first two years of the National Health Service'
AER, May, 1951, 41(2), pp. 652–66.

Principally of historical interest as a survey of the early problems and grouses. The most significant British mistake was seen to be 'the introduction of comprehensive services before the required facilities were available'.

1952

1085 F. ROBERTS, *The Cost of Health*
London: Turnstile Press, 1952, p. 200.

An early study questioning the optimistic view that a free health service simply implies a transfer from direct payment by individuals to indirect payment by society, and that expenditures on health are limited by the existence of some finite amount of treatable disease. The problems of determining the proportion of national income to be devoted to the treatment of ill-health are discussed.

1956

1086 B. ABEL-SMITH, R. M. TITMUSS, *The Cost of the National Health Service in England and Wales*
Cambridge: Cambridge University Press, 1956, pp. xx, 176.

A pioneering study of the National Health Service covering the period 1948 to 1954, prepared for the Guillebaud Committee (a government-appointed inquiry into the total cost of the N.H.S.). The study employed a social accounting framework and broke down expenditures on the N.H.S. into capital and current and central and local government. In examining the rising trend of expenditure, contrary to expectations, the study showed that much of the increase in expenditure could be attributed to higher wages and prices rather than to any increase in the volume of real resources absorbed by the service.

1958

1087 R. M. TITMUSS, *Essays on 'the Welfare State'*
London: George Allen and Unwin Ltd., 1958, p. 262.

A collection of ten lectures, four of which are on health-care topics. Three deal with the various aspects of the National Health Service and provide useful background material. They are: 'Some aspects of structure', 'Some facts about general practice', and 'Science and the sociology of medical care'. The fourth essay on a health topic, 'The hospital and its patients', is a series of reflections on the hospital environment.

1960

D. S. LEES, 'The economics of health services'
LBR, 1960, 56, pp. 26–40.
See 985.

1961

J. JEWKES, S. JEWKES, *The Genesis of the British National Health Service*
Oxford: Basil Blackwell, 1961, pp. xii, 68.

The paper examines the British National Health Service, the arguments in favour of establishing the N.H.S., the scale and distribution of medical facilities before and after the Second World War, and speculation on the likely state of medical services in Britain if the N.H.S. had not been established.

D. S. LEES, *Health Through Choice*
London: Institute of Economic Affairs, Hobart Paper No. 14, 1961.
See 986.

1962

D. S. LEES, 'The logic of the British National Health Service'
JLE, October, 1962, 5, pp. 111–18.
See 988.

D. MIRFIN (ed.) *Buying Better Health*
London: The Acton Society Trust, 1962, pp. v, 98.

A colloquium examining the development and likely role of private health insurance within the British National Health Service. Participants included doctors, hospital and medical administrators, university academics and politicians. The discussion is centred around three main topics: the impact of BUPA and similar schemes on the market for medical care; the effect of increased finance from sources other than the state on quality of service provided; and the effect of increased finance from sources other than the state on planning and administration.

1093   OFFICE OF HEALTH ECONOMICS, *Studies on Current Health Problems*
London: Office of Health Economics, 1962–
See 4.

1963

1094   M. S. FELDSTEIN, 'Developments in health services administration and financial control'
MC, 1963, pp. 171–7.

A brief survey of the developments in financial administration and control in the early years of the British National Health Service, and of the first steps to secure greater efficiency in the use of resources with the development of costing schemes.

1095   J. JEWKES, S. JEWKES, *Value for Money in Medicine*
Oxford: Basil Blackwell, 1963.

The pamplet examines the argument that increased spending on health services increases production and reduces medical costs. In particular, arguments concerning reduced absence from work due to sickness and increased working lifetimes are examined and found wanting, at least at the present time though having possible validity in the earlier years of the twentieth century.

1964

1096   S. E. HARRIS, *The Economics of American Medicine*
New York: The Macmillan Company, 1964, pp. xvi, 508.
See 6.

1097   D. S. LEES, M. H. COOPER, 'Payment per-item-of-service. The Manchester and Salford experience 1913–28'
MC, 1964, 2(3), pp. 151–6.

Traces the experience with fee for service in Manchester and Salford from 1913–1928, the only rival experience to capitation since the introduction of state health insurance in the U.K. It is concluded on the basis of this experience, that any attempt to move to a fee-per-item-of-service system with a fixed pool available for payment, and no direct payment by patients, would be doomed to failure like the Manchester and Salford system.

A. LINDSEY, 'The British National Health Service, its organisation and financing'
In S. J. Mushkin (Chairman) *The Economics of Health and Medical Care*, pp. 48–59 (8).
An enthusiastic view of the British National Health Service, its foundation and history.

G. McLACHLAN (ed.) *Problems and Progress in Medical Care, Essays on Current Research, First to Ninth Series*
London: Oxford University Press, for Nuffield Provincial Hospitals Trust, 1964–1973.
Nine volumes dealing with a large number of socio-medical issues. The study base of most of the papers is the British National Health Service. In particular, the sixth and eighth series examine the role and programme of the Department of Health and Social Security in health services research.
See 7, 13, 16, 20, 24, 25, 30, 37, 38.

1965

J. M. BUCHANAN, *The Inconsistencies of the National Health Service*
London: Institute of Economic Affairs, Occasional Paper No. 7, 1965, p. 24.
The source of the internal conflict in the British National Health Service, it is argued, is the fact that the individual demands more services privately than he will supply publicly. Reform of the N.H.S. must involve the combination of these separate decisions into a single decision, either by moving to a private market for medical care, or by collective decision as to the total supply of health care available and its distribution between individuals.

1966

D. C. PAIGE, K. JONES, *Health and Welfare Services in Britain in 1975*
Cambridge: Cambridge University Press for the National Institute of Economic and Social Research, Occasional Papers 22, 1966, p. 142.
A comprehensive set of projections of future expenditure, numbers of staff and stock of buildings required in the health and welfare services in Britain up to 1975. The development and administration of the health and welfare services and likely changes in administration are outlined. Projections are provided for

the family practitioner services, general hospitals, care of mothers and children, mental health services, care for the aged and handicapped, and total staff requirements.
See 77.

1102 R. STEVENS, *Medical Practice in Modern England*
New Haven: Yale University Press, 1966, pp. xiv, 401.
Sub-titled 'The impact of specialization, and state medicine', the study examines the development of the medical profession in Great Britain from 1700 to the recent period, and the impact of the profession on the National Health Service, and of the National Health Service on the profession.

1967

1103 BRITISH MEDICAL ASSOCIATION, *Is There an Alternative?*
London: British Medical Association, 1967, p. 74.
See 998.

1104 M. S. FELDSTEIN, *Economic Analysis for Health Service Efficiency*
Amsterdam: North-Holland Publishing Company, 1967, p. xi, 322.
See 392.

1968

1105 P. BIERMAN, E. J. CONNORS, E. FLOOK, R. R. HUNTLEY, T. McCARTHY, P. J. SANAZARO, 'Health services research in Great Britain'
MMFQ, January, 1968, 46(1 part 1), pp. 9–102.
An outline is provided of the background to health services research in Great Britain. The majority of the work surveyed is in social medicine, operations research and social administration. The final section of the paper compares the status and content of health services research in Great Britain and the U.S.A. A substantial bibliography is provided.

1106 A. SELDON, *After the NHS: Reflections on the Development of Private Health Insurance in Britain in the 1970s*
London: Institute of Economic Affairs, Occasional Paper No. 21, 1968, p. 43.

An analysis of the scope for extension of private insurance in Britain as the N.H.S. exhibits strains accompanying growing deficiencies of tax finance. *See 1114.*

R. M. TITMUSS, *Commitment to Welfare*
London: George Allen and Unwin Ltd., 1968, p. 272.

A collection of twenty-one essays, a number of which deal with aspects of the National Health Service. Of particular interest are: 'Planning for ageing and the health and welfare services', 'The role of the family doctor today in the context of Britain's social services', and 'Trends in social policy: health'. A number of the essays examine the rationale for state provision of health services: chapter 12 is a reprint of *Choice and 'the Welfare State'*, the paper that began the controversy about the supply of blood for transfusion. *See 1003.*

1969

C. M. LINDSAY, 'Medical care and the economics of sharing'
EC, November, 1969, 36(144), pp. 351–62. Also in M. H. Cooper, A. J. Culyer (eds.) *Health Economics*, pp. 75–89 (33).
See 1006.

M. S. REES, 'The inflation of National Health Service registers of patients, and its effect on the remuneration of general practitioners'
JRSS A, 1969, 132(4), pp. 526–42.

An estimate is made of the total size and distribution of the excess of patient registrations with general practitioners over the number of bona fide N.H.S. patients in the population. A figure of 4.1 per cent of the population of England and Wales is arrived at. This is estimated to have cost £2¼ million in 1968 in excess payments to G.Ps.

1970

J. R. ASHFORD, N. G. PEARSON, 'Who uses the health services and why?'
JRSS A, 1970, 133(3), pp. 295–357.
See 91.

1111   BRITISH MEDICAL ASSOCIATION, *Health Services Financing*
London: BMA, 1970, pp. xvi, 605.

The volume is divided into two sections. The first section considers the history of the health services in Great Britain, and looks at major current issues in the N.H.S. It also contains a proposal to increase the total finance available for health services by drawing on private consumption expenditure, primarily by making available voluntary health insurance which would give access to higher benefits than those received by the poorer sections of the population who would be compulsorily insured. The second section consists of seventeen papers: a paper by Cooper and Culyer on the National Health Service, papers by Peacock and Wiseman and by Seldon looking at alternative sources of finance for medical care in Great Britain, and a further fourteen papers examining the finance and organisation of health services in other developed nations.
See 1065, *1112, 1113, 1114.*

1112   M. H. COOPER, A. J. CULYER, 'An economic assessment of some aspects of the operation of the National Health Service'
Appendix A of British Medical Association, *Health Services Financing*, pp. 187–250 (1111).

The degree to which the National Health Service has succeeded in achieving geographical equality in the availability of health manpower and facilities was assessed by means of 27 indices based mainly on doctors–population ratios, beds–population ratios, and costs per inpatient-week. Intraregional as well as interregional variations in provision were investigated. More relative variation was found to exist within than between regions.

1113   A. T. PEACOCK, J. WISEMAN, 'Public expenditure as a source of finance for medical care in Britain'
Appendix B of British Medical Association, *Health Services Financing*, pp. 251–71 (1111).

The paper contains several public expenditure projections for the period 1965/66 to 1986, and within that, separate projections of health service expenditure on a variety of assumptions about likely levels of provision. The projections are compared to those made by Paige and Jones and to projections in the National Plan. The concluding section of the paper discusses the implications of the projections for future financial arrangements, and in particular considers which alternative sources of revenue would most easily provide for the 'desired' growth in health expenditures.

A. SELDON, 'Private expenditure as a source of finance for medical care in Britain'
Appendix C of British Medical Association, *Health Services Financing*, pp. 273–307 (1111).
The paper examines the scope for drawing additional finance for medical care from private household expenditure. Three techniques are used to estimate the potential growth of private expenditure: statistical projections, international comparisons, and inter-income comparisons (comparisons between income, occupational and socio-economic groups).
See 1106.

R. M. TITMUSS, *The Gift Relationship: from Human Blood to Social Policy*
London: George Allen and Unwin Ltd., 1970, p. 339.
See 1013.

1971

M. H. COOPER, 'How to pay for the health service'
JRSH, 1971, 91(5), pp. 217–21.
See 1016.

M. H. COOPER, A. J. CULYER, 'An economic survey of the nature and intent of the British NHS'
SSM, February, 1971, 5(1), pp. 1–13.
An outline of the background and objectives of the National Health Service. While the price barrier to access to services has been removed, other barriers to equality remain. The failure to bring about equality between regions in the provision of services is discussed.

A. J. CULYER, 'Medical care and the economics of giving'
EC, August, 1971, 38(51), pp. 295–303.
See 1018.

R. HARRIS, A. SELDON, *Choice in Welfare 1970*
London: The Institute of Economic Affairs, 1971, p. 84.
The third report in a series that set out 'to test public response to questions designed to elicit the broad order of magnitude of the preferences between state and private welfare services'. The study looks at preferences in medical care,

education and pensions. The two earlier reports in the series were published by the IEA in 1963 and 1965.

1120 R. F. L. LOGAN, 'National health planning. An appraisal of the state of the art'
IJHS, February, 1971, 1(1), pp. 6–17.

Reviews the failure of the British National Health Service to deal with inequities in the distribution of health resources. Reasons are suggested for these failures, which are seen to result from the difficulties in the implementation of health planning. Plans at least in the short term may be more useful in providing a forum for discussion than for their practical effect.

1121 G. MCLACHLAN (ed.) *Challenges for Change, Essays on the Next Decade in the National Health Service*
London: Oxford University Press, 1971, pp. xxi, 301.

A symposium of nine papers presented by experts in various fields outlining what they see to be the main problems facing the National Health Service in the 1970s, including in their comments speculation on the effects of health service reorganisation. The papers consider the quality of care, organisation of consultant services, general practice, community medicine, use of information within the health services, the implications of some of the proposed structural changes in the organisation of health services, and the problems of staffing.

1122 A. K. MAYNARD, 'Regional inequalities in psychiatric care'
BHJ, September 11th, 1971, 81(4247), pp. 1861–2.

A review of the regional inequalities in the distribution of psychiatric facilities in England and Wales, and changes in these inequalities over the period 1963–7.

1123 M. V. PAULY, *Medical Care at Public Expense, A Study in Applied Welfare Economics*
New York: Praeger Publishers, 1971, pp. xvi, 160.
See 1025.

1124 G. A. POPOV, *Principles of Health Planning in the U.S.S.R.*
Geneva: World Health Organisation, Public Health Papers No. 43, 1971, p. 172.
See 1401.

S. M. SHORTELL, G. GIBSON, 'The British National Health Service: issues of reorganisation'
HSR, Winter, 1971, 6(4), pp. 316–36.

The history and development of the N.H.S. is outlined, and the reorganisation discussed in this light. The authors' basic conclusions are that the re-organisation involves little more than attaching new labels to old containers and that while the goals of the reorganisation have been stated the indicators of performance to monitor progress towards these goals have not.

1972

A. L. COCHRANE, *Effectiveness and Efficiency: Random Reflections on Health Services*
London: The Nuffield Provincial Hospitals Trust, 1972, pp. xii, 92.
See 730.

M. H. COOPER, A. J. CULYER, 'Equality in the National Health Service: intentions, performance, and problems in evaluation'
In M. M. Hauser (ed.) *The Economics of Medical Care*, pp. 47–57 (28).

A study to determine how far the National Health Service has gone towards fulfilling its original equity objectives, with a look in some detail at how far it has fulfilled one particular objective, that of geographical equality in the availability of medical resources. Considerable regional variations were found, and no evidence was found to suggest that deficiencies in the availability of some resources were compensated by extras elsewhere; the poorly off regions were poorly off in all resources. See also the comment by G. R. Ford, pp. 58–60.

A. J. CULYER, 'The "market" versus the "state" in medical care – a minority report on an empty academic box'
In G. McLachlan (ed.) *Problems and Progress in Medical Care, Essays on Current Research, Seventh Series*, pp. 1–31.
See 1030.

A. J. CULYER, 'On the relative efficiency of the National Health Service'
Kyklos, 1972, 25(2), pp. 266–87.
See 1029.

1130   A. J. CULYER, P. JACOBS, 'The war and public expenditure on mental health care in England and Wales – the postponement effect'
SSM, February, 1972, 6(1), pp. 35–56.

The paper examines trends in public expenditure on mental health care in England and Wales between 1920 and 1960. The rising trend of expenditures was broken by the Second World War, and, more puzzling, the rising trend was not resumed until some time after the war. The effect was particularly marked for capital expenditures. The paper examines the possible explanations for the path of expenditures. It is concluded that there was a 'postponement effect' in health and mental care provision and that this was a product of two factors: the war and the post-war institutional reorganisation.

1131   R. KLEIN, 'The political economy of national health'
PI, Winter, 1972, 26, pp. 112–25.

A review of some of the strengths and weaknesses of the British National Health Service.

1132   M. S. LEVITT, 'Problems of efficiency'
In M. M. Hauser (ed.) *The Economics of Medical Care*, pp. 33–41.
See 1032.

1133   OPEN UNIVERSITY, *Health* (Block V, Parts 1–5)
Bletchley, Bucks: The Open University Press, 1972, p. 197.

Part of the Open University course 'Decision making in Britain', this is a carefully structured study guide examining the British National Health Service. The course looks at four major topics: regional disparities in the health sector, current issues in the National Health Service, interest groups and their significance for decision-taking, and finally a section entitled 'authority and the negotiated order in hospitals', which examines processes of decision-making within the health services. Guides to further reading and self-assessment exercises are also included in the volume.

1134   W. RUDOE, 'Allocation of resources within the health and welfare services'
In M. M. Hauser (ed.) *The Economics of Medical Care*, pp. 25–30 (28).

A brief review of a number of resource allocation problems in the National Health Service, the questions that must be tackled and the conditions such as the absence of prices, output measures and clear objectives, that make answers difficult to obtain.

1135   H. C. SALTER, 'Public expenditure and the health and welfare services'
In M. M. Hauser (ed.) *The Economics of Medical Care*, pp. 17–24 (28).

An outline of the problems facing an administrator in the National Health

Service. The paper suggests areas in which economic analysis is likely to be useful. It is however pointed out that both the need to make decisions quickly and public pressure will continue to lead to discussions that may not accord with the results of a more careful economic analysis.

E. M. SUTCLIFFE, 'The social accounting of health'
In M. M. Hauser (ed.) *The Economics of Medical Care*, pp. 238–56 (28).
The uses of social accounts and the problems arising in the construction of a social accounting framework for the health sector are discussed. A framework for health, similar to that used by Peacock, Glennester and Lavers for education, is outlined. The final section of the paper discusses an attempt to fit existing data for the U.K. into the proposed framework. See also the comment by D. S. Lees, pp. 257–8.

1973

M. H. COOPER, 'Rationing and financing health care resources'
In N. Hunt, W. D. Reekie (eds.) *Management and the Social Services*, London: Tavistock Publications, 1973, pp. 11–34.
With need continually in excess of the available supply of resources, rationing has been undertaken implicitly and not necessarily consistently or efficiently by doctors. Instead of careful scrutiny of the use of available funds and manpower most of the response to unmet need has been mistakenly directed towards pressure for increased funds, and schemes for raising non-tax funds that would undermine the principle of the Health Service as originally conceived and bring with them many new problems.

O. GISH, 'Resource allocation, equality of access and health'
IJHS, Summer, 1973, 3(3), pp. 399–412.
An examination of the system of health care provision in Tanzania.
See 958, 1372.

S. B. RIFKIN, R. KAPLINSKY, 'Health strategy and development planning: lessons from the People's Republic of China'
JDS, January, 1973, 9(2), pp. 213–32.
See 976.

P. A. WEST, 'Allocation and equity in the public sector: the hospital revenue allocation formula'
AE, September, 1973, 5(3), pp. 153–66.

The 1971 formula introduced by the Department of Health to reduce discrepancies in expenditure per head between the regions is examined with the aid of a simple dynamic analysis. It was found that the formula would tend to move funds from richer to poorer regions, but the possible effects on quality of care do not make equity judgements unambiguous.

1974

1141   M. H. COOPER, 'Economics of need: the experience of the British Health Service'
In M. Perlman (ed.) *The Economics of Health and Medical Care*, pp. 89–107 (44).

It is argued that the rationing of medical care has been left to the medical profession, who, claiming complete clinical freedom to act in the interests of their patients, ration only implicitly. This results in inconsistencies, and has exacerbated the inequalities that existed before the N.H.S. As needs defined by the profession are limitless, the service has claimed that there are shortages of resources rather than critically examine the current deployment of resources. The process by which the 'need' for medical care is determined is examined.

1142   A. J. CULYER, J. G. CULLIS, 'Private patients in N.H.S. hospitals: waiting lists, and subsidies'
In M. Perlman (ed.) *The Economics of Health and Medical Care*, pp. 108–16 (44).

It is shown that on fairly optimistic assumptions removal of private practice from N.H.S. hospitals would result in only a one or two per cent reduction in waiting lists. Evidence is presented to show that private patients do not pay the full cost of their care.

1143   M. KASER, 'Choice of technique'
In M. Perlman (ed.) *The Economics of Health and Medical Care*, pp. 510–27 (44).

The role of the physician in the choice of technique of treatment is examined, and the sorts of information needed in the light of this to guide a National Health Service type system towards a cost minimand are discussed.

1144   R. KLEIN, 'Policy making in the National Health Service'
PS, 1974, 22(1), pp. 1–14.

An examination of policy areas and policy outputs in the National Health

Service. Three main areas are examined: the distribution of resources, the reorganisation of the health service, and the pay of doctors. The explanatory power of three models of the decision-taking process, the Rational Actor Model, the Organisational Process Model, and the Governmental Politics Model, is examined.

R. KLEIN, J. BARNES, M. BUXTON, E. CRAVEN, *Social Policy and Public Expenditure, 1974*
London: The Centre for Studies in Social Policy, 1974, p. 94.

An examination of the changing pattern over time of public expenditure in the United Kingdom. A short section is included on health and personal social services with a breakdown between capital and current of these expenditures over the period 1968/69–1977/78.

K. LEE, 'Assessing the economics of [NHS] reorganisation: will it pay?' In D. Macmillan, K. Barnard, K. Lee (eds.) *NHS Reorganisation: Issues and Prospects*, pp. 94–115 (1147).

The objectives underlying the reorganisation of the health service are examined, and criteria are presented (of efficiency, effectiveness and equity) by which improvement in the reorganised N.H.S. may be gauged over a period of years. Any firm conclusions about the desirability or otherwise of the reorganisation must at this stage rest on personal value judgements.

D. MACMILLAN, K. BARNARD, K. LEE (eds.) *NHS Reorganisation: Issues and Prospects*
Leeds: Nuffield Centre for Health Service Studies, 1974, p. 143.

A collection of seven papers examining the context in which the N.H.S. operates, its underlying philosophy, and the implications and prospects for development rendered by reorganisation. The papers in the volume are as follows:
D. Macmillan, 'The infinity of demand: a case for integration'.
J. Halles, 'New structures for old'.
K. Palmer, 'The implications of change for NHS personnel'.
R. Gourlay, 'Team and consensus management: hearse or camel?'
M. Johnson, 'Whose stranger am I? Or patients really are people'
K. Lee, 'Assessing the economics of reorganisation: will it pay?'
K. Barnard, 'Health planning – the last of the panaceas'
See 1146.

J. NOYCE, A. H. SNAITH, A. J. TRICKEY, 'Regional variations in the allocation of financial resources to the community health services'
Lancet March 30th, 1974, pp. 554–7.

A study of the regional distribution of expenditure within the U.K. National Health Service in 1971–2 showed that the variations were greater in the hospital than the community sector, and greater among health authorities than for local authorities expenditure for all purposes.

1149   P. TOWNSEND, 'Inequality and the health service'
Lancet, June 15th, 1974, 1(7868), pp. 1179–89.

An evaluation of the British National Health Service by systematic application of the comparative method. Cross-national comparisons, cross-regional comparisons, statistics of mortality and morbidity of different social classes and socio-economic groups are used to examine the performance of the health service and to assess major needs. It is concluded that 'the right of the sick to free access to health care, irrespective of class or income, remains to be firmly established'.

1150   P. WILLMOTT, 'Health and welfare'
In M. Young (ed.) *Poverty Report 1974*, London: Temple Smith, 1974, pp. 194–217.

This chapter of the report examines geographical inequalities in health and welfare services in the United Kingdom, inequalities between social classes in sickness and receipt of services, and inequalities between different sectors of the health service. One change, or beginning of a change, noted is the attempt to improve the lot of mental patients.

(iii)   *Insurance Systems*

1951

1151   F. GOLDMANN, 'Major areas of achievement and deficiency'
AER, May, 1951, 41(2), pp. 626–32.

Chiefly of historical interest, providing an outline of the arrangements for financing medical care in the U.S.A. in the late 1940s and 1950.

1152   C. A. KULP, 'Voluntary and compulsory medical care insurance'
AER, May, 1951, 41(2), pp. 667–75.

An early discussion of possible ways of financing medical care in the U.S.A. The problem is seen to be one of achieving a suitable balance between compulsory and voluntary insurance. Approaches to defining the respective spheres of operation of the two types of insurance are classified into those that represent horizontal, and those that represent vertical divisions between the two types of insurance.

1952

R. R. CAMPBELL, W. G. CAMPBELL, 'Compulsory health insurance: the economic issues'
QJE, February, 1952, 66(1), pp. 1–24.
The issues are considered in the light of Bill S. 1679, at that time going before Congress. The two issues identified as the key to the discussion are: will compulsory health insurance remedy the low level of health in areas where there is a poor distribution of medical manpower and facilities; and is the comprehensive programme the most economical way of remedying the deficiencies. The paper goes on to consider the objections voiced against compulsory health insurance, and some possible alternative programmes. The overall conclusion drawn about compulsory health insurance is a negative one. The paper stimulated replies and the Campbells produced a counter-reply. See also: I. S. Falk, 'The economic issues of compulsory health insurance: comment', *QJE*, November, 1952, 66(4), pp. 572–86; D. Netzer, 'Further comment', *QJE*, November, 1952, 66(4), pp. 586–91; R. R. Campbell, W. G. Campbell, 'The economic issues of compulsory health insurance: reply', *QJE*, February, 1953, 64(1), pp. 125–35.
See 1154.

I. S. FALK, 'The economic issues of compulsory health insurance: comment'
QJE, November, 1952, 66(4), pp. 572–86.
The paper disputes the conclusions reached by the Campbells, and argues that they omit from consideration the major argument for comprehensive insurance, that it is necessary in order to give people 'protection against the uneven, unpredictable, and—for most families—unbudgetable costs of medical care'.
See 1153.

1954

E. GINZBERG, 'What every economist should know about health and medicine'
AER, March, 1954, 44(1), pp. 104–19.
A review of the findings, recommendations and underlying philosophy of the Commission on the Health Needs of the Nation set up in 1951 by President Truman. The Commission produced a five volume report entitled *Building America's Health* (Washington: 1953) covering America's health status, needs and resources, and examining the finance of health care.

1958

1156 P. M. DENSEN, E. BALAMUTH, S. SHAPIRO, *Prepaid Medical Care and Hospital Utilization*
Chicago: American Hospital Association, 1958.
See 1425.

1961

1157 H. M. SOMERS, A. R. SOMERS, *Doctors, Patients and Health Insurance*
Washington D.C.: The Brookings Institution, 1961, pp. xx, 576.
See 3.

1962

1158 P. A. BRINKER, B. WALKER, 'The Hill–Burton Act: 1948–1954'
Rev.Econ.Stats., May, 1962, 44(2), pp. 208–212.
See 353.

1159 V. CARLSON, *Economic Security in the United States*
New York: McGraw-Hill Book Company, 1962, pp. xii, 225.
Most areas of social policy are examined in this volume: public assistance, unemployment compensation, old age and disability insurance, family allowances. One short chapter is included on the allocation of medical services, the issues surrounding compulsory health insurance, and the attitudes of doctors and the public to such insurance examined.

1160 W. J. MCNERNEY and Study Staff, *Hospital and Medical Economics: A Study of Population, Services, Costs, Methods of Payment, and Controls.*
Chicago: Hospital Research and Educational Trust, 1962, p. 1492 (2 vols).
A massive research report which sprang from the Governor's Study Commission on Prepaid Hospital and Medical Care Plans which in turn had been appointed as a result of a request from the Blue Cross Plan serving the State of Michigan for a large increase in rates. The study consists of a

population survey to determine patterns of health care and their financing, five papers on the providers of care, four studies of different types of insurance, and one on the role of government in health care finance, and finally a paper on controls within the voluntary system.

1963

K. J. ARROW, 'Uncertainty and the welfare economics of medical care' *AER*, December, 1963, 53(5), pp. 941–73. Also in M. H. Cooper, A. J. Culyer (eds.) *Health Economics*, pp. 13–48 (33).

A thorough examination of the characteristics of the market for medical services. The market for medical services is considered by comparison to the behaviour of the competitive model under certainty, and the ideal competitive market under uncertainty. It is demonstrated that the market will fail to provide insurance against a number of risks but that 'the special structural characteristics of medical care are largely attempts to overcome the lack of optimality due to the non-marketability of the bearing of suitable risks and the imperfect marketability of information'. In particular, the market for medical services has seen the development of social institutions, such as personal relationships being formed between physicians and families, that give guarantees of behaviour in situations that would otherwise be afflicted with excessive uncertainty.
See 1170, 1173, 1185, 1220, 1244.

H. E. KLARMAN, 'Effect of prepaid group practice on hospital use' *PHR*, November, 1963, 78(11), pp. 955–65.

A survey of work carried out in the 1950s and early 1960s on the impact of prepaid group practice on hospital use.

H. E. KLARMAN, *Hospital Care in New York City, the Roles of Voluntary and Municipal Hospitals*
New York: Columbia University Press, 1963, pp. xxxii, 573.
See 358.

A. QUERIDO, *The Efficiency of Medical Care*
London: H. E. Stanfert Kroese N.V., 1963, p. 288.

An outline of the early work of the Office of Public Health Care in the Municipality of Amsterdam in the field of planning and development of health services.

1964

1165   D. S. Lees, M. H. Cooper, 'Payment per-item-of-service. The Manchester and Salford experience 1913–28'
MC, 1964, 2(3), pp. 151–6.
See 1097.

1166   D. M. MacIntyre, 'Pricing health insurance'
In S. J. Mushkin (Chairman) *The Economics of Health and Medical Care*, pp. 148–69 (8).

A review of the development of health insurance in the United States, the organisation of the market, the forms of insurance available, and the system of rating and the fixing of rates.

1167   N. Piore, 'Metropolitan areas and public medical care'
In S. J. Mushkin (Chairman) *The Economics of Health and Medical Care*, pp. 60–71 (8).

An examination of the health and medical services provided or purchased by government in New York City, and the questions for management of public funds that the large-scale involvement implies. Comment by R. J. Lampman, pp. 71–4.

1168   M. Roberts, 'Trends in the organisation of health services: the private sector'
In S. J. Mushkin (Chairman) *The Economics of Health and Medical Care*, pp. 23–41 (8).

A review of trends in the organisation of health services in the United States. See also the comment by I. M. Labovitz pp. 42–7.

1169   Royal Commission on Health Services, Canada
Ottawa: Queens Printer, 1964, 1965, 1966.

A massive report on the Canadian health services. As well as the discussion in the main document, the Commission arranged for the preparation of 26 independent studies, a high proportion of which deal with manpower problems. The full list of studies appears in Appendix B, pp. 886–7 of the report of the Royal Commission. Some of the major ones are annotated elsewhere in the bibliography.
See 182, 562, 1171.

1965

70 K. J. ARROW, 'Uncertainty and the welfare economics of medical care: reply (the implications of transactions costs and adjustment lags)'
AER, March, 1965, 55(1), pp. 154–8.

A reply to the comment of Lees and Rice on an earlier paper by Arrow. It is pointed out that it is not only the existence of transactions costs that is important but whether or not they are more or less available under different institutional arrangements. The argument that free markets will eventually produce the right types of health insurance is held to be misdirected as other types of institutional arrangement may produce the desired results more quickly. Lees and Rice are really arguing the value judgement that free markets are a 'better' form of organisation.
See 1161, 1173.

71 C. H. BERRY, *Voluntary Medical Insurance and Prepayment*
Ottawa: Queens Printer, Royal Commission on Health Services, 1965, pp. xii, 255.

The study is divided into two parts. The first part examines existing voluntary medical insurance and prepayment in Canada. The second part considers the influence of prepayment or insurance coverage on family expenditure for medical care.
See 1169.

72 E. GINZBERG, 'The political economy of health'
Bull.N.Y.Acad.Med., October, 1965, 41(10), pp. 1015–36.

Major propositions about health care on which the Committee of Social Policy for Health Care reached consensus are set out. These propositions relating to availability, cost and quality of care in the U.S.A. are examined in the light of health economics to identify more clearly the critical issues and to judge the appropriateness of suggested social policy solutions.

73 D. S. LEES, R. G. RICE, 'Uncertainty and the welfare economics of medical care'
AER, March, 1965, 55(1), pp. 140–54.

The paper takes up some points made by Arrow about the market for medical insurance. It is argued here that the absence of insurance policies for certain risks may in fact be a requirement for optimality because of the existence of transactions costs. The second part of the paper argues that Arrow ignored the fact that it would take time for new types of health insurance to develop and for markets to grow. This case is supported by reference to the development of

health insurance in the United States between 1948 and 1963.
See 1161, 1170.

1174   M. Lerner, S. W. Fitzgerald, 'A comparative study of three major forms of health care coverage: a review'
Inquiry, June, 1965, 2(1), pp. 37–60.

1175   L. S. Reed, 'Hospital utilization under the Canadian national hospital insurance programme'
AJPH, March, 1965, 55(3), pp. 435–45.
See 1436.

1966

1176   C. P. Hall, 'Deductibles in health insurance'
JRI, June, 1966, 33(2), pp. 253–63.
A brief review of evidence on the effects of coinsurance and deductible provisions on utilization of health services and the forms of treatment received.

1177   D. C. Riedel, M. Lerner, 'The impact of prepayment on the economics of dental care'
JADA, April, 1966, 72(4), pp. 874–88.
Background information on expenditures for dental care, dentists' incomes, the supply and geographical distribution of dentists, and utilization of dental services, is provided as a basis for assessing the likely effects of the growth of prepayment for dental care. Higher prices, higher dental incomes, and a concentration of dentists in the midwest and north east of the U.S.A. are seen as likely outcomes of the increased demand resulting from the growth of prepayment.

1178   R. Williams, 'A comparison of hospital utilization and costs by types of coverage'
Inquiry, September, 1966, 3(3), pp. 28–42.
The study examines data on utilisation and length of stay drawn from different types of coverage within geographically homogeneous Blue Cross Plans. Deductibles had a minimal effect in reducing utilisation and practically no

effect in reducing the amount of benefits paid by the plans involved. With copayment average utilisation and the amount of benefits paid by plans were lower, but there was no effect on length of stay.

1967

J. S. DEEBLE, 'The costs and sources of finance of Australian health services'
ER, 1967, 43(4), pp. 518–43.

The social accounting framework developed by the WHO is used to look at health service expenditures and sources of finance for financial years 1960–1 and 1963–4. Comparisons are made with the WHO study of U.S.A., Israel, Canada, Chile, Sweden and the U.K. The main aim of the article is to provide basic statistics on Australian health service expenditures and sources of finance. A number of specific problems are considered: the high expenditure on medicaments, the cost of voluntary insurance, and the likely costs resulting from the lack of co-ordination within the Australian health system.

R. B. SCOTTON, 'Voluntary insurance and the incidence of hospital costs'
AEP, 1967, 6(9), pp. 171–91.

Argues that the pre-Nimmo voluntary insurance system in Australia, with its associated non-insurance, under-insurance, and with uniform contributions and income tax allowances, led to a regressive pattern of health-care finance. *See 1007, 1187, 1188, 1198, 1199.*

1968

O. W. ANDERSON, *The Uneasy Equilibrium: Private and Public Financing of Health Services in the United States, 1875–1965*
New Haven, Conn.: College and University Press, 1968.

W. G. BOWEN, F. H. HARBISON, R. A. LESTER, H. M. SOMERS, *The American System of Social Insurance, its Philosophy, Impact and Future Development*
New York: McGraw-Hill Book Company, 1968, pp. xi, 255.
See 1285.

1183 P. A. BRINKER, *Economic Insecurity and Social Security*
New York: Appleton-Century-Crofts, 1968, p. 566.

Provides a lot of detail on the major public and private social security programmes in the U.S.A. including the health insurance and disability compensation schemes.

1184 M. R. GREENLICK, A. V. HURTADO, C. R. POPE, E. W. SAWARD, S. S. YOSHIOKA, 'Determinants of medical care utilization'
HSR, Winter, 1968, 3(4), pp. 296–315.

See 1445.

1185 M. V. PAULY, 'The economics of moral hazard: comment'
AER, June, 1968, 58(3), pp. 531–7.

It is demonstrated that even if all individuals are risk-averters, insurance against some events may be non-optimal. The case is developed with reference to medical coinsurance. The cases in which insurance is non-optimal are the result of 'moral hazard'. It is argued that it is possible that 'the loss due to "excess" use under insurance may exceed the welfare gain from insurance for one individual but fall short of it for another individual'. See also the comment by K. J. Arrow, pp. 537–9.
See 1161.

1186 V. N. RAJAN, 'Medical care under social insurance in India'
ILR, July, 1968, 98(2), pp. 141–56.

A description of the Employees' State Insurance Corporation (E.S.I.C.) which administers the only scheme of compulsory social insurance in India. Details of the coverage, sources of contribution, benefits, types of care available and likely future development are provided.

1187 R. B. SCOTTON, 'Voluntary health insurance in Australia'
Aus.Ec.Rev., 1968, 2nd Quarter, pp. 37–44.

An extended critique of the pre-Nimmo voluntary insurance system in Australia.
See 1007, 1180, 1188, 1198, 1199.

1188 R. B. SCOTTON, J. S. DEEBLE, 'Compulsory health insurance for Australia'
Aus.Ec.Rev., 1968, 4th Quarter, pp. 9–16.

Proposes a compulsory health insurance plan to replace the 'deficiencies, contradictions and complexities' of the then existing Australian system. The chief issues in the controversy are reviewed.
See 1007, 1180, 1187, 1198.

A. SELDON, *After the NHS: Reflections on the Development of Private Health Insurance in Britain in the 1970s*
London: Institute of Economic Affairs, Occasional Paper No. 21, 1968, p. 43.
See 1106, *1114*.

U.S. DEPARTMENT OF HEALTH, EDUCATION AND WELFARE, *Reimbursement Incentives for Hospital and Medical Care: Objectives and Alternatives*
Washington D.C.: USDHEW, Research Report No. 26, U.S. Govt. Printing Office, 1968, pp. vii, 103.

A collection of five papers: one historical paper examining hospital cost reimbursement from 1920 to the present time; one paper examining reimbursement plans in terms of incentives, quality and efficiency of care; and three papers looking at particular reimbursement proposals in greater depth.

1 I. Wolkstein, 'The legislative history of hospital cost reimbursement', pp. 1–21.
2 P. J. Feldstein, 'An analysis of reimbursement plans', pp. 23–54.
3 S. Waldman, 'Average increase in costs – an incentive reimbursement formula for hospitals', pp. 55–69.
4 R. M. Sigmond, 'Capitation as a method of reimbursement to hospitals in a multi hospital area', pp. 71–86.
5 P. J. Feldstein, 'A proposal for capitation reimbursement to medical groups for total medical care', pp. 87–103.

1969

T. S. BODENHEIMER, 'Regional Medical Programmes: no road to regionalisation'
MCR, December, 1969, 26(11), pp. 1125–66.

A discussion of Regional Medical Programmes and the reasons for their failure to generate comprehensive regionalisation in the U.S.A., in the sense of providing a mechanism to allocate resources within a region, rather having satisfied themselves with establishing limited affiliations among health institutions. A large bibliography is included.

M. CREW, 'Coinsurance and the welfare economics of medical care'
AER, December, 1969, 59(5), pp. 906–8.

It is demonstrated that monopoly and coinsurance can lead to an optimum output of medical care, while competition and coinsurance or insurance cannot (in the absence of perfectly inelastic demand). The former solution, however, has distributional consequences in that it transfers resources to the rich, i.e. the medical profession.

1193　A. DONABEDIAN, 'An evaluation of prepaid group practice'
Inquiry, September, 1969, 6(3), pp. 3–27.

A review of mainly published work on the performance of prepaid group practice plans as compared to performance and delivery of care under other organisational arrangements. The aspects of performance examined include subscriber choice of plan and satisfaction with the plan, the use of services within and outside the plan, in particular the effects of hospital utilisation, the effect on the levels of expenditure for care, the productivity of prepaid group practice and the quality of care provided.
See 1257.

1194　E. GINZBERG, M. OSTOW, *Men, Money and Medicine*
New York: Columbia University Press, 1969, pp. xii, 291.

The book examines the changing structure of health services in the United States in the post-1945 period. The opening section of the book examines the important financial and manpower changes in the United States health system. The second and third sections deal with manpower problems. The final section examines the problems of persons suffering from chronic conditions, mental handicap, mental illness and tuberculosis.
See 218.

1195　H. E. KLARMAN, 'Reimbursing the hospital – the differences the third party makes'
JRI, December, 1969, 36(5), pp. 553–66.

Examines the effects of third-party payment, the implications of the characteristics of health services and their organisation for third-party payment, the problem of different reimbursement mechanisms existing simultaneously and the advent of the government into the field. The major inadequacies are seen to lie in the weaknesses of incentives to efficiency. See also the comment by H. Malisoff, *JRI*, March, 1971, 38(1), pp. 137–9, and the reply by Klarman, pp. 139–41.

1196　M. V. PAULY, 'A measure of the welfare cost of health insurance'
HSR, Winter, 1969, 4(4), pp. 281–92.

Adopts Harberger's formula for the welfare cost of a set of excise taxes to measure the effect of excess usage of insured services on welfare. It is concluded that no *a priori* case can be made for increasing, or restricting, insurance coverage as a means for reducing excess usage costs. Better estimates of demand elasticities will, however, allow prediction of the effect of any health insurance package on welfare. Estimates based on demand elasticity estimates, available in the United States, suggest that the welfare cost is 10 per cent of the total cost of insurance.

K-K. Ro, R. Auster, 'An output approach to incentive reimbursement for hospitals'
HRS, Fall, 1969, 4(3), pp. 177–87.

A reimbursement formula based upon defining a standard cost for an episode of illness (average cost for an area plus or minus a number of standard deviations) is outlined. The amount of reimbursement is based on a weighted average of the standard cost and the actual cost of the case to the hospital, the weighting factor being chosen to produce the desired degree of incentive.

R. B. Scotton, 'Membership of voluntary health insurance'
ER, March, 1969, 45(109), pp. 69–83.

Survey data were analysed to estimate the extent of non-insurance among the Australian population. Three factors (migrant origin, anti selection by good risks and low income) accounted for a high proportion of the 15–17 per cent of the population without insurance coverage.

R. B. Scotton, J. S. Deeble, 'The Nimmo Report'
ER, June, 1969, 45(110), pp. 258–75.

A review of the report of the Nimmo Committee, which was set up to assess the Australian Voluntary Health Insurance scheme, an integral part of the Australian social welfare system. The findings of the committee, it is concluded, would reduce the cost and complexity of health insurance.

I. Wolkstein, 'Incentive reimbursement plans offer a variety of approaches to cost control'
Hospitals, June 16th, 1969, 43, pp. 63–7.

A brief review of incentive reimbursement schemes that have been tried or suggested in the U.S.A.

1970

C. W. Baird, 'A proposal for financing the purchase of health services'
JHR, Winter, 1970, 5(1), pp. 89–105.

The case for collective action in the health-care market is investigated. A proposal for tax credits against personal income tax for 75–80 per cent of health-care expenditures other than the initial physician visit is developed, which is effectively a health insurance policy with deductible and coinsurance clauses. Estimates are made of how the burden of the costs of the proposal would be distributed. It is argued that the proposal is better able to redistribute towards the poor than existing arrangements. See also a comment by J. H. Weiss, *JHR*, Winter, 1971, 6(1), pp. 123–4, and the reply by Baird, *JHR*, 6(1), pp. 125–9.

1202　R. J. BLENDON, 'Policy issues in financing medical care'
HA, Spring, 1970, 15(2), pp. 46–59.

A survey of the issues that should be considered in a choice between private insurance and welfare or social insurance as the means of financing medical care provision.

1203　BRITISH MEDICAL ASSOCIATION, *Health Services Financing*
London: BMA, 1970, pp. xvi, 605.
See 1065, 1111.

1204　C. P. HARDWICK, H. WOLFE, 'Incentive reimbursement'
MC, May–June, 1970, 8(3), pp. 173–88.

The paper presents details of three experiments testing different reimbursement systems in W. Pennsylvania. See also the comment by J. Rafferty, *MC*, November–December, 1971, 9(6), pp. 518–20.
See 493, 1205.

1205　C. P. HARDWICK, H. WOLFE, 'Incentive reimbursement'
Hospitals, September 16th, 1970, 44(18), pp. 45–8.

A target model of incentive reimbursement is outlined. An incentive bonus is paid on the difference between estimated and actual costs for the current year. In addition a bonus is paid for past cost reductions at a rate that is lower the further into the past the cost savings took place.
See 493, 2004.

1206　C. C. HAVIGHURST (ed.) *Health Care*
Part I, *Law Contemp.Probl.*, Spring, 1970, 35(2).
Part II, *Law Contemp.Probl.*, Autumn, 1970, 35(4).
See 1297.

C. M. LINDSAY, J. M. BUCHANAN, 'The organisation and financing of medical care in the United States'
Appendix Q of British Medical Association, *Health Services Financing*, pp. 535–85 (1065).

The first part of the paper traces the development of medical care in the United States. Sections are included on physicians, hospitals and the role of government in medical care provision.
See 1012.

J. P. NEWHOUSE, V. TAYLOR, 'The subsidy problem in hospital insurance: a proposal'
JB, October, 1970, 43(4), pp. 452–6.

A proposal for the adoption of variable cost insurance by government health insurance plans in the U.S.A., insurance payments to the sick being independent of the hospital used and fixed according to the 'average' cost hospital in each community. See also the comment by M. Schnabel, *JB*, April, 1972, 45(2), pp. 302–4.

M. V. PAULY, D. F. DRAKE, 'Effect of third-party methods of reimbursement on hospital performance'
In H. E. Klarman (ed.) *Empirical Studies in Health Economics*, pp. 297–314.
See 437.

M. V. PAULY, 'The welfare economics of community rating'
JRI, September, 1970, 37(3), pp. 407–18.

It is demonstrated that community rating is inefficient because it inserts a wedge into the price structure of insurance in the same way as a partial excise tax. If other forms of insurance exist, problems are created for community rating as low risk individuals will be attracted out of the community scheme. The paper goes on to examine the relationship between different types of insurance and the existence of moral hazard. It is concluded that indemnity plans would eliminate certain types of moral hazard but that such plans are unlikely to emerge in a competitive system.

M. V. PAULY, 'Efficiency, incentives and reimbursement for health care'
Inquiry, March, 1970, 7(1), pp. 114–31.

The incentives to consumers in three broad categories of health insurance (cost average, indemnity based on illness, and indemnity per unit of service) to modify the quantity and mix of medical care they purchase are outlined.

1212   A. P. RUDERMAN, 'Task Force Reports on the cost of health services in Canada. A review article'
CJPH, July–August, 1970, 61(4), pp. 321–4.

A guide to the three volume set of Task Force Reports on the Cost of Health Services in Canada (Department of National Health and Welfare, Ottowa, November, 1969). A summary is provided of the reports that were commissioned to provide, 'recommendations that would yield short-run returns in providing health services of acceptable quality and quantity to the Canadian people at less-rapidly-rising cost'.

1213   J. B. STOLTE, 'Health services in the Netherlands'
W. Hosp., 1970, 6(3), pp. 147–56.

A description of health services in the Netherlands. The general social context and the health status of the population are outlined as a background to a description of the availability, structure and method of financing of health services.

1214   R. M. TITMUSS, *The Gift Relationship: from Human Blood to Social Policy*
London: George Allen and Unwin Ltd., 1970, p. 339.
See 1013.

1215   R. ZECKHAUSER, 'Medical insurance, a case study of the trade-off between risk spreading and appropriate incentives'
JET, March, 1970, 2(1), pp. 10–26.

A medical insurance model based on individual utility maximisation is presented (the individual's utility is a function of the levels of medical expenditure on his behalf and his wealth). The model is used to examine insurance plans with different coinsurance provisions, from a plan that pays no attention to medical condition (the same expense sharing regardless of medical condition) to a plan with a different expense sharing provision for each medical condition. The model illustrates the importance of the trade-off between risk-spreading and incentives in the designing of insurance plans.

1971

1216   H. R. BOWEN, J. R. JEFFERS, *The Economics of Health Services*
New York: General Learning Press, 1971, p. 24.
See 22.

17 R. R. CAMPBELL, *Economics of Health and Public Policy*
Washington D.C.: American Enterprise Institute for Public Policy Research, 1971, p. 108.
See 23.

18 M. S. FELDSTEIN, 'Hospital cost inflation: a study of non-profit price dynamics'
AER, December, 1971, 61(5), pp. 835–72.
See 447.

19 I. G. GREENBERG, M. L. RODBURG, 'The role of prepaid group practice in relieving the medical care crisis'
HLR, February, 1971, 84(4), pp. 887–1001.

An extensive study of prepaid group practice to examine the role it might play in overcoming some of the difficulties facing the health care system in the U.S.A. The principles of operation and characteristics of prepaid group practice are outlined, and an assessment is made of the performance (economic and medical), the ability to provide care to various sections of the population and the acceptability of such care. Barriers to the development of prepaid group practice are also examined, as is the policy of Federal Government to prepaid group practice.

20 H. G. GRUBEL, 'Risk, uncertainty, and moral hazard'
JRI, March, 1971, 38(1), pp. 99–106.

Moral hazard is viewed as a natural result of economically rational behaviour on the part of individuals confronted by a lowered price for a service. Attempts to change the attitudes of the public seem unlikely to reduce the extent of moral hazard in the long run. It is demonstrated, however, that under certain circumstances compulsory insurance raises public welfare even when moral hazard exists – a result of differences in private and public administrative and selling costs, and the existence of external and income redistributive effects.
See 1161.

21 T. L. HALL, S. DIAZ, 'Social security and health care patterns in Chile'
IJHS, November, 1971, 1(4), pp. 362–77.

Traces the development of health care under social security in Chile from 1918 to the present day. Data on utilisation of physician, dentist and hospital services, from a 1968 sample survey are presented.
See 1462.

1222   J. E. HASTINGS, 'Federal–provincial insurance for hospital and physician's care in Canada'
IJHS, November, 1971, 1(4), pp. 398–414.

A descriptive survey of the health services and the evolution of social insurance in Canada. The impact of the social insurance programmes is discussed in terms of their effects on financing and costs, manpower and facilities, and planning and organisation.

1223   T. H. HIBBARD, 'Insurance and the optimal distribution of medical care'
WEJ, September, 1971, 9(3), pp. 231–41.

A critical examination of Arrow's suggestion for complementing insurance with non-price demand controls. It is concluded that while such control mechanisms may enable the attainment of an optimal level and distribution of care, they should not be used to duplicate the demand pattern that would have been forthcoming in the absence of insurance. It is demonstrated that the differences in optimal care with and without insurance could be substantial.

1224   R. S. KAPLAN, L. B. LAVE, 'Patient incentives and hospital insurance'
HSR, Winter, 1971, 6(4), pp. 288–300.

The moral hazard problem associated with full coverage medical insurance is outlined. A number of studies that have been carried out on the effects of hospital utilisation of deductibles and copayment are discussed. Two more radical schemes of insurance reform (variable cost insurance and payment) are examined.

1225   J. P. NEWHOUSE, V. TAYLOR, 'How shall we pay for hospital care?'
PI, Spring, 1971, 23, pp. 78–92.
See 1226.

1226   J. P. NEWHOUSE, V. TAYLOR, 'A new type of hospital insurance'
JRI, December, 1971, 38(4), pp. 601–12.

Variable cost insurance (insurance for which the household chooses the type of hospital it will use for treatment and then the insurance premium is fixed according to the costliness of the hospital chosen) is discussed, the problems of implementation are outlined and an experiment to demonstrate the viability of the VCI suggested.

1227   J. P. NEWHOUSE, V. TAYLOR, 'Financing health care: here's a fresh solution'
ME, October 25th, 1971, 48(23), pp. 244–57.

The case for variable cost insurance as a means for combating the rising cost of health care is developed.

M. V. PAULY, 'Indemnity insurance for health care efficiency'
EBB, Fall, 1971, 24(1), pp. 53–9.

Develops a case for indemnity insurance to cover the treatment of at least some types of medical conditions. Indemnity insurance provides an incentive to consumers to consider costs of treatment, overcoming the moral hazard problem. It is least satisfactory in situations where 'medically necessary' procedures to treat a condition are not clear or subject to varying interpretations by different physicians.

M. V. PAULY, *Medical Care at Public Expense, A Study in Applied Welfare Economics*
New York: Praeger Publishers, 1971, pp. xvi, 160.
See 1025.

C. M. STEVENS, 'Physician supply and national health care goals'
IR, May, 1971, 10(2), pp. 119–44.
See 267.

R. STEVENS, *American Medicine and the Public Interest*
New Haven: Yale University Press, 1971, pp. xiv, 572.

A comprehensive study looking at the evolving patterns of medical practice in the United States. The study centres around the impact of specialisation on the organisation and politics of health services. The study is divided into five parts, the first three parts looking at the development of specialties from colonial times to 1950, the last two parts examining the recent period, trends in the profession, and government involvement in the health-care system.

1972

R. R. ALFORD, 'The political economy of health care: dynamics without change'
Politics and Society, Winter, 1972, 3, pp. 127–64.
See 1314.

S. E. BERKI, *Hospital Economics*
Lexington, Massachusetts: Lexington Books, D. C. Heath and Company, 1972, pp. xxi, 270.

The literature on pricing, reimbursement and incentives is reviewed in chapter

seven. The discussion has generally been in terms of the applicability and desirability of marginal cost and peak load pricing with some more recent work on aspects of fixed price contracts such as prospective budgeting or capitation prepayment.
See 462.

1234 S. E. BERKI, A. W. HESTON (eds). 'The Nation's Health: Some Issues' *AAAPSS*, January, 1972, 399, pp. 100–74.

A collection of sixteen papers by social scientists and doctors on various aspects of the U.S. situation.

D. Mechanic, 'Human problems and the organisation of health care', pp. 1–11.

M. W. Herman, 'The poor: their medical needs and the health services supplied them', pp. 12–21.

I. Leveson, 'The economics of health services for the poor', pp. 22–9.

R. E. Stevenson, R. R. Howell, 'Some medical and social aspects of the treatment for genetic-metabolic diseases', pp. 30–7.

C. G. Sheps, C. Seipp, 'The medical school: its products and its problems', pp. 38–49.

D. Neuhauser, F. Turcotte, 'Costs and quality of care in different types of hospitals', pp. 50–61.

R. Anderson, J. J. May, 'Factors associated with the increasing cost of hospital care', pp. 62–72.

T. E. Chester, 'United States hospital costs in international perspective', pp. 73–81.

M. Lynch, 'The physician "shortage": the economists' mirror', pp. 82–8.

R. N. Grosse, 'Cost–benefit analysis of health service', pp. 89–99.

M. R. Greenlick, 'The impact of prepaid group practice on American medical care: a critical evaluation', pp. 100–13.

H. N. Newman, 'Medicare and Medicaid', pp. 114–24.

S. E. Berki, 'National health insurance: an idea whose time has come?' pp. 125–44.

B. C. Stuart, 'Who gains from public health programmes?' pp. 145–50.

W. L. Kissick, S. P. Martin, 'Issues of the future in health', pp. 151–9.

A. R. Somers, 'The Nation's health: issues for the future', pp. 160–74.
See 284, 459, 486, 737, 1315, 1324.

1235 K. DAVIS, 'Community hospital expenses and revenues: pre-Medicare inflation'
SSB, October, 1972, 35(10), pp. 3–19.
See 445, 466, 468, 502, 503, 529.

6 R. G. EVANS, *Price Formation in the Market for Physician Services in Canada 1957–1969*
Ottawa: Queens Printer, 1972, pp. vi, 131.
See 276.

7 V. R. FUCHS, M. J. KRAMER, *Determinants of Expenditures for Physicians' Services in the United States 1948–68*
Washington D.C.: U.S. Department of Health, Education and Welfare, National Center for Health Services, Research and Development, DHEW, Publication No. (HSM) 73–3013, December 1972, p. 63.
See 120.

8 P. B. GINSBURG, 'Resource allocation in the hospital industry: the role of capital financing'
SSB, October, 1972, 35(10), pp. 20–30.
See 475.

9 A. S. HARO, T. PUROLA, 'Planning and health policy in Finland'
IJHS, February, 1972, 2(1), pp. 23–34.

0 H. JOSEPH, 'Hospital insurance and moral hazard'
JHR, Spring, 1972, 7(2), pp. 152–61.
An examination of the hypothesis that the existence of third-party reimbursement increases length of stay. For seven out of twenty-two diagnoses examined, length of stay was influenced by insurance status, moral hazard occurring mainly with less serious cases. For most diagnoses low elasticities of demand were computed, suggesting the limited usefulness of coinsurance schemes for those diagnoses.

1 H. JOSEPH, 'The measurement of moral hazard'
JRI, June, 1972, 39(2), pp. 257–62.
Insurance data, in which the proportion of loss borne by individuals differs, are used to estimate price elasticities of demand for medical care, providing an indication of moral hazard. It is shown that the amount of moral hazard varies significantly with age, class, type of illness, type of accommodation and whether there were complications, but not with the sex of the patient.

1242   K. KIIKUNI, 'Health insurance programmes in Japan'
Inquiry, March, 1972, 9(1), pp. 16–23.
A description of the development and present state of social insurance programmes in Japan.

1243   J. R. LAVE, S. LEINHARDT, 'The delivery of ambulatory care to the poor: a literature review'
MS, December, 1972, 19(4), pp. 78–99.
Work on the availability of health care to the poor in the U.S.A. and on various attempts – emergency and outpatient departments, neighbourhood health centres, satellite clinics, and the use of paramedics – to increase availability of care to the poor is reviewed. A proposal involving a three-level system involving a central hospital, neighbourhood clinics and satellite storefronts is outlined.
See 122.

1244   J. D. LONG, 'Risk, uncertainty, and moral hazard: comment'
JRI, March, 1972, 39(1), pp. 130–5.
Provides a useful brief survey of the Arrow, Lees, Rice, Pauly, Grubel debate on the welfare economics of compulsory medical insurance. It is argued that the Pauly (*AER*, 1968) criticism is not refuted by Grubel (*JRI*, 1971) unless compensation is actually being made to low risk individuals rather than being hypothetically made.
See 1161.

1245   C. E. PHELPS, J. P. NEWHOUSE, 'Effects of coinsurance: a multivariate analysis'
SSB, June, 1972, 35(6), pp. 20–8.
A different statistical methodology from that used by Scitovsky and Snyder (pp. 3–19) is used to examine the same data. Both studies reach essentially the same conclusions, involving a decline in the number of visits and average expense.
See 1247.

1246   D. S. SALKEVER, 'A microeconometric study of hospital cost inflation'
JPE, November–December, 1972, 80(6), pp. 1144–66.
See 491.

1247   A. A. SCITOVSKY, N. M. SNYDER, 'Effect of coinsurance on use of physician services'
SSB, June, 1972, 35(6), pp. 3–19.

A study of the impact of the introduction of a 25 per cent coinsurance provision on the demand for physician and outpatient ancillary services under a comprehensive prepaid medical care plan offered by Stanford University to its full-time employees. The number of physician services used per capita fell by 24.1 per cent, and per capita cost fell by 23.8 per cent. It appeared that coinsurance reduced the demand for care for minor illnesses by considerably more than the demand for medical care for other conditions.
See 1245.

48 J. T. WARD, P. M. TATCHELL, 'Health expenditures in New Zealand'
ER, December, 1972, 48(124), pp. 500–16.

The social accounting framework developed by the WHO is used to estimate the national expenditure and sources of finance for health services in New Zealand in 1968–9. Estimates are also made for 1960–1 to establish trends over time, and to allow comparison with WHO studies.

49 J. H. WEISS, L. BRODSKY, 'An essay on the national financing of health care'
JHR, Spring, 1972, 7(2), pp. 139–51.
See 1325.

1973

0 R. G. BECK, 'Economic class and access to physican services under public medical care insurance'
IJHS, Summer, 1973, 3(3), pp. 341–55.

A study of Saskatchewan revealed that the introduction of public medical care insurance has reduced the disparity in access to physicians' services between low and high income classes, but has not eliminated it. The disparity has decreased over time but there is indication of a levelling off at present levels of inequality.

51 M. S. FELDSTEIN, 'The welfare loss of excess health insurance'
JPE, March–April, 1973, 81(2 part 1), pp. 251–80.

The paper specifies and estimates a structural equation for the demand for health insurance. The parameter estimates indicate that an increase in the price of hospital care causes a substantial increase in the demand for insurance (and more insurance increases the price of care – although the system is dynamically stable). The final section estimates the welfare gains that would result from an increase in the average coinsurance rate from 0.33 to 0.5 or 0.67; the most likely values imply net gains of the order of $4,000 million per year.

1252   P. J. FELDSTEIN, *Financing Dental Care: An Economic Analysis*
Lexington: D. C. Heath and Company, 1973, pp. xvii, 260.
See 36.

1253   P. FISHER, 'Major social security issues: Japan'
SSB, March, 1973, 36(3), pp. 26–38.

A descriptive survey providing information on the two major health insurance schemes.

1254   B. FRIEDMAN, 'Consumer response to incentives under alternative health insurance programmes'
Inquiry, September, 1973, 10(3), pp. 31–5.

A discussion of some of the economic issues in improving the design of the United States health insurance system. It is concluded that expanded non-price rationing of care would be required if lower copayment ceilings were set for families already having health insurance. For families at the lower end of the medical expenditure spectrum it is concluded that eliminating copayment altogether is unlikely to eliminate the lags between the appearance of symptoms and the treatment of serious illness, and that insurance would have to be supplemented by specific detection programmes.

1255   M. I. KAMIEN, N. L. SCHWARTZ, 'Payment plans and the efficient delivery of health care services'
JRI, September, 1973, 40(3), pp. 427–36.

In providing complete health care to a given population there is a problem of achieving an economically efficient mix of preventive care and treatment for illness. A model is constructed to devise a payment plan that will induce the recipients of health care to seek this economically efficient mix. In a wide range of circumstances a suitable copayment rate will achieve this result. Conditions under which complete prepayment or fee for service are preferable are also specified.

1256   T. PUROLA, E. KALIMO, K. NYMAN, K. SIEVERS, 'National sickness insurance in Finland: its impact and evaluation'
IJHS, Winter, 1973, 3(1), pp. 69–80.

A review of the objectives and findings of a national health interview survey conducted in Finland in 1964, prior to the introduction of national health insurance, and in 1968, four years after the implementation of the scheme.

M. I. ROEMER, W. SHONICK, 'HMO performance: the recent evidence'
MMFQ, Summer, 1973, 51(3), pp. 271–317.

An examination of the evidence on Health Maintenance Organisation's performance that has become available since Donabedian's 1969 study. Evidence on performance is classified under seven categories: subscriber composition, participation of physicians, utilisation rates, quality assessments, costs and productivity, health status outcomes, and patient attitudes. *See 1193.*

R. N. ROSETT, L. HUANG, 'The effect of health insurance on the demand for medical care'
JPE, March–April, 1973, 81(2 part 1), pp. 281–305.

The paper uses data from the 1960 U.S. Survey of Consumer Expenditures to estimate price and income elasticities of the demand for hospitalization and physicians' services. The estimated demand curve is then used to compute the increase in expenditure due to ownership of an insurance policy and to divide that increase into two parts: its worth to the consumer, and the excess of cost over its worth.

H. S. RUCHLIN, D. C. ROGERS, *Economics and Health Care*
Springfield, Illinois: Charles C. Thomas Publisher, 1973, pp. xvii, 317.

Macro and micro aspects of financing health care in the U.S.A. are examined, deficiencies particularly in the method of reimbursing providers of health care are noted, and several alternative schemes of reimbursement that have been suggested are reviewed. *See 39.*

D. A. STEWART, 'The history and status of proprietary hospitals'
BCRRS, March, 1973, 9, pp. 2–9.
See 520.

D. WHIPPLE, 'A voucher plan for financing health care delivery'
Soc.-Econ.Plan.Sciences, December, 1973, 7(6), pp. 681–6.

An explanation of some of the operational characteristics of a voucher system to provide full premium payment for membership in a comprehensive prepaid health plan in a specified period, or to pay a predetermined amount towards a health insurance premium. The voucher would be implemented on an area basis. An analytical model of the decision process of regional voucher boards is developed. Optimal selection of voucher redemption levels and capital subsidy programmes are calculated.

1974

1262   R. C. AUGER, V. P. GOLDBERG, 'Prepaid health plans and moral hazard'
PP, Summer, 1974, 22(3), pp. 353–97.

The concept of the prepaid health plan is outlined. The nature of moral hazard is explored and the distinction is made between consumer moral hazard and provider-originated moral hazard. It is argued that prepaid health plans will have their most significant effect on provider-originated moral hazard, and evidence on utilisation and the incidence of surgery bears out this view.

1263   R. G. BECK, 'The effect of co-payment on the poor'
JHR, Winter, 1974, 9(1), 129–42.

Examination of information on the introduction of copayment in Saskatchewan suggests a reduction of about 18 per cent in consumption of medical services by the poor, compared to 6–7 per cent for the whole population, with patient elective services declining more than physician elective services.

1264   W. L. DOWLING, 'Prospective reimbursement of hospitals'
Inquiry, September, 1974, 11(3), pp. 163–80.

Examines the characteristics and possible impacts (on admissions, length of stay, complexity, intensity of service, scope of service, quality of service) of prospective reimbursement (prepayment) as a means of paying hospitals.

1265   M. S. FELDSTEIN, 'Econometric studies of health economics'
In M. D. Intriligator, D. A Kendrick (eds.) *Frontiers of Quantitative Economics*, Vol. 2, pp. 377–447, Amsterdam: North Holland, 1974.

Looks at work on the demand for health insurance, the effect of health insurance on the quantity and price of health services and its welfare effects, and finally at work on national health insurance.
See 42.

1266   B. FRIEDMAN, 'Risk aversion and the consumer choice of health insurance option'
Rev.Econ.Stats., May, 1974, 56(2), pp. 209–14.

Develops a model of consumers' choice between alternative health insurance options based on the theory of expected utility maximisation. The model is tested with reference to permanent federal employees' choice of health insurance option.

V. R. FUCHS, *Who Shall Live? Health, Economics and Social Choice*
New York: Basic Books Inc., 1974, pp. vii, 168.
See 43.

C. C. HAVIGHURST (ed.) *Regulating Health Facilities Construction*
Washington D.C.: American Enterprise Institute for Public Policy
Research, 1974, p. 314.
The proceedings of a conference centred around 'Certificate-of-need' laws –
state laws prohibiting construction or expansion of medical facilities without a
prior certification of 'need' by a state agency. The concept of 'certificate-of-
need' is borrowed from public utility regulation and the intention is usually to
treat health-care providers as public utilities. The conference proceedings are
divided into four parts. Part one deals with 'Health planning and health
planners: forerunners of certificates of need'. Part two is entitled 'Health
facilities planning with "teeth": certificate-of-need laws', part three 'Non-profit
monopolies in health care: controlling the progeny of certificate-of-need laws',
and part four, 'National health policy directions: the future of certificate-of-
need laws and health planning'. Twelve papers are included together with
commentaries on the papers and reports of the discussions they provoked.
See 546, 548, 1045, 1343, 1344, 1421.

T. HIGUCHI, 'Medical care through social insurance in the Japanese rural
sector'
ILR, March, 1974, 109(3), pp. 251–74.
A historical study outlining the development of social insurance in the rural
sector in the last 35 years, its coverage, benefits and finance.

T. KAWAKAMI, 'The system of medical care in Japan and its problems'
In M. Perlman (ed.) *The Economics of Health and Medical Care*, pp.
41–56 (44).
Traces the development of the Japanese medical care system. The major
problem is seen to be that the public provision for medical care has been
debated so far only in relation to the payment system, without considering the
institutions of medical care, delivery, medical education and medical supplies.

A. I. KISCH, 'The health care system and health: some thoughts on a
famous misalliance'
Inquiry, December, 1974, 11(4), pp. 269–75.
It is argued that leaving control of the direction of health services in the hands
of physicians in the U.S. has a distinctly negative effect on health care – an
overconcentration on curative rather than preventive care and a manipulation
of the system for their own ends.

1272   J. KRIZAY, A. WILSON, *The Patient as Consumer: Health Care Financing in the United States*
Lexington, Massachusetts: Lexington Books, D. C. Heath, 1974, pp. xxii, 229.

A major study tracing the development of the health insurance movement in the U.S.A., examining the effects of health insurance on motivations of consumers, doctors and hospitals, the behaviour of the health insurance bureaucracy of Blue Cross and the private plans, the nature of prepaid group practice, and the present role of the government. The final chapter discusses the requirements that any health insurance reform or national health insurance proposals must try to fulfil.

1273   J. K. KWON, 'On the relative efficiency of health care systems'
Kyklos,1974, 27(4), pp. 821–39.
See 542.

1274   J. P. NEWHOUSE, 'A design for a health insurance experiment'
Inquiry, March, 1974, 11(1), pp. 5–27.

Describes the Rand Health Insurance Study, a study partly experimental, and partly involving an analysis of existing data, designed to measure the effect of various financing provisions on the demand for health services and the effect of financing arrangements on health states, and to test the administrative feasibility of some of the features of national health insurance proposals. See also in the same issue of *Inquiry* papers by L. L. Orr, 'The Health Insurance Study: experimentation and health financing policy', pp. 28–39; by A. I. Kisch and P. R. Torrens, 'Health status assessment in the Health Insurance Study', pp. 40–52; and by J. Hester and I. Leveson, 'The Health Insurance Study: a critical appraisal', pp. 53–60, which comment on the Rand Study.

1275   J. P. NEWHOUSE, C. E. PHELPS, 'Price and income elasticities for medical care services'
In M. Perlman (ed.) *The Economics of Health and Medical Care*, pp. 139–61.
See 56.

1276   M. V. PAULY, 'Overinsurance and public provision of insurance'
QJE, February, 1974, 88(1), pp. 44–62.

Examines the problems presented to attainment of optimal insurance provision by moral hazard and adverse selection. Compulsory provision is discussed as a means for overcoming these problems. Alternatives to compulsory provision involving either facing buyers with premium rates that rise along with the size of purchases of insurance, or insurers fixing a quantity and a price of insurance, are also discussed.

C. E. PHELPS, J. P. NEWHOUSE, 'Coinsurance, the price of time, and the demand for medical services'
Rev.Econ.Stats., August, 1974, 56(3), pp. 334–42.

On the assumption that consumers maximise a utility function in 'other goods' and health status, subject to a budget constraint, the relationships between demand for medical care and various price components, including time inputs, are specified. The authors then go on to estimate average arc elasticities in the range 0 to 25 per cent coinsurance using a variety of data sources not previously exploited. The data generally support the hypotheses about the demand for care: services with a relatively high time price (especially physician office visits) exhibit relatively low average elasticities, and relatively high time price elasticities; services with a high money price show considerably higher own price elasticities. Money prices appear to fall with coinsurance rates. The findings are compared with those found in other studies.

G. RUFFOLO, 'Health and insanity: an improbable system'
Rev.Econ.Cond.Italy, January, 1974, 28(1), pp. 28–45.

A general review of health care in Italy. The health status of the nation and the characteristics of the health-care system, its financing, staffing, and the nature and distribution of hospitals, are outlined. A 'National Health Service' with equality of access to all, with public control of the health-care system's principal functions is canvassed as an alternative to the present structure with its disorganisation and financial troubles.

(iv)   *Medicare, Medicaid*

1952

R. R. CAMPBELL, W. G. CAMPBELL, 'Compulsory health insurance: the economic issues'
QJE, February, 1952, 66(1), pp. 1–24.
See 1153.

1964

1280   S. E. HARRIS, *The Economics of American Medicine*
New York: The Macmillan Company, 1964, pp. xvi, 508.
See 6.

1966

1281   E. FEINGOLD, *Medicare: Policy and Politics*
San Francisco: Chandler Publishing Company, 1966, pp. xvi, 318.

A study of the political and economic issues surrounding the establishment of Medicare. A large number of comments and short articles are reproduced in the book representing a wide variety of interests and specialisms. The book is divided into six sections: medical care for the general population, the special problem of the aged, the legislative history of Medicare, alternative solutions for the aged, financing medical care, and the role of government. Substantial bibliographies are provided, as are details of various bills and a summary of the medical care portions of the 1965 legislation.

1967

1282   E. A. JOHNSON, 'Cost calculations show where Medicare reimbursement formula fails'
Hospitals, March 1st, 1967, 41, pp. 42–7.

Medicare's reimbursement formula is examined using a hypothetical set of hospital accounts. Inadequate allowance for capital costs seem likely to restrict hospital expansion in the future.

1283   H. M. SOMERS, A. R. SOMERS, *Medicare and the Hospitals, Issues and Prospects*
Washington D.C.: The Brookings Institution, 1967, pp. xvi, 303.

The book is concerned to a large extent with the environment into which Medicare was introduced, Medicare being viewed as likely to accelerate or make evident existing problems rather than simply generating entirely new ones.
See 397.

1968

O. W. ANDERSON, *The Uneasy Equilibrium: Private and Public Financing of Health Services in the United States, 1875–1965*
New Haven, Conn.: College and University Press, 1965.

W. G. BOWEN, F. H. HARBISON, R. A. LESTER, H. M. SOMERS, *The American System of Social Insurance, its Philosophy, Impact and Future Development*
New York: McGraw-Hill Book Company, 1968, pp. xi, 255.

A symposium held at Princeton University in 1967. Eight papers – some on specific social insurance programmes, some on the overall philosophy of social insurance, and some on problems of financing the system.

W. J. Cohen, 'Federalism and social insurance', pp. 1–21.
R. A. Musgrave, 'The role of social insurance in an overall programme of social welfare', pp. 23–46.
O. Eckstein, 'Financing the system of social insurance', pp. 47–76.
R. J. Myers, 'The past and future of old-age, survivors and disability insurance', pp. 77–118.
H. M. Somers, 'Medicare and the cost of health services', pp. 119–52.
R. A. Lester, 'The uses of unemployment insurance', pp. 153–86.
R. Tilove, 'The impact of social insurance on the development of private benefit plans', pp. 187–212.
G. V. Rimlinger, 'American social security in a European perspective', pp. 213–40.

P. A. BRINKER, *Economic Insecurity and Social Security*
New York: Appleton-Century-Crofts, 1968, p. 566.
See 1183.

P. J. FELDSTEIN, S. WALDMAN, 'Financial position of hospitals in the early Medicare period'
SSB, October, 1968, 31(10), pp. 18–23.

The authors found an improvement, particularly in the first year of Medicare, in the financial position of all types of hospitals. The biggest change was the increase in the level of hospital charges. Brief explanations for the changes are suggested.

1969

1288   A. DONABEDIAN, J. A. THORBY, 'The systematic impact of Medicare'
MCR, June, 1969, 26(6), pp. 567–85.

The authors assess the effect so far and the likely future impact of Medicare. A large number of studies are surveyed, covering the degree of public acceptance, effects on utilisation of various health services, and the degree of health insurance coverage. Most of the studies relate to the first two years of Medicare.

1289   R. ELLIOTT, R. ROSS, F. VAN DYKE, 'Medicare and the hospital-based specialist: pathologists' and radiologists' arrangements with hospitals 1965–68'
Inquiry, March, 1969, 6(1), pp. 49–59.

An examination of the effects of Medicare upon the salary arrangements of these hospital based specialists. An increase in the amount of direct billing of patients was noted, but this has levelled off in the last year. The shift to direct billing was larger for radiologists.

1290   P. J. FELDSTEIN, S. WALDMAN, 'The financial position of hospitals in the first two years of Medicare'
Inquiry, March, 1969, 6(1), pp. 19–27.

Examination of net revenue ratios indicates a significant improvement in the financial position of hospitals in the first two years of Medicare, with small and medium sized hospitals showing the greatest gains. The authors suggest reasons for the improvement.

1291   E. GINZBERG, M. OSTOW, *Men, Money and Medicine*
New York: Columbia University Press, 1969, pp. xii, 291.
See 218, 1194.

1970

1292   O. W ANDERSON, 'Universal and compulsory health insurance the last alternative'
HA, Summer, 1970, 15(3), pp. 35–53.

A survey paper examining the issues that arise in considering the implementation of universal health insurance in the U.S.A. The reasons for the growing demand for such insurance are discussed as are the problems involved in deciding sources of funds, administration, increasing manpower resources, the nature of the benefit package and its distribution, the method of payment of providers of care, and the problem of managing quality.

C. B. CHAPMAN, J. M. TALMADGE, 'Historical and political background of Federal health care legislation'
Law Contemp.Probl., Spring, 1970, 35(2), pp. 334–47.

A brief history of the development of U.S. health legislation from 1793 to the present day. The authors conclude that 'the legislative end results have been determined by a mix of pragmatism, political opportunism, the pressure of special interest groups, health crises, technologic factors, and genuine concern for the public "good"'. The constitutional and political issues relating to national health insurance are viewed as having being settled by earlier decisions, and only legislative and administrative details remain to be worked out.

I. S. FALK, 'National health insurance: a review of policies and proposals'
Law Contemp.Probl., Autumn, 1970, 35(4), pp. 669–96.

A review of the American 'medical care crisis' and seven competing proposals put forward to deal with it. All of the proposals contemplate increased government intervention in design and financing of the system but none envisage government ownership, operation or provision of health services.

R. FEIN, 'What direction for national health insurance?'
Hosp.Pract., August, 1970, 5(3), pp. 67–72.

A discussion of the issues that must be faced, and decisions made, in the introduction of national health insurance – how to finance the proposals, how they will affect the delivery system. A major contention is that supply should be allowed to expand to meet the resulting increased demand, rather than supply expanded over the next decade in preparation for introducing national health insurance proposals with rationing devices other than price being adopted in the interim.

C. C. HAVIGHURST, 'Health maintenance organisations and the market for health services'
Law Contemp.Probl., Autumn, 1970, 35(4), pp. 716–95.

It is argued that HMOs operating against a background of a functioning health-care market place could provide protection against excessive costs to government, and would not remain providers of second class care for the poor. This view of the HMO operating in a free market is evaluated in the light of worries about the effect of the profit motive on health care, and the problems of preventing the development of monopolistic elements.

1297　C. C. HAVIGHURST (ed.) *Health Care*
Part I, *Law Contemp.Probl.*, Spring, 1970, 35(2).
Part II, *Law Contemp.Probl.*, Autumn, 1970, 35(4).

A symposium on the American medical care system and the problems it is facing. Sixteen papers are presented by representatives from a number of disciplines.
Part I
D. Mechanic, 'Problems in the future organisation of medical practice', pp. 233–51.
J. R. Lave, L. B. Lave, 'Medical care and its delivery: an economic appraisal', pp. 252–66.
R. Kessel, 'The A.M.A. and the supply of physicians', pp. 267–83.
M. I. Roemer, 'Controlling and promoting quality in medical care', pp. 284–304.
W. Worthington, L. H. Silver, 'Regulation of quality of care in hospitals: the need for change', pp. 305–33.
C. B. Chapman, J. M. Talmadge, 'Historical and political background of federal health care legislation', pp. 334–47.
R. Stevens, 'Medicaid: anatomy of a dilemma', pp. 348–425.
Part II
I. S. Falk, 'National health insurance: a review of policies and proposals', pp. 669–96.
I. Wolkstein, 'Medicare 1971: changing attitudes and changing legislation', pp. 697–715.
C. C. Havighurst, 'Health maintenance organisations and the market for health services', pp. 716–95.
J. Phelan, R. Erickson, S. Fleming, 'Group practice prepayment: an approach to delivering organised health services', pp. 796–816.
B. Steinwald, D. Neuhauser, 'The role of the proprietary hospital', pp. 817–38.
A. J. G. Priest, 'Possible adaptation of public utility concepts in the health care field', pp. 839–48.
R. J. Carlson, 'Health manpower licensing and emerging institutional responsibility for the quality of care', pp. 849–78.
J. E. Ludlam, 'Physician-hospital relations: the role of staff privileges', pp. 879–900.
N. L. Canter, 'The law and poor people's access to health care', pp. 901–22.
See 233, 239, 441, 443, 1293, 1294, 1296.

1298　R. J. MYERS, *Medicare*
Homewood, Illinois: R. D. Irwin Inc., 1970, pp. xvi, 352.

A study of Medicare and to a lesser extent Medicaid – the evaluation, the provisions, the costs, the experience gained on a variety of issues, and possible future trends.

G. F. ROHRLICH (ed.) *Social Economics for the 1970s*
New York: Dunellen Publishing Company, 1970, p. 189.
See 21.

S. WALDMAN, 'Tax credits for private health insurance: cost estimates for alternative proposals for 1970'
MC, September–October, 1970, 8(5), pp. 353–67.
An estimate is made of the total cost of four tax credit proposals: a hypothetical plan providing tax credits for only those with low incomes, a proposal by Rashi Fein, a bill (H.R.9835) introduced by Representative Fulton, and the A.M.A.'s 'Medicredit' plan. The plans are costed on the assumption of a tax credit of equal size.

1971

S. E. BERKI, 'Economic effects of national health insurance'
Inquiry, June, 1971, 8(2), pp. 37–55.
A framework is presented within which to consider national health insurance proposals. Such proposals, it is argued, have a much more pervasive effect than simple cost measures indicate. As an illustration the 1970 Fannin Bill (variation on Medicredit), a tax credit mechanism, is considered.

H. R. BOWEN, J. R. JEFFERS, *The Economics of Health Services*
New York: General Learning Press, 1971, p. 24.
See 22.

E. M. BURNS, 'A critical review of national health insurance proposals'
HSMHA Health Rep., February, 1971, 86(2), pp. 111–20.
A discussion of the proposals for reform of the health care structure in the United States (eleven proposals are considered).

R. R. CAMPBELL, *Economics of Health and Public Policy*
Washington D.C.: American Enterprise Institute for Public Policy Research, 1971, p. 108.
See 23.

1305   M. S. FELDSTEIN, 'A new approach to national health insurance'
PI, Spring, 1971, 23, pp. 93–105.

Six criteria by which to judge any proposed system for financing health care are set out. The present U.S. system and several proposed reforms fail on one or several of these criteria. A proposal for major risk insurance and government guaranteed postpayment loans is put forward. Such insurance would eliminate financial hardship by meeting all expenses above some defined annual sum, and provision of loans would allow spreading of expenditures below this limit.

1306   M. S. FELDSTEIN, 'An econometric model of the Medicare system'
QJE, February, 1971, 85(1), pp. 1–20.

A model of the Medicare system is constructed to examine the interstate variation in five key variables: the proportion of enrollees with supplementary medical insurance, the hospital and extended care admission rates, and the average levels of hospital and medical insurance benefits. The model is estimated by instrumental variables. It explains a substantial proportion of the variation in terms of demographic and economic characteristics of the population, state health policy variables, and local health care system characteristics. One problem revealed by the analysis is that the use of hospital care by the aged population is much less sensitive than use by the non-aged population to interstate differences in the availability of hospital beds. This suggests the need for replacement of the present uniform Medicare system with a system that tailors incentives to local conditions.
See 1332.

1307   I. G. GREENBERG, M. L. RODBURG, 'The role of prepaid group practice in relieving the medical care crisis'
HLR, February, 1971, 84(4), pp. 887–1001.
See 1219.

1308   S. KELMAN, 'Toward the political economy of medical care'
Inquiry, September, 1971, 8(3), pp. 30–8.

An examination of the dialectical relationship between technology, market and social structure, in the development of the American medical care system in the twentieth century. The analysis indicates that the prepaid group practice can develop institutionally into an industrial monolith similar to other industries, with the insurance companies and banks in an advantageous position.

1309   R. LOEWENSTEIN, 'Early effects of Medicare on the health care of the aged'
SSB, April, 1971, 34(4), pp. 3–20.

A report of the major findings of a two part survey, carried out in April and

May of 1966 and November and December 1967, to determine the effects of Medicare on health care received by the over-65s. Evidence was found of substantially increased days of hospital care and substantial reductions in the proportion of out-of-pocket outlays for hospital care, although because of price rises out-of-pocket payments for all services declined by only 15 per cent.

0 J. P. NEWHOUSE, V. TAYLOR, 'How shall we pay for hospital care?'
PI, Spring, 1971, 23, pp. 78–92.
See 1226.

1 M. V. PAULY, 'An analysis of government health insurance plans for poor families'
PP, Summer, 1971, 19(3), pp. 489–521.

An analysis of the Nixon administration's proposal to replace Medicaid for low income families with children by a scheme called the Family Health Insurance Plan. Estimates are made of the cost of the proposal and of some modifications of the scheme.

2 M. V. PAULY, *Medical Care at Public Expense, A Study in Applied Welfare Economics*
New York: Praeger Publishers, 1971, pp. xvi, 160.
See 1025.

3 R. STEVENS, *American Medicine and the Public Interest*
New Haven: Yale University Press, 1971, pp. xiv, 572.
See 1231.

1972

4 R. R. ALFORD, 'The political economy of health care: dynamics without change'
Politics and Society, Winter, 1972, 3, pp. 127–64.

In spite of the expansion of the health-care industry the problems facing the U.S. health service today are virtually the same as those facing it thirty-five years ago – the situation is one of 'dynamics without change'. The various proposals for reform are examined (market reform, bureaucratic reform), as are the various interest groups operating in the health-care field. The absence of change is seen to result from a struggle between major interest groups in the context of a market society.

1315   S. E. Berki, 'National health insurance: an idea whose time has come?' *AAAPSS*, January, 1972, 399, pp. 125–44.

A survey article tracing the history of national health insurance proposals in the U.S.A. Key policy variables are identified, and some criteria for evaluating different aspects of the proposals outlined. Three major proposals current at the time (the Nixon administration proposal, the Kennedy Bill and the American Medical Association proposal) are discussed.
See 1234.

1316   R. Fein, 'On achieving access and equity in health care' *MMFQ*, October, 1972, 50(4 part 2), pp. 157–90.

The reasons for the concern with equity in the area of health care, the equity–equality debate, the present and some suggested future patterns of paying for health care in the U.S.A., and the problems of achieving an adequate spatial distribution of physicians, are among the many issues considered in this paper.

1317   M. S. Feldstein, B. Friedman, H. Luft, 'Distributional aspects of national health insurance benefits and finance' *NTJ*, December, 1972, 25(4), pp. 497–510.

A simulation method for calculating the actuarial value of the benefits of different insurance coverages and different price elasticities of demand is developed, and implemented using Survey of Economic Opportunity data. A standard plan of coverage and financing is evaluated and various modifications considered.

1318   D. Gayer, 'The effects of Medicaid on state and local government finances' *NTJ*, December, 1972, 25(4), pp. 511–19.

Medicaid was found to have stimulated expenditures for medical care for low income individuals, but the increases have not come from state and local funds. Treatment standards and cost burdens have not been equalised between states as a result of the programme; the coefficients of variation have in fact increased. It is concluded that Medicaid has failed to fulfil many of its objectives.

1319   J. M. Glasgow, 'Prepaid group practice as a national health policy: problems and perspectives' *Inquiry*, March, 1972, 9(1), pp. 3–15.

It is argued that the discussion surrounding the financing and delivery of health care has failed to recognise that the proposed changes will not operate in a vacuum but as part of a total system. The article considers the problems of promoting group practice, how large are the benefits from group practice, whether the resources are available, and whether the budget estimates are realistic.

20 J. R. LAVE, S. LEINHARDT, 'The delivery of ambulatory care to the poor: a literature review'
MS, December, 1972, 19(4), pp. 78–99.
Literature is reviewed on attempts in the U.S.A. to increase health care available to the poor, involving both financing and programmes to provide facilities.
See 122, 1243.

21 L. G. SGONTZ, 'The economics of financing medical care: a review of the literature'
Inquiry, December, 1972, 9(4), pp. 3–19.
See 1034.

22 H. M. SOMERS, A. R. SOMERS, 'Major issues in national health insurance'
MMFQ, April, 1972, 50(2 part 1), pp. 177–210.
The various proposals for national health insurance are grouped into four broad categories: proposals for incentives to stimulate purchase of private health insurance; proposals for the purchase of private insurance by employers for their employees; proposals for a comprehensive federal programme financed by payroll and general taxation; and proposals to extend and strengthen Medicare to the entire population. A set of guidelines for evaluating the various proposals is then applied, and a proposal for a national health insurance programme covering the entire civilian population without distinction as to income or contributions is canvassed.

23 B. C. STUART, 'Equity and Medicaid'
JHR, Spring, 1972, 7(2), pp. 162–78.
An assessment of the distributional impact between states of Medicaid during the fiscal year 1967–8. The test used to examine distributive impact is a comparison of the actual distribution of costs and benefits between states with a hypothetical distribution (burden proportional to per capita state income, benefit proportional to the medical needs of the poor of the state). The findings suggest that as a between state redistributive mechanism Medicaid is a failure; it even redistributes income from poor to wealthy states, and the gap between the welfare payments received by the poor in the wealthy states and the poor in

the poor states has widened. Maldistribution of benefits was found to be responsible for more of the distributive inequities than was maldistribution of costs.

1324   B. C. STUART, 'Who gains from public health programmes?'
AAAPSS, January, 1972, 399, pp. 145–50.
The distributional implications of various proposals for national health insurance in the light of experience with Medicare and Medicaid.

1325   J. H. WEISS, L. BRODSKY, 'An essay on the national financing of health care'
JHR, Spring, 1972, 7(2), pp. 139–51.
Four major problems of the American health-care system are identified: maldistribution of services, high costs and poor quality control, rising prices of care, and inadequate catastrophic health insurance for most Americans. The paper looks at possible choices of health insurance schemes to combat these problems, while recognising that the objectives they imply conflict. A number of questions are asked on basic strategy, questions related to coverage, reimbursement of providers, incentives to efficiency, and financing of the plan. The Kennedy Plan is then examined with regard to its ability to combat the four problems identified, and its political feasibility. The direction of the effect, on the problems, of many of the items is uncertain. The plan, it is concluded, is likely to fail in the anti-inflation goal, and is probably too destructive of the present system to be politically feasible.

1973

1326   R. M. BALL, 'Social security amendments of 1972: summary and legislative history'
SSB, March, 1973, 36(3), pp. 3–25.
Detailed summary of the major amendments to the social security system in the U.S.A., which included substantial modifications of Medicare, extending its coverage and attempting to improve its effectiveness.

1327   E. M. BURNS, *Health Services for Tomorrow, Trends and Issues*
New York: Dunellen, 1973, pp. xiv, 226.
A survey of the organisation and functioning of the U.S. health-care system, the development of Medicare and Medicaid and the policy issues to which they gave rise, and various proposals for compulsory health insurance and their likely impact. A good bibliography is provided.

28 K. DAVIS, 'Hospital costs and the Medicare programme'
SSB, August, 1973, 36(8), pp. 18–36.
See *466, 468, 502, 503, 529.*

29 P. J. FELDSTEIN, *Financing Dental Care: An Economic Analysis*
Lexington: D. C. Heath and Company, 1973, pp. xvii, 260. *See 36.*
See 36.

30 M. E. GRANFIELD, S. L. CONRAD, M. J. OEHM, 'Toward better analysis of
social programmes'
Inquiry, December, 1973, 10(4), pp. 24–33.
An examination of the distributional effects of Medi-Cal (California
Medicaid), looking at the dollar value rather than the quantity and quality of
services rendered.

31 U. E. REINHARDT, 'Proposed changes in the organisation of health-care
delivery: an overview and critique'
MMFQ, Spring, 1973, 51(2), pp. 169–222.
A review of a large range of empirical evidence (on factor substitution,
economies of scale, the effects of different methods of payment for health
services) suggests that many proposals for reform of the American system of
health-care delivery, and in particular the proposal for a nationwide network of
HMOs, are based more on faith than on sound empirical evidence.

32 L. B. RUSSELL, 'An econometric model of the Medicare system'
QJE, August, 1973, 87(3), pp. 482–9.
The paper re-examines some of the ground covered by Feldstein on the effect of
extended care facilities available through Medicare on the total cost of
institutional care. Feldstein concluded that the net effect of extended care
facilities is to raise cost per hospital episode. Russell, with data on Medicare
patients as opposed to Feldstein's data on all patients, reaches the opposite
conclusion. See also the reply by Feldstein, pp. 490–4.
See 1306.

33 L. B. RUSSELL, 'The impact of the extended-care facility benefit on
hospital use and reimbursements under Medicare'
JHR, Winter, 1973, 8(1), pp. 57–72.
Regression analysis using data from 48 states revealed that including use of
extended-care facilities under Medicare reduced average length of hospital stay
by 1.4 days in 1967 and 1.8 days in 1968. The savings in hospital reimbursements were also substantially greater than outlays for ECF use.

1334   B. C. Stuart, R. Stockton, 'Control over the utilization of medical services'
MMFQ, Summer, 1973, 51(3), pp. 341–94.

Five methods of controlling utilisation of medical services are examined: supply limitations, financial disincentives, authorisation requirements, review mechanisms, and legal action. Most existing forms of control in the United States are seen to suffer from ambiguity of purpose. The best hope for the longer term is seen to be the changing of the incentive structure for both providers and users, e.g. the prepaid health centre. A substantial bibliography is provided.

1335   R. J. Vogel, J. F. Morrall, 'The impact of Medicaid on state and local health and hospitals expenditure, with special reference to blacks'
JHR, Spring, 1973, 8(2), pp. 202–11.

A single equation supply and demand model explained over 80 per cent of the variations in state and local health and hospital expenditures per capita. Medicaid was found to have had a significant and favourable impact on the provision of health care for the needy, and especially blacks.

1974

1336   W. J. Baumol, 'An overview of the results on consumption, health, and social behaviour'
JHR, Spring, 1974, 9(2), pp. 253–64.
See 1473.

1337   L. Breslow, 'Quality and cost control: Medicare and beyond'
MC, February, 1974, 12(2), pp. 95–114.

Reviews the development of views on cost and quality controls between the inception of Medicare and the present time and makes some suggestions for future action.

1338   E. W. Brian, S. F. Gibbens, *California's Medi-Cal Copayment Experiment*
MC, December, 1974, 12(12 Supplement), p. 303.

A description of the experiment that introduced low charges for medical services for Medicaid recipients. The results, showing the effect on utilization of different services by the different welfare aid groups, are tabulated.

9   B. FRIEDMAN, 'A test of alternative demand-shift responses to the Medicare programme'
In M. Perlman (ed.) *The Economics of Health and Medical Care*, pp. 234–47.
See 150.

0   J. HESTER, E. SUSSMAN, 'Medicaid prepayment: concept and implementation'
MMFQ, Fall, 1974, 52(4), pp. 415–44.
Examines the advantages that are claimed for prepayment for health services in providing health care for the poor, in the light of experience in converting a New York City Neighbourhood Health Center to prepayment for Medicaid patients and of results from large-scale prepayment experiments in New York City and California.

1   H. E. KLARMAN, 'Major public initiative in health care'
PI, Winter, 1974, 34, pp. 106–23.
The development and the problems of Medicare, Medicaid, Regional Medical Care Programs, Comprehensive Health Planning, and Health Maintenance Organisations (HMOs) are discussed. It is suggested that major improvements in the system of care could be achieved by changes such as movement away from cost reimbursement, or by reducing the supply of beds. Politicians and health administrators have preferred sharp breaks with the existing system to new institutions like HMOs.

2   J. KRIZAY, A. WILSON, *The Patient as Consumer: Health Care Financing in the United States*
Lexington, Massachusetts: Lexington Books, D. C. Heath, 1974, pp. xxii, 229.
See 1272.

3   J. R. LAVE, L. B. LAVE, 'The supply and allocation of medical resources: alternative control mechanisms'
In C. C. Havighurst (ed.) *Regulating Health Facilities Construction*, pp. 163–81.
An examination of the difficulties facing the United States health-care industry and the attempts and suggestions that have been made in the last decade to deal with these problems.
See 1268.

1344 J. P. NEWHOUSE, J. P. ACTON, 'Compulsory health planning laws and national health insurance'
In C. C. Havighurst (ed.) *Regulating Health Facilities Construction*, pp. 217–31.

It is argued that advocacy of compulsory planning stems from the consequences of reimbursement insurance. The likely effectiveness of regulation, alternative forms of health insurance as a basis of national health insurance, and the cream-skimming argument in favour of controlling entry into the health industry, are examined.
See 1268.

1345 H. A. PALLEY, 'Policy formulation in health – some considerations of governmental constraints on pricing in the health delivery system'
Am.Beh.Scientist, March–April, 1974, 17(4), pp. 572–84.

Traces the development of the government's role in influencing the price of medical care in the period after the introduction of Medicare.

1346 D. E. YETT, L. DRABEK, M. D. INTRILIGATOR, L. J. KIMBELL, 'Econometric forecasts of health services and health manpower'
In M. Perlman (ed.) *The Economics of Health and Medical Care*, pp. 459–69.
See 1424.

(c) Consequences of Different Systems of Provision for Labour Force Participation, Health Preservation, Compensation and Specific Redistribution

---

The length of the title is due more to the heterogeneity of the subject-matter than to its central importance. A consequence of the choice of health-care system is that the material welfare of particular groups may be differentially affected. The relevant groups and effects are diverse: the major topics covered by our references are disability, control of disease-inducing work conditions, and accident compensation.

It should be observed that such studies might also have been included as fringe items in a section concerned with income redistribution through health delivery systems, which in turn necessitates the observation that no such section in fact appears in the bibliography. The reason for this is that, while some work on redistribution does exist, it is normally incorporated in studies with other, or broader objectives. Specifically, some of the studies of Medicare and Medicaid, cited at (b) (iv) above, are concerned with questions of redistribution (see Feldstein, Friedman and Luft, 1317; and Stuart, 1323).

1963

7 M. S. GORDON, *The Economics of Welfare Policies*
New York: Columbia University Press, 1963, pp. xii, 159.

A brief outline of welfare programmes in the U.S.A., some international comparisons of various social welfare expenditures, and some information on income-redistribution effects of welfare programmes are presented in the first three chapters of the book. The major part of the book is devoted to an examination of the effects of the Old-age, Survivors, and Disability Insurance Programme (OASDI), and unemployment insurance.

1964

8 A. F. CONARD, J. MORGAN, R. PRATT, C. VOLTZ, R. BOMBAUGH, *Automobile Accident Costs and Payments – Studies in the economics of Injury Reparation*
Ann Arbor: University of Michigan Press, 1964, pp. xxviii, 506.

Information is provided on the system of reparation of victims of automobile accidents in the U.S.A., the size and sources of compensation they receive, and the economic losses they suffer as a result of the accident. The operation of the system of reparation is discussed and compared with systems of reparation for automobile injuries in England, Sweden, France and Germany.
See 825.

1965

9 R. W. CONLEY, *The Economics of Vocational Rehabilitation*
Baltimore: The Johns Hopkins Press, 1965, pp. xii, 177.
See 652.

1967

1350   O. E. WILLIAMSON, D. G. OLSON, A. RALSTON, 'Externalities, insurance, and disability analysis'
EC, May, 1967, 34(134), pp. 235–53.
A demonstration that externality analysis is an appropriate vehicle with which to study disability problems. The implications of the availability of insurance for the results, and the problems of estimating damages and determining appropriate insurance rates where the former are not objectively specified and insurance not administratively costless, are spelled out. Applications and limitations of the analysis are illustrated by reference to the cases of automobile injury, radiation injury and workmen's compensation.

1968

1351   W. G. BOWEN, F. H. HARBISON, R. A. LESTER, H. M. SOMERS, *The American System of Social Insurance, its Philosophy, Impact and Future Development*
New York: McGraw-Hill Book Company, 1968, pp. xi, 255.
See 1285.

1352   P. A. BRINKER, *Economic Insecurity and Social Security*
New York: Appleton-Century-Crofts, 1968, p. 566.
See 1183.

1969

1353   R. W. CONLEY, 'A benefit–cost analysis of the vocational rehabilitation programme'
JHR, Spring, 1969, 4(1), pp. 226–52.
Apart from the benefits to the disabled, estimates are also made of the benefits to taxpayers from the reduction in their tax liability due to a decrease in tax-supported payments for the maintenance and care of the disabled, and the increased tax payments of rehabilitants.
See 652, 687.

M. Crew, 'Coinsurance and the welfare economics of medical care'
AER, December, 1969, 59(5), pp. 906–8.
See 1192.

1970

M. Berkowitz, W. G. Johnson, 'Towards an economics of disability: the magnitude and structure of transfer and medical costs'
JHR, Summer, 1970, 5(3), pp. 271–97.
An examination of the rationale of various parts of the whole transfer programme, short-term, long-term, public and private devoted to the problem of what the authors term the 'workman's disability income system'. Details are provided of the size and distribution of the various payments to those of labour force age, the total amounting to 13.7 billion dollars in 1967.
See 693.

G. Calabresi, *The Costs of Accidents: A Legal and Economic Analysis*
New Haven: Yale University Press, 1970, pp. x, 340.
See 694.

1971

A. I. Harris, J. R. Buckle, C. R. W. Smith, E. Head, E. Cox, *Handicapped and Impaired in Great Britain*
London: HMSO, Office of Population Censuses and Surveys, Parts I and II, 1971, Part III, 1972, p. 600.
See 891.

M. V. Pauly, *Medical Care at Public Expense, A Study in Applied Welfare Economics*
New York: Praeger Publishers, 1971, pp. xvi, 160.
See 1025.

1972

1359   W. J. DRAYTON, 'The tar and nicotine tax: pursuing public health through tax incentives'
YLJ, July, 1972, 81(8), pp. 1487–516.

Arguing that previous government efforts to discourage smoking have harried the cigarette smoker but have not changed smoking patterns, it is argued that a useful task would be to try and reduce the harmfulness of what is being smoked. The case for a federal tax fixed according to the tar and nicotine content of cigarettes is developed.
See 761, 792, 793.

1360   I. GARFINKEL, 'Equal access, minimum provision, and efficiency in financing medical care'
JHR, Spring, 1972, 7(2), pp. 242–9.

Demonstrates, using a simple partial equilibrium analysis, that the efficient method of financing medical care depends upon which of two alternative objectives a government pursues. For achieving equal access to health care irrespective of income, the appropriate system is a subsidy to the poor and an excise tax on the rich man's medical care consumption, although political realities probably dictate comparison of the relative inefficiencies of pure subsidy and free provision. Ensuring that all individuals attain some minimum level of care requires a pure price subsidy; a nationalised free health service is inappropriate.

1973

1361   R. W. CONLEY, *The Economics of Mental Retardation*
Baltimore: The Johns Hopkins Press, 1973, pp. xiii, 377.
See 769.

1362   L. D. HABER, 'Social planning for disability'
JHR, 1973, 8(Supplement), pp. 33–55.

The article examines the findings of the Social Security Survey of Disabled Adults, a sample of non-institutionalised disabled adults aged 18–64 years in the U.S.A. The implications for social planning are discussed, and the need to fit the disabled into the workforce is stressed. It is concluded that co-ordination of compensation and rehabilitation programmes is necessary for maximum

effect; separately, the rigid disability criteria for compensation may lead to disincentives for rehabilitation.
See 916.

3   D. S. LEES, N. DOHERTY, 'Compensation for personal injury'
LBR, April, 1973, 108, pp. 18–32.
The effects of the major schemes of accident compensation and their implications for efficiency and the distribution of compensation are outlined. The deficiencies of the tort system are examined. In addition to the usual criticisms it is shown that the tort system hinders the ability of the remaining systems to distribute compensation so as to maximise economic welfare.

4   S. SAINSBURY, *Measuring Disability*
London: Occasional Papers on Social Administration No. 54, G. Bell and Sons Ltd., 1973, p. 125.
See 930.

1974

5   R. L. AKEHURST, 'Optimal control of disease-inducing work conditions'
In A. J. Culyer (ed.) *Economic Policies and Social Goals*, pp. 199–215 (41).
Discusses the present methods of fixing industrial hygiene standards in the U.K. and then discusses the information needed for designing an optimal policy for controlling industrial disease.
See 790, 791.

6   H. BOLDERSON, 'Compensation for disability'
JSP, July, 1974, 3(3), pp. 193–211.
Examines the difficulties encountered in making transfers to disadvantaged individuals, and looks at the historical development of compensation schemes in the United Kingdom. An as-of-right payment for all disabled people, with some supplement for functional limitation based on a disability measure, is seen as a potentially fruitful line of development.

7   A. J. CULYER, 'Economics, social policy and disability'
In D. S. Lees, S. Shaw (eds.) *Impairment, Disability and Handicap*, pp. 17–29.
See 801.

1368 N. DOHERTY, D. S. LEES, 'Damages for personal injury: some economic issues'
In D. S. Lees, S. Shaw (eds.) *Impairment, Disability, and Handicap*, pp. 56–78 (809).

The paper examines the allocative, distributive and organisational implications of the tort system of damages, and presents a numerical picture of how the system works in the United Kingdom. It is pointed out that if the fault system is replaced, any new scheme must also contain incentives for accident avoidance.

1369 R. KIDNER, K. RICHARDS, 'Compensation to dependants of accident victims'
EJ, March, 1974, 84(1), pp. 130–42.

The deficiencies of the present system of compensation to dependants of accident victims, actuarial defects, and problems of inflation and expectations of rising real income, are discussed. An alternative approach taking into account these defects is suggested; this approach would result in significantly higher settlements. The no-fault system of compensation used in New Zealand is also considered.

1370 J. WISEMAN, J. G. CULLIS, 'Social policy towards disabled workers'
In A. J. Culyer (ed.) *Economic Policies and Social Goals*, pp. 138–70 (41).

Develops a rationale for policy toward the disabled, first of all in a competitive labour market, and then recognising existing labour market imperfections. Existing policy in the U.K. is considered, and a shift to a policy of subsidies to compensate employers for higher costs of training, permanently reduced productivity or a higher cost working environment, is recommended.

6 Planning Whole Systems

'Whole systems' studies are defined as those that attempt to embrace all the relationships of a health-care system (demand, supply, output) within a comprehensive model. There are essentially three types of study: descriptive, systems analysis (OR), and econometric. An illustration of the descriptive approach is provided by Titmuss *et al.* (1372). Systems analysis is used by Navarro (1384, 1385, 1391, 1392) and by Crombie (1404). The econometric approach to modelling health-care systems has been used by Feldstein (1380, 1381, 1388, 1389), by Yett *et al.* (1403, 1411, 1424), and by Lave, Lave and Leinhardt (1422).

1957

1 S. SWAROOP, K. UEMURA, 'Proportional mortality of 50 years and above: a suggested indicator of the component "health, including demographic conditions" in the measurement of levels of living'
WHO Bulletin, 1957, 17, pp. 439–81.
See 845.

1964

72 R. M. TITMUSS (Chairman), B. ABEL-SMITH, G. MACDONALD, A. W. WILLIAMS, C. H. WOOD, *The Health Services of Tanganyika, A Report to the Government*
London: Pitman Medical Publishing Co. Ltd., 1964, pp. xiii, 265.
A comprehensive report on the existing health services and health needs of Tanganyika, and a suggested plan for the development of these services over the period to 1980. The main emphasis in suggested developments is on 'the balanced development of health services within an overall national plan'. Detailed proposals are put forward, implicit in which is a shift in emphasis from curative to preventive medicine. An annual increase of 4 per cent in health expenditure was assumed in the plan.

1965

1373   CENTRE FOR DEVELOPMENT STUDIES OF THE CENTRAL UNIVERSITY OF VENEZUELA, CARACAS IN CO-OPERATION WITH THE PAN AMERICAN SANITARY BUREAU, *Health Planning: Problems of Concept and Method* Washington D.C.: Pan American Health Organisation and World Health Organisation, 1965, pp. v, 77.
See 953.

1374   C. L. CHIANG, *An Index of Health: Mathematical Models* Washington D.C.: USDHEW, Public Health Service, National Center for Health Statistics, Series 2, No. 5, 1965, p. 19.
See 852.

1966

1375   D. C. PAIGE, K. JONES, *Health and Welfare Services in Britain in 1975* Cambridge: Cambridge University Press for the National Institute of Economic and Social Research, Occasional Papers 22, 1966, p. 142.
See 77, 1101.

1376   G. C. WIRICK, 'A multiple equation model of demand for health care' *HSR*, Winter, 1966, 1(3), pp. 301–46.
A simultaneous equation model of the demand for health care is constructed and tested. Five fundamental factors – need, realisation of need, financial resources, motivation to obtain care and availability of services – are viewed to have an effect on the consumption of hospital care, doctor care, dental care and prescribed medicines.

1967

1377   B. ABEL-SMITH, *An International Study of Health Expenditure, and its Relevance for Health Planning* Geneva: World Health Organisation, Public Health Papers, No. 32, 1967, p. 127.
See 1057.

8 R. BARLOW, 'The economic effects of malaria eradication'
AER, May, 1967, 57(2), pp. 130–48.
See 664, 672.

9 H. CORREA, 'Health planning'
Kyklos, 1967, 20(4), pp. 909–23.
After considering several possible objective functions for health planners, mortality data are chosen as an index of output of health services. Two planning problems are considered using simple static models: the problem of allocating resources between preventive and curative care for a particular disease, and the problem of allocation of resources among several diseases. A statistical example of the first problem is presented, the case of whooping cough in Chile. The possibility of a dynamic approach to allocation problems is also briefly discussed.

0 M. S. FELDSTEIN, 'An aggregate planning model of the health care sector'
MC, November–December, 1967, 5(6), pp. 369–81. Also in M. H. Cooper, A. J. Culyer (eds.) *Health Economics*, pp. 210–29 (33).
A six equation model of the health-care sector is constructed. The concepts behind such a model and its properties are discussed. The uses to which such a model might be put are considered. As an illustration Feldstein uses the model to examine the relationship between the supply and demand for hospital inpatient care in the United States.
See 1381.

1 M. S. FELDSTEIN, *Economic Analysis for Health Service Efficiency*
Amsterdam: North-Holland Publishing Company, 1967, pp. xii, 322.
A nine equation model of the health-care system is constructed. The model allows examination of the inter-relationships between hospital, local authority and general practitioner services, as well as the effects on these health sector activities of the demographic and social characteristics of the population. The model is estimated using cross-section data for 1960.
See 392, 1380.

2 WORLD HEALTH ORGANISATION, *National Health Planning in Developing Countries*
Geneva: World Health Organisation, Technical Report Series No. 350, 1967, p. 40.
The report of a WHO Expert Committee, making recommendations on the organisation of health planning and its place in national development planning.

1969

1383   V. NAVARRO, 'Planning for the distribution of personal health services'
PHR, July, 1969, 84(7), pp. 573–81.

Examines six methods that have been used or suggested in the literature to plan the level and type of provision of medical care. The methods discussed are based upon morbidity, mortality and utilisation data, upon the distribution of population and facilities, upon the performance of health systems, and upon the structure of the health system.

1384   V. NAVARRO, 'A systems approach to health planning'
HSR, Summer, 1969, 4(2), pp. 96–111.

Presents a stochastic model involving a Markov chain that integrates the component parts of a health-care system (defining the transitional probabilities of individuals moving from one state and part of the system to another). Applications of the model are then outlined (giving numerical examples) in prediction, straightforward extrapolation to determine resources required, simulation to examine the effect of changing parameters, and meeting specified objective functions optimally.

1385   V. NAVARRO, 'Systems analysis in the health field'
Soc.-Econ.Plan.Sciences, 1969, 3, pp. 179–89.

A survey of approaches to health planning. The paper examines the nature of the health-care system, models of the system (structure), and indicators of performance.

1386   D. H. STIMSON, 'Utility measurement in public health decision-making'
MS, 1969, 16(2), pp. B-17–B-30.
See 865.

1970

1387   J. R. ASHFORD, N. G. PEARSON, 'Who uses the health services and why?'
JRSS A, 1970, 133(3), pp. 295–357.
See 91.

1388   M. S. FELDSTEIN, 'Health sector planning in developing countries'
EC, May, 1970, 37(146), pp. 139–63.

A linear programming model is developed for the allocation of health sector resources between and within disease control programmes. An illustrative application of the model to tuberculosis control planning is provided. Seven types of benefits from tuberculosis activities were identified: economic benefits (reduced income losses), reduced number of deaths in four age groups, reduced permanent impairments and reduced short-term disabilities, the weights attached to the different benefits to be decided by politically responsible officials. The differences between the linear programming optimisation and cost–benefit analysis are outlined, and the problems of the extension of the optimisation to a number of periods and the incorporation of uncertainty are discussed.

9 P. J. FELDSTEIN, S. KELMAN, 'A framework for an econometric model of the medical care sector'
In H. E. Klarman (ed.) *Empirical Studies in Health Economics*, pp. 171–90 (18).
A model of the medical care sector of the United States is formulated and specified in equation form. The areas to which such a model might be put are outlined but no empirical results are presented in the paper. Most of the paper is concerned with elaborating the determination of output in the five institutional settings considered in the model: acute hospital and nursing homes have a stock-adjustment model; outpatient clinics, doctors' offices, and the patient's home are explained by more conventional demand and supply equations.

0 J. E. MILLER, 'An indicator to aid management in assigning programme priorities'
PHR, August, 1970, 85(8), pp. 725–31.
See 868.

1 V. NAVARRO, 'Methodology on regional planning of personal health services: a case study: Sweden'
MC, September–October, 1970, 8(5), pp. 386–94.
An outline is provided of the methods used in Sweden to estimate future demand for care, the resources required to meet this demand in each region, and the methods used to determine the size of the regions.

2 V. NAVARRO, R. PARKER, K. L. WHITE, 'A stochastic and deterministic model of medical care utilization'
HSR, Winter, 1970, 5(4), pp. 342–57.
See 1460.

1393   R. ZEMACH, 'A model of health-service utilization and resource allocation'
OR, November–December, 1970, 18(6), pp. 1071–86.

A discrete time macro-model is constructed describing the total utilisation of health and medical services by the population of a region, the allocation of resources to provide these services, and the costs of health and medical care derived from the prevailing costs of resources. A simplified illustrative example is provided.

1971

1394   C. J. AUSTIN, 'Selected social indicators in the health field'
AJPH, August, 1971, 61(8), pp. 1507–13.
See 873.

1395   M. S. FELDSTEIN, 'An econometric model of the Medicare system'
QJE, February, 1971, 85(1), pp. 1–20.
See 1306.

1396   J. T. GENTRY, 'The planning of community health services: facilitating rational decision making'
Inquiry, September, 1971, 8(3), pp. 4–21.

An assessment of the nature and usefulness of information available in the U.S.A. for health planning. Information is given on health promotion, primary disease prevention, secondary disease prevention, tertiary disease prevention, quantity and quality of medical treatment and the distribution of these services, rehabilitation, manpower and facility resources, and morbidity and mortality and their associated costs.

1397   H. E. HILLEBOE, A. BARKHUUS, 'Health planning in the United States: some categorical and general approaches'
IJHS, May, 1971, 1(2), pp. 134–48.

Four areas of categorical planning and one of general planning are discussed with a view to providing lessons for the development of comprehensive health policies. The categorical areas discussed are the Hill–Burton programme, the heart, cancer, stroke and kidney disease programmes, mental health planning, and American Indian health. The general area discussed is that of comprehensive health planning (state and area wide) as enacted in Public Law 89–749 in 1966.

8   S. LITSIOS, 'The principles and methods of evaluation of national health plans'
IJHS, February, 1971, 1(1), pp. 79–85.

Seven questions to be used as a basis for evaluating health plans are set out, relating to the nature of the plan, the nature of the planning process and the results achieved following plan implementation.

9   R. F. L. LOGAN, 'National health planning. An appraisal of the state of the art'
IJHS, February, 1971, 1(1), pp. 6–17.
See 1120.

0   J. P. NEWHOUSE, 'Allocation of public sector resources in medical care: an economist looks at health planning'
EBB, Winter, 1971, 23(2), pp. 8–12.

Two approaches are outlined that may be used by governments to plan health services: the market signal approach, involving the estimation of demand and cost curves for particular medical services; and the production function approach, involving the equalisation of marginal product/marginal cost ratios (marginal product being defined by using health status as the output of the production function). The problems associated with each approach are discussed, and the way in which a policy maker might best use information provided by the approaches is suggested.

1   G. A. POPOV, *Principles of Health Planning in the U.S.S.R.*
Geneva: World Health Organisation, Public Health Papers No. 43, 1971, p. 172.

A description of the system of health planning in the U.S.S.R. The planning is based on estimates of need, determined by experts. The health system of the U.S.S.R. emphasises outpatient care and maternal and child health services.

2   L. J. SHUMAN, J. P. YOUNG, E. NADDOR, 'Manpower mix for health services: a prescriptive regional planning model'
HSR, Summer, 1971, 6(2), pp. 103–19.
See 265.

3   D. E. YETT, L. DRABEK, M. D. INTRILIGATOR, 'A macro-econometric model for regional health planning'
EBB, Fall, 1971, 24(1), pp. 1–21.

A model designed to assist comprehensive health planning agencies is con-

structed. At present the model is limited to personal health services, excluding mental health, drugs and dental services. For each category of health service a demand and a supply equation are used to explain utilisation rate and price. The sum of the quantities of health services produced is used in determining the demands for each type of health manpower. These demand equations in conjunction with health manpower supply equations yield the market wage rates. The intention is that the model will allow examination of long-run as well as short-run impacts of changes, and permit analysis of the effects of policy instruments as they simultaneously act on different groups. Some preliminary empirical results are presented. The variables and the relationships between them in the model are set out in appendices.
See 111, 270, 458, *1411, 1424.*

1972

1404   D. L. CROMBIE, 'A model of the medical care system: a general systems approach'
In M. M. Hauser (ed.) *The Economics of Medical Care*, pp. 61–98 (28).

A large number of aspects of the medical care system are discussed. Central to the discussion is the problem of the correct division between curative and preventive care, and the division of responsibility between the various elements in the health service system particularly the division between general practice and the hospital services. Determination of the correct balance between the various elements is hampered by a lack of basic information, and the need for a standardised information system is outlined. The paper also examines the role of the primary assessor of patients' problems. It is argued that the general practitioner offers greater value in this area than other providers of medical care.

1405   P. DRAPER, 'Some technical considerations in planning for health'
JSP, April, 1972, 1(2), pp. 149–61.

A variety of approaches to health planning are discussed, recent approaches in the United Kingdom which have their origin in social medicine, approaches which concentrate on inputs, approaches based on utilisation of consumption of services, and an outcome measuring approach. While an outcome approach is regarded as desirable it will for some time be applicable in only a limited number of areas. A number of suggestions are made for improving technical planning in the interim.

1406   B. S. HETZEL, 'The implications of health indicators: a comment'
IJE, December, 1972, 1(4), pp. 315–18.
See 893.

H. E. HILLEBOE, A. BARKHUUS, W. C. THOMAS, *Approaches to National Health Planning*
Geneva: World Health Organisation, Public Health Papers No. 46, 1972, p. 108.

The paper examines planning approaches and techniques used in developed and developing countries. Chapters are included on planning in developing countries, planning in India, health manpower planning in Peru, Taiwan and Turkey, and on the PAHO-CENDES method of planning. Planning in the developed world is examined by reference to the United States, Sweden and the U.S.S.R.

O. G. KENNEDY, B. B. HAMILTON, J. GALLIERS, 'A conceptual model for planning the delivery of rehabilitation services'
APMR, October, 1972, 53(10), pp. 461–9.

A combination of management science and economic techniques are used to plan the provision of medical–vocational rehabilitation services at a community level. The approach has two main components: a demand model to estimate the numbers who will seek care, and a delivery model to generate and test alternatives for the delivery of care and to allocate scarce resources to the alternatives in an efficient manner.

R. L. PARKER, A. K. MURTHY, J. C. BHATIA, 'Relating health services to community health needs'
Indian J.Med.Res., 12th December, 1972, 60(12), pp. 1835–48.
See 126.

J.-E. SPEK, 'On the economic analysis of health and medical care in a Swedish health district'
In M. M. Hauser (ed.) *The Economics of Medical Care*, pp. 261–8.
See 128.

D. E. YETT, L. DRABEK, M. D. INTRILIGATOR, L. J. KIMBELL, 'Health manpower planning: an econometric approach'
HSR, Summer, 1972, 7(2), pp. 134–7.

Two econometric models under development at the Human Resources Research Center of the University of Southern California are described. Both are models of the entire health-care system, dealing with demand and supply of health services and health manpower. The first model is a macro-econometric model utilising aggregate data, the second is a micro-simulation model dealing

with the behaviour of a representative sample of individual consumers and institutions.
See 290, *1403*.

1973

1412   J. R. ASHFORD, G. FERSTER, D. M. MAKUC, 'An approach to resource allocation in the reorganised National Health Service'
In G. McLachlan (ed.) *The Future – and Present Indicatives, Problems and Progress in Medical Care, Essays on Current Research, Ninth Series,* pp. 57–90 (38).
The use of a mathematical programming approach to resource allocation is outlined. The basic concepts concern the classification of the population served by the health system, the sectors of the health services, the types of care dealt with by particular sectors, the alternative procedures available for particular types of care, the associated costs and benefits, and resources required. The best opportunity for using the techniques is seen to be in situations in which alternative procedures are available to treat the same type of case. The costs and benefits of health services are discussed. The application of the techniques is illustrated by reference to the provision of maternity care in a district.

1413   C. L. CHIANG, R. D. COHEN, 'How to measure health: a stochastic model for an index of health'
IJE, March, 1973, 2(1), pp. 7–13.
See 910.

1414   A. DONABEDIAN, *Aspects of Medical Care Administration: Specifying Requirements for Health Care*
Cambridge, Massachusetts: Harvard University Press, 1973, p. 649.
See 35.

1415   M. S. FELDSTEIN, M. A. PIOT, T. K. SUNDARESAN, *Resource Allocation Model for Public Health Planning: A Case Study of Tuberculosis Control*
Geneva: World Health Organisation, 1973, p. 110.
See 771.

P. J. FELDSTEIN, *Financing Dental Care: An Economic Analysis*
Lexington: D. C. Heath and Company, 1973, pp. xvii, 260.
See 36.

C. HIMATSINGANI, 'Approaches to health and personal social services
planning in the National Health Service and the place of health indices'
IJE, March, 1973 2(1), pp. 15–21.

Methods of planning health services based on both input and output concepts
are reviewed, and a way forward for the British National Health Service
outlined.
See 917.

1974

D. F. BERGWALL, P. N. REEVES, N. B. WOODSIDE, *Introduction to Health
Planning*
Washington D.C.: Information Resources Press, 1974, pp. vii, 231.

A textbook designed principally for students of health-care administration and
comprehensive health planning. There are chapters on the history of health
planning in the United States, current United States planning programmes,
forecasting techniques, the formulation of goals and objectives, spatial aspects
of health planning, manpower planning, determining requirements, cost–
benefit analysis and evaluation. Bibliographies of additional reading are
included for each chapter.
See 312.

J. P. DUPUY, 'On the social rationality of health policies'.
In M. Perlman (ed.) *The Economics of Health and Medical Care*, pp.
481–509.
See 936.

R. FEIN, 'Priorities and decision making in health planning'
IJMS, 1974, 10(1–2), pp. 67–80.

Discusses at a general level the problems of health planning, from the stage of
analytical framework and theoretical structure to the problems of plan
implementation.

1421   C. C. HAVIGHURST (ed.) *Regulating Health Facilities Construction*
Washington D.C.: American Enterprise Institute for Public Policy
Research, 1974, p. 314.

Of particular interest are the papers by:
S. R. Gottlieb, 'A brief history of health planning in the United States',
pp. 7–25.
R. N. Grosse, 'The need for health planning', pp. 27–31.
J. J. May, 'The planning and licensing agencies', pp. 47–67.
See 1268.

1422   J. LAVE, L. B. LAVE, S. LEINHARDT, 'Modelling the delivery of medical
services'
In M. Perlman (ed.) *The Economics of Health and Medical Care*, pp.
326–51 (44).

A model of health-care delivery is constructed. Medical care is delivered in a
primary care station, clinic or hospital; individuals make the decision to seek
care on the basis of their current symptoms. Complete specification requires the
addition of information on the health status of the population, the efficiency of
the medical care system, and the willingness of the patient to comply with the
treatment recommended. The model is simulated to investigate cost/health
status trade-offs.

1423   E. LEVY, 'Health indicators and health systems analysis'
In M. Perlman (ed.) *The Economics of Health and Medical Care*, pp.
377–401.
See 940.

1424   D. E. YETT, L. DRABEK, M. D. INTRILIGATOR, L. J. KIMBELL, 'Econometric
forecasts of health services and health manpower'
In M. Perlman (ed.) *The Economics of Health and Medical Care*, pp.
459–69 (44).

An outline is presented of the Human Resources Research Center macro-
econometric model of the health-care system of the United States. Two uses of
the model are illustrated: structural analysis (examining the estimated coefficients of the model where it is shown that Medicare exerts a substantial
influence on the demand for medical services); and policy evaluation (two types
of policy initiatives are considered, the effects of particular features of national
health insurance proposals, and policies designed to increase the total number
of physicians).
See 1403.

7 Utilisation Studies

Most of the studies in this section are studies of hospital resource utilisation: there are close links with some of the studies classified under 2(b) and 3(c)(i).

A number of the studies deal with the relations between utilisation and financial provision (particularly insurance provision): Densen *et al.* (1425), Weisbrod and Fiesler (1428), Reed (1436), Rodman (1437), Ferber (1439) and Alexander (1441). Studies examining a broader range of factors affecting utilisation include Rosenthal (1438), White (1447), Picken and Ireland (1455), Navarro, Parker and White (1460) and J. G. Anderson (1468, 1463). Cross-national studies of utilisation include Anderson, Smedby and O. W. Anderson (1458), Bice and White (1461) and Kalimo, Kohn and Bedenic (1466).

The remainder of the studies in this section constitute a heterogeneous group including such delicacies as the influence of smoking and of a negative income tax.

1958

P. M. DENSEN, E. BALAMUTH, S. SHAPIRO, *Prepaid Medical Care and Hospital Utilization*
Chicago: American Hospital Association, 1958.

P. M. DENSEN, E. W. JONES, E. BALAMUTH, S. SHAPIRO, 'Prepaid medical care and hospital utilization in a duel choice situation'
AJPH, November, 1960, 50(11), pp. 1710–26.

P. M. DENSEN, S. SHAPIRO, E. W. JONES, I. BALDINGER, 'Prepaid medical care and hospital utilization'
Hospitals, November 16th, 1962, 36, pp. 63–8, 138.

A series of articles comparing hospitalisation experiences of pairs of population groups. One group in all three studies was covered under the Health Insurance Plan of Greater New York and the other group was covered by a different plan in each study.

1961

1426   M. I. ROEMER, 'Bed supply and hospitalization: a natural experiment'
Hospitals, November 1st, 1961, pp. 35–42.
See 350.

1427   M. I. ROEMER, 'Hospital utilization and the supply of physicians'
JAMA, December 9th, 1961, 178(10), pp. 989–93.
See 351.

1428   B. A. WEISBROD, R. J. FIESLER, 'Hospitalization insurance and hospital utilization'
AER, March, 1961, 51(1), pp. 126–32.

A comparison was made of the hospitalisation experience of two large groups of subscribers to Blue Cross Hospital Care plans, before and after the extension of a more comprehensive insurance plan to one of the groups. Utilisation did increase relatively for the group with the additional coverage but the increase was concentrated among females over 55 years of age.

1963

1429   U.S. DEPARTMENT OF HEALTH, EDUCATION AND WELFARE, *Conference on Research in Hospital Use*
Washington D.C.: USDHEW, Public Health Service Publication No. 930–E–2, 1963; pp. viii, 148.

Report of a conference that brought together persons from a broad range of disciplines. Chiefly of use as a review of early work in the U.K. and the U.S.A. on hospital utilisation.

1964

1430   R. L. DURBIN, G. ANTELMAN, 'A study of the effects of selected variables on hospital utilization'
HM, August, 1964, 98(2), pp. 57–60.

An examination of the relationship between admission rates and length of stay, and the number of beds, physicians, health insurance coverage and per capita income. Length of stay was found to increase as each of the four variables increased. Admission rates increased with the number of beds, decreased with the number of physicians and with higher average income and were little affected by insurance coverage. G. D. Rosenthal 'A critical comment: A study of the effects of selected variables on hospital utilization', *HM*, October, 1964, 98(3), pp. 67–8, disagrees with the specification of the problem and the choice of variables by Durbin and Antelman.

T. B. FITZPATRICK, D. C. RIEDEL, 'Some general comments on methods of studying hospital use'
Inquiry, January, 1964, 1(2), pp. 49–68.

G. D. ROSENTHAL, *The Demand for General Hospital Facilities*
Chicago: American Hospital Association, Hospital Monograph Series No. 14, 1964, p. 101.
See 66.

1965

M. S. FELDSTEIN, 'Hospital bed scarcity: an analysis of the effects of inter-regional differences'
EC, November, 1965, 32(128), pp. 393–409.
See 362.

P. J. FELDSTEIN, J. J. GERMAN, 'Predicting hospital utilization: an evaluation of three approaches'
Inquiry, June, 1965, 2(1), pp. 13–36.

J. E. OSBORNE, 'Characteristics of hospital utilization in Canada'
AJPH, March, 1965, 55(3), pp. 446–52.

Information is presented on the utilisation of hospital services in Canada by age, sex and diagnoses. Utilisation rates of hospital care are concluded to be higher than in the U.S.A. because care for the chronically ill is included in the Canadian hospital insurance programme.
See 1436.

1436 L. S. REED, 'Hospital utilization under the Canadian national hospital insurance programme'
AJPH, March, 1965, 55(3), pp. 435–45.

A survey of the utilisation of hospital services in Canada before and after the extension of federal government aid to provincial programmes of hospital insurance. Comparisons with the U.S.A. indicate that utilisation rates have been higher in Canada from before the programme, and were rising before its introduction, but since the introduction the rise in admissions and days of care has continued at an accelerated rate. Further information on utilization by age, sex and diagnosis is provided by J. E. Osborne, 'Characteristics of hospital utilization in Canada', *AJPH*, March, 1965, 55(3), pp. 446–52.
See 1435.

1437 A. C. RODMAN, 'Comparison of Baltimore's utilization rates under two physician-payment systems'
PHR, June, 1965, 80(6), pp. 476–80.

A study of the effects on the utilisation of physician services and hospital clinic utilisation of a change from a capitation to a fee-for-service system of payment. Physician utilisation was found to have increased, clinic utilisation to have decreased, with overall utilisation having increased, after the introduction of fee for service.
See 1441.

1438 G. D. ROSENTHAL, 'Factors affecting the utilization of short-term general hospitals'
AJPH, November, 1965, 55(11), pp. 1734–40.

Principal components analysis is used in an examination of the factors that affect utilisation of general hospitals. The analysis suggests that population characteristics affecting utilisation may be grouped in five components: income, marital status and sex, age, housing and education. The model could not predict admissions nearly as well as length of stay and a number of other aspects of treatment.

1966

1439 B. FERBER, 'The relationship of multiple health insurance coverage and hospital utilization'
Inquiry, December, 1966, 3(4), pp. 14–27.

An attempt to discover the relationship between type and extent of hospital use and insurance coverage. It was found that more with multiple insurance coverage had private rooms than those with a single insurance, but there was no evidence that they used the hospital more extensively.

0 E. R. WEINERMAN, R. S. RATNER, A. ROBBINS, M. A. LAVENHAR, 'Determinants of use of hospital emergency services'
AJPH, July, 1966, 56(7), pp. 1037–56.
A study of visits to an emergency service which examines socio-economic and demographic characteristics of the patients in relation to the urgency of the condition for which they are using the services. The population using the emergency facility for non-urgent conditions tended to be young, male, unmarried, central urban and relatively poor.

1967

1 C. A. ALEXANDER, 'The effects of change in method of paying physicians: the Baltimore experience'
AJPH, August, 1967, 57(8), pp. 1278–88.
Analysis of the effects of a changeover from capitation to fee for service as the method of paying physicians caring for the indigent in Baltimore. Changes in the utilisation of physicians' services, clinics and hospitalisation are examined. *See 1437.*

2 O. W. ANDERSON, P. B. SHEATSLEY, *Hospital Use – A Survey of Patient and Physician Decisions*
Chicago: University of Chicago, Center for Health Administration Studies, Research Series No. 24, 1967.

3 S. SHAPIRO, 'End result measurement of quality of medical care'
MMFQ, 1967, 45(2), pp. 7–30.
See 857.

1968

4 R. ANDERSEN, *A Behavioural Model of Families' Use of Health Services*
Chicago: University of Chicago, Center for Health Administration Studies, Research Series No. 25, 1968, pp. xi, 111.

1445   M. R. GREENLICK, A. V. HURTADO, C. R. POPE, E. W. SAWARD, S. S. YOSHIOKA, 'Determinants of medical care utilization'
HSR, Winter, 1968, 3(4), pp. 296–315.

A study of the patterns of utilisation in a prepaid group practice plan providing comprehensive medical care. Preliminary findings are presented on the characteristics of the sample population, patterns of medical care utilisation, and utilisation for different types of sickness. Of the total registered population, 77 per cent used the facilities at least once during the year, and 95 per cent of the services were provided during clinic hours.

1446   A. H. PACKER, 'Applying cost-effectiveness concepts to the community health system'
OR, March–April, 1968, 16(2), pp. 227–53.
See 682.

1447   E. WHITE, 'A graphic presentation of age and income differentials in selected aspects of morbidity, disability and utilization of health services'
Inquiry, March, 1968, 5(1), pp. 18–30.

Data collected in a continuing health interview survey conducted by the U.S. National Center for Health Statistics are presented. Information is provided on the prevalence of chronic conditions, use of physician services, use of dental services, use of hospital services and out-of-pocket expenses for health, by each age and income group.

1969

1448   R. ANDERSEN, J. T. HULL, 'Hospital utilization and cost trends in Canada and the United States'
HSR, Fall, 1969, 4(3), pp. 198–222.

A descriptive study looking at the reasons for rising hospital utilisation in the period 1950–67.

1449   T. W. BICE, K. L. WHITE, 'Factors related to the use of health services: an international comparative study'
MC, March–April, 1969, 7(2), pp. 124–33.

Data on use of physicians' services from areas in England, the U.S.A. and Yugoslavia were analysed using multivariate techniques. Differences in the levels of perceived morbidity accounted for the greatest amount of the variance in utilisation between the areas.

0   A. DONABEDIAN, 'An evaluation of prepaid group practice'
    Inquiry, September, 1969, 6(3), pp. 3–27.
    See 1193, *1257*.

1   H. R. GARLAND, 'Hospital utilization by characteristic of industry in South Western Ohio'
    Inquiry, March, 1969, 6(1), pp. 60–71.
    An examination of the relationship between age and income, and the utilisation of hospitals for particular medical incidents by employees from ten industry groups.

2   A. V. HURTADO, M. R. GREENLICK, E. W. SAWARD, 'The organisation and utilization of home-care and extended-care-facility services in a prepaid comprehensive group practice plan'
    MC, January–February, 1969, 7(2), pp. 30–40.
    A preliminary report on a project to provide home-care and extended-care facilities of Medicare to a well-defined population of more than 100,000 people. Estimates are made of the costs of providing such services and their effects in reducing the use of acute hospital facilities.

3   J. W. KOVNER, L. B. BROWNE, A. I. KISCH, 'Income and the use of outpatient medical care by the insured'
    Inquiry, June, 1969, 6(2), pp. 27–34.
    An examination of the relationship between income and use of medical services by subscribers to two insurance plans. For insured services, income and use of services were found to be independent; for uninsured services, use was correlated with income for only one of the plans.

4   M. KRAMER, 'Statistics of mental disorders in the United States: current status, some urgent needs and suggested solutions'
    JRSS A, 1969, 132(3), pp. 353–407.
    An outline is provided of available sources of data on the patterns of utilisation of the mental health services. Necessary improvements in the data for evaluative purposes, international comparisons and determination of the relationship between morbidity and social and economic factors are discussed.

1455   B. PICKEN, G. IRELAND, 'Family patterns of medical care utilization: possible influences of family size, role, and social class on illness behaviour'
JCD, August, 1969, 22(3), pp. 181–91.

This is a study of a Scottish general practice. No significant relationship was found between social class or family size and the level of consultations of fathers and mothers. Children from upper social class families and from smaller families were found to consult more often than other children. Patterns of concordance in consultation were shown to exist for fathers and sons from larger families, for lower social class families, and for mothers and daughters in certain family groupings.

1456   M. REIN, 'Social class and the utilization of medical care services'
Hospitals, July 1st, 1969, 43(13), pp. 43–54.

Information is presented on the utilisation of services and consultation for a variety of diagnoses by different social classes under the British National Health Service.

1457   K-K. RO, 'Patient characteristics, hospital characteristics, and hospital use'
MC, July–August, 1969, 7(4), pp. 295–312. Also in V. R. Fuchs (ed.) *Essays in the Economics of Health and Medical Care*, pp. 69–96.
See 418.

1970

1458   R. ANDERSEN, B. SMEDBY, O. W. ANDERSON, *Medical Care Use in Sweden and the United States: A Comparative Analysis of Systems and Behaviour*
Chicago: University of Chicago, Center for Health Administration Studies, Research Series, No. 27, 1970, pp. xii, 174.
See 1064.

1459   J. R. ASHFORD, N. G. PEARSON, 'Who uses the health services and why?'
JRSS A, 1970, 133(3), pp. 295–357.
See 91.

V. NAVARRO, R. PARKER, K. L. WHITE, 'A stochastic and deterministic model of medical care utilization'
HSR, Winter, 1970, 5(4), pp. 342–57.

A model is presented that brings into consideration the deterministic process of ageing as it affects the demographic structure of the population, and also the stochastic processes of birth and death and the stochastic process of health services utilisation by different age groups. A numerical illustration is given.

1971

T. W. BICE, K. L. WHITE, 'Cross-national comparative research on the utilization of medical services'
MC, May–June, 1971, 9(3), pp. 253–71.

The conceptual issues underlying utilisation research are discussed. The most fruitful comparative utilisation research is seen to be that which examines how forms of organisation, financing and modes of medical practice affect rates and patterns of utilisation. A taxonomy of four types of cross-national utilisation studies is developed.

T. L. HALL, S. DIAZ, 'Social security and health care patterns in Chile'
IJHS, November, 1971, 1(4), pp. 362–77.

Data on the utilisation of physician, dentist and hospital services by different sections of the population are presented. A strong positive correlation was found between social security coverage and utilisation of medical and dental services, along with an inverse correlation between coverage and unmet demand.
See 1221.

A. H. RAPHAELSON, S. HENEMIER, 'A model for the distribution of hospital services in Pennsylvania'
EBB, Fall, 1971, 24(1), pp. 60–7.

A multiple regression model of the intrastate geographic distribution of the use of hospital services is developed. Four main categories of variables are used to predict the average daily census of hospitals in 67 counties in Pennsylvania: demographic factors, factors relating to the general economic condition of the population, public expenditure relevant to health care, and insurance activity relevant to health care.

1972

1464   T. W. BICE, R. L. EICHHORN, P. D. FOX, 'Socio-economic status and use of physician services: a reconsideration'
MC, May–June, 1972, 10(3), pp. 261–71.

The conceptual and methodological problems of utilisation studies are reviewed. A survey of a number of major studies revealed that the relationship between family income and physician use has diminished substantially over the last 40 years. Few studies were found that lent support to social–psychological or cultural explanations of differences in use between socio-economic groups.

1465   A. V. HURTADO, M. R. GREENLICK, 'The utilization and cost of home care and extended care facility services in a comprehensive, prepaid group practice programme'
MC, January–February, 1972, 10(1), pp. 8–16.

A study examining the effects of making home-care and extended-care facility services available to a population under 65 years of age. The use of the acute hospital was only 87 per cent of that which might have been expected without the services, and 74 per cent for the Medicare population.

1466   E. KÄLIMO, R. KOHN, B. BEDENIC, 'Interrelationships in the use of selected health services: a cross-national study'
MC, March–April, 1972, 10(2), pp. 95–108.

A study using household survey data to determine the correlation between the use of different components of health services by the adult population. The data for the study were collected from 12 areas within seven countries: Canada, the United States, the United Kingdom, Argentina, Finland, Poland and Yugoslavia. The hope of possibly providing a unidimensional measure of overall medical care use was not fulfilled; the average correlation among variables of use in all the study areas was only 0.14.

1973

1467   R. ANDERSEN, J. F. NEWMAN, 'Societal and individual determinants of medical care utilization in the United States'
MMFQ, Winter, 1973, 51(1), pp. 95–124.

A framework for studying health services utilisation is developed. The framework shows how societal determinants of utilisation and the health services system interact with individual determinants in producing health services utilisation. Some empirical findings are then examined to illustrate the use of the framework in explaining trends in utilisation.

8   J. G. ANDERSON, 'Demographic factors affecting health services utilization: a causal model'
MC, March–April, 1973, 11(2), pp. 104–20.

In areas where alternative health services are lacking, an increase in the supply of beds was found significantly to alter both the admission rate and the average length of stay. Hospital utilisation was found to be highly sensitive to changes in age structure. Increased usage was also associated with urbanisation.

9   J. G. ANDERSON, 'Health services utilization: framework and review'
HSR, Fall, 1973, 8(3), pp. 184–99.

Identifies five approaches that have been used to study the utilisation of health services: socio-cultural, social–demographic, social–psychological, organisational, social systems. Review of these approaches suggests that the last named is potentially the most fruitful.

0   T. W. BICE, D. L. RABIN, B. H. STARFIELD, K. L. WHITE, 'Economic class and the use of physician services'
MC, July–August, 1973, 11(4), pp. 287–96.

Multivariate analysis of Baltimore data revealed that changing the net price of services had a greater effect on the utilisation of services by the poor than by the rich. Non-economic predisposing factors were found to have a greater effect on the use of preventive services than on all forms of physician use taken together.

1   L. B. RUSSELL, 'The impact of the extended-care facility benefit on hospital use and reimbursement under Medicare'
JHR, Winter, 1973, 8(1), pp. 57–72.
See 1332, 1333.

B. C. STUART, R. STOCKTON, 'control over the utilization of medical services'
MMFQ, Summer, 1973, 51(3), pp. 341–94.
See 1334.

1974

1473 W. J. BAUMOL, 'An overview of the results on consumption, health, and social behaviour'
JHR, Spring, 1974, 9(2), pp. 253–64.

Part of a symposium examining the effects of the New Jersey–Pennsylvania negative income tax experiment. No significant effects on health or on the utilisation of health services were observed with the introduction of negative income tax.

1474 F. CORDLE, H. A. TYROLER, 'The use of hospital medical records for epidemiologic research. I. differences in hospital utilization and in-hospital mortality by age – race – sex – place of residence and socio-economic status in a defined community population'
MC, July, 1974, 7(7), pp. 596–610.

This study of a county in South Carolina revealed an admission rate for whites 1.8 times that for blacks, but low income blacks shared the highest admission rates with low income whites. Blacks experienced an in-hospital mortality 8 times that of whites.

1475 T. W. OAKES, G. D. FRIEDMAN, C. C. SELTZER, A. B. SIEGELAUB, M. F. COLLEN, 'Health service utilization by smokers and non-smokers'
MC, November, 1974, 12(11), pp. 958–66.

A study of the differences in utilisation of a variety of health services by smokers, ex-smokers and non-smokers. Health examinations were used least by smokers. Different smoking habits increased utilisation of some services but reduced the use of others.

8 Bibliographies

Entries cover two kinds of publication. First, those that give useful compilations of studies concerned with health economics. Second, those that are concerned with a broader subject-matter, whether in economics or in health, but whose coverage is such that some items of interest to health economists will be covered.

1960

76 NATIONAL LIBRARY OF MEDICINE, *Index Medicus*
Washington D.C.: United States Department of Health, Education and Welfare, Public Health Service, National Institutes of Health, 1960–
Index Medicus appears monthly with a cumulative author and subject edition appearing after the end of each year. The index provides a listing of authors and titles. The items are not annotated. It is compiled from a search of over 2,000 mainly medical journals. A list of the journals searched appears in the January issue each year. There are sections within *Index Medicus* entitled Economics, Economics/Dental, Economics/Hospital, Economics/Medical, Economics/Nursing, Costs and Cost Analysis and Socio-economic Factors, which bring together most of the material of interest to economists. From 1976 a section will be included on Cost–Benefit Analysis.

1961

77 DEPARTMENT OF HEALTH AND SOCIAL SECURITY, *Hospital Abstracts*
London: HMSO, 1961–
A monthly survey of world literature (annotated) prepared by the DHSS. A lot of technical literature and non-English language literature is covered. For economists the sections most likely to contain relevant material are those on organisation and administration.

1963

1478   AMERICAN ECONOMIC ASSOCIATION, *The Journal of Economic Literature*
Evanston, Illinois: American Economic Association, 1963–

The journal appears four times a year in March, June, September and December. The first section of the journal is devoted to surveys of areas of economic analysis. The bibliographical section of the journal is divided into five parts: book reviews, an annotated listing of new books, a listing of the contents of current periodicals, a listing of articles by subjects, and selected article abstracts arranged by subject. A section of the bibliography deals specifically with the economics of health (913).

1964

1479   THE COOPERATIVE INFORMATION CENTER FOR HOSPITAL MANAGEMENT STUDIES, *Abstracts of Hospital Management Studies*
Michigan: The University of Michigan, 1964–

An annotated bibliography appearing quarterly with an annual cumulated edition appearing in June of the following year. The material is arranged in over forty sections. Each section contains a list of the other sections likely to be of interest to the enquirer. The mainstream economic journals are not covered but the major medical, social-medical, health administration and OR journals are included, as are U.S. doctoral and Master's theses. Most of the material in the bibliography can be obtained on Xerox or microfilm direct from the Information Center.

1966

1480   M. BLAUG, *Economics of Education: A Selected Annotated Bibliography*
Oxford: Pergamon Press Ltd., 1966, pp. xiv, 190.

A major bibliography of a closely related field. Nearly 800 items are included. The volume is divided into two main parts: developed countries, and developing countries. The items within the two sections are arranged under seven heads:
1   General Surveys of the Subject
2   The Economic Contribution of Education
3   The Economic Aspects of Education
4   Educational Planning

5   Manpower Forecasting
6   Social Mobility and Reserves of Talent
7   The Politics of Education
In the second edition (Pergamon, 1970) 1,350 items are annotated.
See 17.

1969

81   R. T. FLINT, K. C. SPENSLEY, 'Recent issues in nursing manpower: a review'
NR, May–June, 1969, 18(3), pp. 217–29.
A bibliography of 398 books and articles appearing in the period 1956–68. The bibliography is organised under ten sub-headings:
1   Overview: summaries and projections
2   Analytical studies
3   Sociological and psychological studies
4   Education
5   Refresher training
6   Recruitment
7   Utilization
8   Supportive personnel
9   Innovations
10   Attrition and turnover

1970

82   W. D. WOOD, H. F. CAMPBELL, *Cost–Benefit Analysis and the Economics of Investment in Human Resources – An Annotated Bibliography*
Kingston, Ontario: Industrial Relations Centre, Queen's University, 1970, pp. viii, 211.
A bibliography of 389 items arranged under eight headings:
1   Human Capital
2   Theory and Application of Cost–Benefit Analysis
3   Theoretical Problems in Measuring Benefits and Costs
4   Investment Criteria and the Social Discount Rate
5   Schooling
6   Training, Retraining and Mobility
7   Health
8   Poverty and Social Welfare

1971

1483 INTERNATIONAL MEDICAL ABSTRACTING SERVICE, *Excerpta Medica*
(Section 36, Health Economics and Hospital Management)
Amsterdam: The International Medical Abstracting Service. Published
with the aid of the Ministry of Public Health and Environmental
Hygiene, The Hague, 1971–

A massive bibliography in which the items are annotated. The bibliography
covers most of the well-known journals in economics and also a large number
in operations research, social medicine, medicine and health-care administration. The volume for 1974 had 1,980 entries. The material is arranged under
eight section headings and these sections are further subdivided.

1 General Aspects of Health Care
2 Health Care Organisations
3 Macro-economics
4 Input of Health Care Systems, Running Costs
5 Output of Health Care Systems
6 Prevention
7 Insurance
8 Hospital Management and Organisation.

1972

1484 S. E. BERKI, *Hospital Economics*
Lexington, Massachusetts: Lexington Books, D. C. Heath and
Company, 1972, pp. xxi, 270.

An excellent bibliography of 446 items is included, covering health economics
rather than just hospital economics. Most of the material in the bibliography is
American.
See 462.

1485 J. M. GLASGOW, 'The economics of health: a review of the literature in the
last decade'
Choice, March, 1972, pp. 33–42.

A brief review of most of the major areas that have concerned health
economists and the way they have been treated in the American literature.

6 J. D. HENNES, 'The measurement of health'
MCR, December, 1972, 29(11), pp. 1268–88.
See 892.

7 P. QUAETHOVEN, 'Health organisation in the European Economic Community, an annotated bibliography'
IJHS, November, 1972, 2(4), pp. 513–24.
A bibliography of 41 publications divided into five sections:
1 General
2 Costs
3 Social security
4 Professional staff
5 National health care
The bibliography includes some non-English language material.

8 L. D. WILCOX, R. M. BROOKS, G. M. BEAL, G. E. KLONGLAN, *Social Indicators and Societal Monitoring*
Amsterdam: Elsevier Scientific Publishing Company, 1972, p. 464.
See 901.

1973

9 A. DONABEDIAN, *Aspects of Medical Care Administration: Specifying Requirements for Health Care*
Cambridge, Massachusetts: Harvard University Press, 1973, p. 649.
Extensive bibliographies accompany each section of the book. Useful references to United States statistical sources are included.
See 35.

0 R. KOHN, S. RADIUS, 'International comparison of health service systems, an annotated bibliography'
IJHS, Spring, 1973, 3(2), pp. 295–309.
A bibliography of 70 items up to 1970, divided into cross-national and national studies.

1974

1491 J. RAFFERTY (ed.) *Health Manpower and Productivity*
Lexington, Massachusetts: D. C. Heath and Company, 1974, pp. xxiv,
228.
A collection of seven papers with extensive bibliographies.
See 329.

Author Index

The alphabetical author index identifies by number the entries attributed to the author concerned. Numbers refer to entries and not to page numbers. Where a publication is listed in more than one Section (and hence has more than one number), the contents may not be described in more than one entry. The numbers of unannotated entries are in bold type in the index.